# Evidence-Based Cancer Care and Prevention

## Behavioral Interventions

**Charles W. Given, PhD,** is a Professor in the Department of Family Practice at Michigan State University and Senior Scientist at the Walther Cancer Institute, where he received the Distinguished Faculty Award in 1997. Given is actively involved in research in home care for chronic illness including cancer, focusing on symptom clusters, health service issues, and physical function. Having received funding for 23 consecutive years from the NIH, intervention trials have been a recent focus on his research. Given is a reviewer for numerous professional journals and has served as a grant reviewer for the Agency for Healthcare Research and Quality, the National Cancer Institute, the National Institute of Nursing Research, the Department of Defense, and the National Institute on Aging.

**Barbara Given, RN, PhD, FAAN,** is a University Distinguished Professor in the College of Nursing and Senior Scientist of the Institute for Health Care Studies at Michigan State University. She has been actively involved in federally funded research in chronic illness and family care for over 5 years; intervention trials have been the focus of her recent research and funding. She is active in Sigma Theta Tau, the Oncology Nursing Society, and serves on the Expert Panel of Aging in the American Academy of Nursing and continues to be active in Policy Panels at the State and National levels. Given is a reviewer for numerous professional journals, and is currently serving on the editorial board for *Research in Nursing & Health* and *Cancer Nursing*. Recent awards include the McWilliams Award for Excellence in Research (2001) and Friends of National Institute for Nursing Research Pathfinder Distinguished Researcher Award (2001).

**Victoria L. Champion, DNS, RN, FAAN,** is Distinguished Professor and Associate Dean for Research at Indiana University School of Nursing; Director of Cancer Control, Indiana University Cancer Center, and; Research Director for the Center for Excellence in Women's Health. Champion's current research focus is promoting behaviors that will allow for the discovery of breast cancer at a state at which complete cure is possible. Her most recent funding includes a National Cancer Institute grant to tailor her interventions to a low-income African-American sample. In 2001, Dr. Champion received the Lifetime Achievement Award for Oncology Research from the Oncology Nursing Society. She is the author of numerous articles. Her national commitments have included chairing the behavorial study section for the American Cancer Society, the integration panel for the Department of Defense breast cancer project, the executive committee of Great Lakes Division of the American Cancer Society, and numerous NIH review and consensus panels.

**Sharon Kozachik, MSN, RN, MS,** is a research assistant with the Family Care Research Program at Michigan State University and the Walther Cancer Institute.

**Dànielle Nicole DeVoss, PhD,** is an Assistant Professor in the Department of American Thought and Language at Michigan State University. Her work has most recently appeared in the *Writing Center Journal, CyberPsychology and Behavior,* the *Journal of Business and Technical Communication,* and *Moving a Mountain: Transforming the Role of Contingent Faculty in Composition Studies and Higher Education* (2001 E.E. Schell and P. Stock, Eds.). DeVoss teaches composition, professional writing, Web development, and rhetoric courses.

# Evidence-Based Cancer Care and Prevention

## Behavioral Interventions

**Charles W. Given,** PhD
**Barbara Given,** RN, PhD, FAAN
**Victoria L. Champion,** DNS, RN, FAAN
**Sharon Kozachik,** MSN, RN, MS
**Dànielle Nicole DeVoss,** PhD

**Editors**

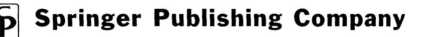 Springer Publishing Company

Springer Publishing Company, Inc.
536 Broadway
New York, NY 10012-3955

*Acquisitions Editor: Ruth Chasek*
*Production Editor: Matt Fenton*
*Cover design by Joanne Honigman*

03 04 05 06 07 / 5 4 3 2 1

**Library of Congress Cataloging-in-Publication Data**

Evidence-based cancer care and prevention : behavioral interventions / [edited by] Charles
    W. Given . . . [et al.].
        p. ; cm.
    Includes bibliographical references and index.
    ISBN 0-8261-1574-8
        1. Cancer—Psychological aspects. 2. Health behavior. 3. Cancer—Prevention. 4.
    Evidence-based medicine. I. Given, Charles W.
        [DNLM: 1. Neoplasms—prevention & control. 2. Behavioral Therapy—methods. 3.
    Evidence-Based Medicine. 4. Neoplasms—therapy. 5. Self Care. 6. Smoking Cessation. QZ
    200 E936 2003]
    RC262.E95 2003
    616.994'4'0019—dc21

                                                                                2003041527

Printed in the United States of America by Maple Vail.

# Contents

# Contributors

**Barbara L. Andersen, PhD**
Department of Psychology
The Ohio State University
Columbus, OH

**Marylin J. Dodd, RN, PhD, FAAN**
Center for Symptom Management
School of Nursing
University of California, San Francisco
San Francisco, CA

**Betty Ferrell, PhD**
Department of Nursing Research and Education
City of Hope National Medical Center
Duarte, CA

**R. Brian Giesler, PhD**
Indiana University Cancer Center
Indianapolis, IN

**Ellen R. Gritz, Ph.D.**
Department of Behavioral Science
The University of Texas
MD Anderson Cancer Center
Houston, TX

**Debra Haire-Joshu, PhD, RN**
Department of Behavioral Science
Saint Louis University
School of Public Health
St. Louis, MO

**Barbara Hastie, PhD**
Department of Nursing Research and Education
City of Hope National Medical Center
Duarte, CA

**Amy B. Lazev, PhD**
Department of Behavioral Science
The University of Texas
MD Anderson Cancer Center
Houston, TX

**Christine Miaskowski, RN,
PhD, FAAN**
Department of Physiological
Nursing
School of Nursing
University of California, San
Francisco
San Francisco, CA

**Victoria Mock, DNSc, AOCN,
FAAN**
Johns Hopkins University School
of Nursing
Baltimore, MD

**Marilyn S. Nanney, MS,
MPH, RD**
Senior Research Manager
Saint Louis University School of
Public Health
St. Louis, MO

**Susan M. Rawl, PhD, RN**
School of Nursing
Indiana University
Indianapolis, IN

**Celette Sugg Skinner, PhD**
Duke University Medical Center
Duke University Comprehensive
Cancer Center
Durham, NC

**Damon J. Vidrine, MS, DrPH**
Department of Behavioral Science
The University of Texas
MD Anderson Cancer Center
Houston, TX

**Gwen Wyatt, RN, PhD**
College of Nursing
Michigan State University

# Preface

This book emerged as the result of extended conversations among several of the authors, who recognized that although a considerable number of meta-analyses of behavioral interventions have been completed, few sources were available that described and summarized what we know about behavioral interventions across the cancer care trajectory. The purpose of this book is to synthesize state-of-the-science behavioral interventions. To meet these goals, we enlisted a number of scientists who felt, as we did, that it was time for a compendium to describe the status and science of behavioral interventions across the cancer care trajectory.

In February of 2001, the contributors came together for a daylong working session to define the evaluation criteria for the book and agree on the contents. The authors were dedicated to evaluating and critiquing each other's ideas and suggestions. Authors took on the responsibility of producing a chapter while continuing their own research agendas, teaching courses, advising students, and serving on institutional and national committees. Contributors were asked to review state-of-the-science behavioral interventions in their area of expertise. Each was asked to apply rules of evidence to their summaries. We asked that they give preference to information obtained from randomized clinical trials, and we asked that they pay close attention to variables that might compromise the conclusions of the studies collected for analysis, summary, and inclusion in this book's chapters, such as sample size and possible sources of bias. Most importantly, chapter authors were asked to describe the rationale for the inclusion of patients, the theories used to guide the intervention, attrition from trials, the impact of the intervention on patients, and system-wide intervention outcomes.

The significant effort of each author resulted in a completed book. Readers will find an in-depth examination of the approaches to understanding cancer care at all phases in the cancer trajectory: from prevention and detection to diagnosis and early treatment to survivorship, recurrence, and/or death. This book offers state-of-the-science knowledge to readers interested in exploring the role of behavioral interventions in detecting and treating cancer.

The book begins with prevention studies and concludes with research on end-of-life care. In each chapter, readers will find common elements, including summaries of recent research on cancer-related behavioral interventions supported by literature reviews, discussions of the studies summarized, acknowledgments of intervention limitations, and suggestions for future research.

# Acknowledgments

This book—and the time, energy, and motivation behind it—is a product of collaboration among members of the Behavioral Cooperative Oncology Group (BCOG) of the Mary Margaret Walther Program for Cancer Care Research at the Walther Cancer Institute. Without the leadership of Dr. Victoria Champion, who dedicated a portion of the monetary award she received as the 1999 Walther Cancer Institute Collaborator of the Year, this book would not have been possible. This compendium is a tribute to the collaborative efforts of BCOG scientists. The colleagues who worked tirelessly to produce the chapters on a short deadline once again demonstrated their dedication to the science and to the spirit of collaboration that has enriched our work.

# 1

## Introduction: The State of the Knowledge of Intervention Research in Cancer Care

**Charles W. Given**

Behavioral oncology is a relatively new but rapidly growing body of science that can improve the lives of patients and their families across the cancer trajectory. The goal of behavioral oncology is, first, to understand and explain the role and impact of behaviors on cancer prevention. Second, behavioral oncology strives to develop strategies to help detect the presence of cancer early, to manage symptoms and side effects, to maintain quality of life during treatments, and, ultimately, to assist patients to die with greater calm, peace, and dignity. The goal of this book is to assess the state of the science with regard to the effects of behavioral interventions on

- Understanding complex and often intertwined lifestyle factors—such as smoking, diet, and physical activity—and their impact on cancer risk, incidence, and prevention;
- Recognizing smoking behavior, including cessation, relapse prevention, disease-specific treatment, and sustained cessation;
- Increasing adherence to cancer-screening techniques, especially among vulnerable and hard-to-reach populations;
- Facilitating patient and family decision-making regarding diagnostic and treatment interventions using decision aids;

- Assisting patients and their family caregivers to manage cancer treatment-related symptoms in the home;
- Enhancing the quality of life experienced by cancer patients as they adjust to diagnosis, treatment, survival, and perhaps recurrence of the disease;
- Assessing often severe, disruptive, and distressing symptoms and pain, and effectively tailoring interventions toward patients and their families;
- Supporting family caregivers so that they can assume caregiving roles and negotiate the multiple and challenging demands of caring for a loved one with cancer;
- Teaching providers so that they can best address the physical, psychological, social, and spiritual needs of cancer patients facing the end of life; and
- Implementing complementary and alternative therapies.

Although this list outlines the chapters to follow, this book will not resolve these issues; the debates will continue. However, the authors of these chapters believe strongly that it is time to join the debate and address when, where, and under what circumstances behavioral interventions should be included in the prevention, early diagnosis, treatment, and outcomes of cancer care.

This introductory chapter is organized to provide an overview for the reader. We begin with a brief review of the historical milestones in the development of behavioral oncology. Next, summaries of each chapter are included, organized according to the timeline of the cancer trajectory, beginning with prevention and ending with end-of-life care. Because a primary goal of behavioral oncology is to become better integrated into the care of patients and because we recognize that issues related to the inclusion of behavioral interventions into clinical practice extend beyond the science, this introductory chapter concludes with a brief summary of the precepts of evidence-based medicine. Because a primary goal of behavioral oncology is for behavioral interventions to be better integrated into patient care, and because we recognize that issues related to the inclusion of behavioral interventions into clinical practice extend beyond the current science, this introductory chapter concludes with a brief summary of the precepts of evidence-based medicine.

# A BRIEF HISTORY OF THE DEVELOPMENT OF BEHAVIORAL ONCOLOGY

During the early part of the twentieth century, a cancer diagnosis meant almost certain death. Treatment was usually an attempt to surgically excise the tumor. Because chemotherapy and radiation had not been developed, radical surgery was the only viable solution. Addressing psychosocial needs seemed irrelevant when almost everyone diagnosed with cancer died of the disease.

In 1913, the American Cancer Society (ACS) was organized and began to alter society's view of cancer. A significant part of the ACS mission was to support cancer patients and their families, thus opening a new dimension of cancer care. As science progressed and survival rates improved, the public began to view cancer differently and more interest in psychosocial issues emerged (Holland, 1998). Early work on grief and people's reactions to death opened the door to palliative care (Kubler-Ross, 1975).

In the 1970s, psychosocial research in cancer care began to receive attention and support from the federal government. In 1972, the National Cancer Plan included the Division of Cancer Control and Rehabilitation, which paved the way for research support in behavioral oncology. The first psychosocial research conference was held in 1975, but much of the progress in psychosocial oncology has occurred in the last 20 years.

Several reviews of behavioral research in cancer reveal an increasing number of publications beginning in the early to mid-1980s and growing steadily through the 1990s (Devine & Westlake, 1995; Fawzy, 1999; Fawzy, Cousins, et al., 1990; Fawzy, Fawzy, Arndt, & Pasnau, 1995; Fawzy, Kemeny, et al., 1990; Glanz, 1997; Lewis, 1997; Meyer & Mark, 1995; Redd, Montgomery, & DuHamel, 2001). Support for this research came from the National Cancer Institute (NCI) and the ACS, both of which have committed increasing amounts of money to fund behavioral research. The number of studies of cancer prevention, screening, treatment, and palliative care has increased substantially. For example, once an early detection of cancer was shown to decrease morbidity and mortality (NCI, 1986), funds devoted to research that could improve the rates of screening among the populations and persons at risk increased.

## Behavioral Interventions Across the Cancer Trajectory

As psychosocial issues in oncology have gained wider recognition, the development of a knowledge base to support their inclusion into clinical practice has become more important. Behavioral oncology has followed the cancer trajectory with research on prevention, screening, and early detection through treatment, symptom management, and toward care that extends from diagnosis to the end of life. Four areas along this trajectory represent important concentrations for research. The first of these is prevention and early detection, or primary and secondary prevention. Primary prevention is the implementation of health-promoting behaviors that prevent cancer from occurring. The oldest preventive practices include the NCI's Five-a-Day program, which promotes the consumption of fruits and vegetables. Other primary-prevention behaviors include smoking cessation, skin protection, and exercise. More recently, chemoprevention programs, such as Tamoxifen for the prevention of breast cancer, have undergone large-scale clinical trials.

In Chapter 2, "Behavioral Interventions for Cancer Prevention: Dietary Intake and Physical Activity," Haire-Joshu and Nanney classify the various prevention programs examined by behavioral oncologists related to dietary intake and physical activity. Although the successes and failures of different approaches to preventive behavioral changes are the focus of their chapter, the debate continues as to the efficacy of diet and exercise in the prevention of cancers.

Secondary prevention seeks to detect cancers at the earliest possible stage so that treatments may be more effective. Prospective trials have concluded that screening for breast, cervical, and colorectal cancers result in reduced mortality rates for these diseases. Champion, Rawl, and Sugg Skinner summarize in Chapter 3, "Cancer Screening," the behavioral interventions for screening for these three cancers. Champion and her coauthors approach behavioral interventions from individual and community approaches, and from the perspectives of healthcare systems and care providers.

In Chapter 4, "Smoking Cessation in Cancer Patients: Never Too Late to Quit," Gritz, Lazev, and Vidrine explore smoking cessation interventions, noting that, although most smoking cessation efforts have been aimed at the primary prevention of cancer, smoking has significant effects on cancer treatment and treatment outcomes. Thus, smoking cessation interventions are important both as a preventive strategy and to improve the efficacy of treatment modalities for those with cancer.

With the rapid advances in the therapeutic sciences, patients and their families are faced with a potentially bewildering array of treatment options. Seeking second opinions is becoming ever more common as families attempt to identify treatments that may be most effective, that are likely to be better tolerated, and that fit within the demands of patients' daily schedules. Prostate cancer is an example where alternative treatment options abound, yet none with clearly preferable treatment or survival outcomes. Sugg Skinner and Giesler describe the use of decision aids in Chapter 5, "Decision Aids for Cancer-Related Behavioral Choices," and explore how information on alternative treatments may be more appropriately presented to patients. Decision aids take the form of brochures, video- or audiotapes, interactive media, counseling, or combinations of these strategies. Decision aids can be employed along the cancer trajectory to help persons decide whether or not and at what interval to receive screening, how to select a treatment regime among the many available alternatives, and how to choose among options for palliative care when disease is advanced. Decision aids are clearly different from other behavioral interventions in that they do not attempt to achieve a prespecified outcome. Instead, in the face of uncertainty, they are designed to help patients and families make decisions that are, in the words of Skinner and Giesler, "good decisions" for them.

In Chapter 6, "Psychological Interventions for Cancer Patients," Andersen summarizes the theoretical frameworks that underlie behavioral and psychological interventions related to symptom management and the care of cancer patients. She points to the relatively small number of trials conducted that link theoretical concepts with specific empirical referents and thus are able to adequately test the efficacy of the theory for guiding the intervention in question.

Following this review of the conceptual frameworks that guide interventions are chapters devoted to behavioral strategies for symptom management. In Chapter 7, "The PRO-SELF© Program: A Self-Care Intervention Program," Dodd and Miaskowski review and summarize their program of research, which has extended over 10 years. The PRO-SELF Program seeks to activate and involve patients and their families in the management of symptoms at home, and it has been applied to a number of cancer symptoms. Mock reviews behavioral interventions for the management of fatigue in Chapter 8, "Evidence-Based Interventions for Cancer-Related Fatigue," and Miaskowski focuses on strategies for the management of pain in Chapter 9, "Pain Management."

In Chapter 10, "Complementary and Alternative Therapy Interventions Used by Cancer Patients," Wyatt summarizes what is known about the wide array of complementary and alternative therapies that patients use to support or enhance their conventional care. Many of these therapies have behavioral components because they involve persons administering touch and physical-manipulation interventions.

In Chapter 11, "Family Caregiving Interventions in Cancer Care," Given, Given, Kozachik, and Rawl review behavioral interventions for family caregivers as they assist their patients and adjust to the impact of the cancer experience. The majority of cancer treatments occur in outpatient settings, placing special responsibilities upon families. Such responsibilities include transporting patients, monitoring their symptoms and side effects, and interacting with healthcare professionals and the healthcare system while adjusting to new patterns of role organization within the home and within their workplaces.

Ferrell and Hastie in Chapter 12, "Interventions at the End of Life," review behavioral interventions for patients at the end of life, focusing on the settings where related interventions occur, such as nursing homes and long-term care facilities, and how these settings may impact end-of-life issues, such as the quality of life of both patients who are dying and their family members.

The concluding chapter, "Conclusion: The Future of Behavioral Intervention Research in Cancer Care," analyzes and summarizes the studies presented across the chapters to address recruitment variables, adjustment issues, and outcome measurement—three important foci for future research if behavioral interventions are to be incorporated into standard practice.

## Development and Evaluation of Evidence for Behavioral Interventions

The chapters in this book evaluate intervention research because healthcare practitioners over the past decade have come to demand evidence from research in order to select treatments that demonstrate the highest probability of producing a cure, recovery, or successful disease management (Guyatt & Rennie, 2002). Clinical approaches to evidence-based medicine pose questions that assess the quality of evidence to support, for example, the use of medical versus surgical treatment procedures. This approach to the science of evidence-based medicine began in past decades, has been fully accepted, and is the preeminent paradigm for the delivery of high-quality medical care (see Guyatt and Rennie 2002 for a summary of the development of methods and strategies for translating evidence into practice).

Through the use of carefully constructed review articles and meta-analyses, evidence bearing on a specific clinical question is evaluated and conclusions are reached as to which treatment, among the alternatives, is most likely to produce the desired therapeutic outcome. A continuing challenge facing all evidence-based summaries is how to use evidence obtained through samples of patients to guide the care of any single patient (Guyatt & Rennie, 2002).

Evaluating the quality of evidence for interventions requires using scientific criteria accepted by experts. Evidence regarding the effects of behavioral interventions in cancer care is limited and differs substantially by focus across the cancer trajectory. In general, the quality of evidence supporting behavioral interventions in any area closely parallels the number of studies that employed randomized clinical trials. According to Hadorn, Baker, Hodges, and Hicks (1996), evidence should be judged according to the rigor of the processes employed in its production. The more rigorous the processes employed, the greater the confidence in the reliability and validity of the evidence and that it represents a true effect and not an artifact of other factors or the whim of random occurrence.

Many factors may explain why an observed effect, or lack of one, may be false. The most pervasive is a bias or systematic error in the collection and analysis of data. Hadorn et al. (1996) argued that as research designs move from randomized control trials (RCTs) through cohort or case-control studies to case-series designs, their vulnerability to bias increases. However, a design alone does not eliminate bias. Each study needs to be conducted according to certain standards of scientific inquiry. This has led to the creation of scoring systems to quantify the quality of research studies (Hadorn et al., 1996; Harbour & Miller, 2001).

Although the gold standard for research designs remains the RCT, a number of authors have presented evidence that well-executed observational studies may produce information consistent with that produced by RCTs. Concato, Shah, and Horwitz (2000) and Benson and Hartz (2000) selected a number of topic areas and employed systematic search routines to identify RCTs and observational studies reporting on the same topic; results from studies using the two designs were compared. According to the magnitudes of the treatment effects, each author employed a different strategy to select studies, but invoked similar criteria for RCTs and for the observational studies. Comparisons of the effect sizes for observational versus RCTs for each of the areas under investigation revealed that few differences could be attributed to the design alone.

Concato et al. (2000) indicated that observational studies that included a restricted cohort design, specified criteria for the inclusion and exclusion of subjects, included baseline data collection, adjusted for differences in baseline susceptibility for the outcome of interest, and employed intention-to-treat analyses produced findings comparable to those reported by RCTs. For observational studies, following the rigorous standards defined by RCTs increases the likelihood they will produce results similar to those obtained through RCTs. Cox (1958); Friedman, Furberg, and DeMets (1996); Piantadosi (1997); and Pocock (1983) suggested that methods for the conduct of clinical trials be clear and rigorous, and that they follow relatively strict protocols for implementation. Observational studies that adopt these standardized criteria, even though they may not have included random assignments, are likely to lead to similar conclusions. However, not all investigators who conducted such comparisons arrived at the same conclusions. Ioannidis et al. (2001) found that where treatment effects exceeded chance, treatment benefits were higher in nonrandomized studies. Nonrandomized observational studies often result in greater treatment benefits than RCTs.

In this book, we asked each contributor to emphasize studies involving RCTs in their reviews and to include observational studies only when no trials were available to examine the questions under investigation. Readers will want to scrutinize carefully comparative longitudinal designs that, although not RCTs, may provide important evidence regarding the effects of an intervention or how interventions may interact with patients possessing different risk factors.

## Four Defining Features of Quality Behavioral Interventions

We have chosen to focus on four elements that define the quality of a study. These four elements standardize the conduct of the inquiry, sharpen the comparison, and increase confidence in the conclusions. The four elements are theory, research questions, bias, and precision. To the extent that a study addresses each, it can advance the state of the science. The following summaries describe why we believe these four elements are critical to advancing our knowledge of behavioral interventions.

### DEFINING FEATURES OF QUALITY BEHAVIORAL INTERVENTIONS: THEORY

Theoretical frameworks guide the overall organization of behavioral interventions, specifically which elements will affect the outcomes and establish the findings with a larger body of information. As Piantadosi (1997) suggested, science is more than observation. Theory is essential to organize and frame research questions and to guide what observations are most critical and how the timing of measurements will be set. In the chapters that follow, the specification of theoretical frameworks may differ by topic area. In some areas, theories are implicit and seem to follow a medical model. In other areas, more fully developed models linking psychosocial dispositions with behavioral changes, which in turn lead to actions designed to promote health or reduce the impact of the disease (outcomes), are presented.

More complex theoretical models are used to explain fatigue and to direct interventions for its management. This theory, presented by Mock, begins with deficits in hemoglobin and seeks to demonstrate how moderate exercise may alleviate fatigue. Cognitive-behavioral models are proposed to instill patient belief about how exercise can improve fatigue. A weakness of these behavioral theories is that they fail to incorporate, for example, how growth-stimulating factors or other supportive agents might moderate the biochemical basis for the fatigue. For example, cognitive-behavioral approaches, designed to involve patients with fatigue in a program of exercise, might be enhanced by the use of supportive agents to boost the effect of exercise and thus increase patients' sense of control and efficacy of their actions. Thus, theories need to be expanded and incorporate arguments suggesting how behavioral interventions, in the presence of supportive care medications, may reduce patients' levels of fatigue over and above medical interventions alone. This will be essential if behavioral interventions are to demonstrate their unique value-added benefit for patient-centered care. In summary, theories that guide behavioral interventions need to incorporate clinical or physiological factors into the models in order to better account for observed patient outcomes.

## DEFINING FEATURES OF QUALITY BEHAVIORAL INTERVENTIONS: RESEARCH QUESTIONS

Regardless of the theory presented, the design employed, or the structure of the protocol, the single most important consideration is the research questions being posed (Cox, 1958; Piantadosi, 1997). To quote E. O. Wilson (1992), research questions:

> Spring fresh from a more primitive mode of thought, wherein the hunter's mind weaves ideas from old facts and fresh metaphors and the scrambled crazy images

of things recently seen. To move forward is to concoct new patterns of thought which in turn dictate the design of the models and experiments. (p. 63)

The research question frames the hypothesis and dictates the number of factors in the experiment, the comparisons to be made between or among factors, and the timing and nature of the proximal and more distant endpoints. Because the goal of an RCT is to compare a novel treatment with either conventional care or with another treatment, the research question establishes the conditions under which the comparisons will be made: how treatment factors influence or modify psychological states and hypothesize changes in behaviors and health outcomes. The research question should specify the risk factors that will influence the intensity and duration of the intervention needed, and when an outcome is most likely to be attained. A clearly presented research question clarifies the design by specifying the intervention, indicating the outcomes against which the intervention will be compared, identifying the timing of those comparisons, clarifying how risk factors may necessitate adjustments of the doses, and specifying how these features may affect the timing and probability that the desired outcome will be observed.

In this book, regardless of the behavioral intervention presented, the studies that employed randomized trial designs were more likely to pose more carefully crafted research questions. For example, in the chapter on screening and early detection, the research questions focus on how a behavioral intervention can affect women's stage of change or their perceived self-efficacy to increase the likelihood they will obtain a screening test for breast or other cancers. Research questions seeking to test new behavioral interventions should specify more carefully the dosage of the intervention in relation to the risk factors and how together these features influence the time when an outcome may be observed and the strength of the expected response. Research questions that seek to test behavioral interventions should specify the timing of the intervention and the hypothesized dose–response relationship between that intervention and the desired outcome.

## DEFINING FEATURES OF QUALITY BEHAVIORAL INTERVENTIONS: BIAS

An important reason for implementing an RCT is to reduce bias. Bias defines systematic error (Piantadosi, 1997). It is a systematic, nonrandom deviation of results and inferences from the truth, which can occur during the collection, analysis, interpretation, or publication of data. Types of bias may include selection bias, information bias, and recall bias (Last, 1995).

Numerous types of bias may enter into research and most result from inattention to study design. Bias enters into behavioral interventions when samples are not appropriately framed and when important sources of known variations in the sample are not included. Careful definitions of inclusion and exclusion criteria of participants are essential to assure that only patients with selected characteristics, which the intervention is seeking to address, are entered into trials (Piantadosi, 1997; Sacket, Haynes, Guyatt, & Tugwell, 1991).

Selection bias is a critical and complex feature of behavioral interventions (Piantadosi, 1997). Behavioral trials define inclusion criteria in terms of disease-based or clinical criteria, but they say little about *behavioral* components that might directly affect the outcomes of the research. Only rarely do studies define samples in terms of the intersection of clinical and behavioral characteristics. For example, studies on fatigue include patients with cancer. However, the eligibility criteria were not framed and did not include treatment protocols or the use of supportive drugs, nor did they include emotional distress, which may differentially influence patients' perceptions of fatigue. These two potential sources of bias in the selection and assignment of patients could have an independent effect on patient outcomes and can plausibly interact with the behavioral intervention in unknown ways. Further, studies seeking to reduce the burden of family members caring for cancer patients include family caregivers in the studies, but eligibility based on the level of caregiver burden is not considered in selecting family members.

Trials of behavioral interventions that do not take into account the timing of chemotherapy administration or the timing of the cycles with respect to the dates on which patient observations are made are open to bias. The chemotherapeutic protocol may vary in the types and severity of the symptoms produced. Further, if the timing of the cycles is not considered, then patients may have the behavioral intervention administered at different times in the cycle. Due to the nature of the side effects related to the nadir of the chemotherapy agents administered, some patients might be less eager or able to carry out the assigned interventions. Similarly, observations collected prior to entry into a trial or as proximal or distal endpoints can be biased if some occur close to the nadir of a cycle, while others occur just before the administration of the protocol.

If behavioral interventions are to be fairly assessed, more attention needs to be paid to how clinical factors may create bias in behavioral interventions. Behavioral research needs to consider and adjust for risk factors that may interact with the interventions and thus affect the observed outcomes. For example, women's levels of perceived vulnerability may affect research design. Disease progression (staging) is a risk factor, as are types of treatment protocols for clarifying how the dose of an intervention may differentially affect a specified outcome. Too often, trials of behavioral interventions do not include post-hoc analyses that seek to determine how risk factors (such as patient depression or disease severity) may alter findings. Thus, potential biases in the effect of interventions on outcomes may go unrecognized.

DEFINING FEATURES OF QUALITY BEHAVIORAL INTERVENTIONS: PRECISION

Lack of precision is perhaps the most significant weakness of most clinical trials. Precision describes the sample size considerations in clinical trials. Precision in estimating the outcome of a trial is related directly to the size of the sample. Precision in estimating a mean proportion or difference score depends upon measurement errors relating to person-to-person variations (Piantadosi, 1997). One classic study found that 69 of the 71 nonsignificant trials assessed had inadequate sample sizes to detect significant treatment effects. The calculation of sample size for a trial is complex and, as Friedman, Furberg, and DeMets (1996) indicated, parameter estimates are often calculated on small prior studies that have included populations different from those to be included in a larger study. Small developmental studies often involve receptive intervention patients familiar to the researchers and thus are fraught with self-selection bias.

Precision is frequently lost when investigators fail to appreciate the heterogeneity imposed by varying treatment protocols, people's prior use of the healthcare system, patients' comorbid conditions, and their psychological states, income, and/or education levels. Each of these characteristics may produce larger standard deviations around parameter estimates, which may require larger samples in order to detect a statistically significant effect. Many of the studies reported here have employed small sample sizes, which reduced their ability to detect significant effects of the interventions.

These four components of any RCT will affect the capacity of the researcher to produce and explain results within a framework other researchers can interpret and build upon. Thus, something close to causality can be inferred, and type I and II errors can be set within conventions. We trust readers will consider these criteria of quality as they read the following chapters and examine the presented studies. We believe that a critical review drawing upon these elements to evaluate the framework, the testable questions, the underlying assumptions, and the precision with which they are tested is a significant step in developing a body of evidence regarding the effects of behavioral interventions.

## CONCLUSION

Successful behavioral interventions will be those that add value and quality to the lives of patients. Implementing behavioral interventions in cancer care may add to or lower the costs of care and, in so doing, those costs will have to be assessed against the beneficial *outcomes* they produce. The demand for behavioral interventions may come from a variety of healthcare stakeholders, including insurance companies, insurance payers, clinicians, and/or patients and their families. Increases in the costs of healthcare, combined with an aging population with chronic diseases, may open the doors for the introduction of behavioral interventions to improve quality of life, to detect diseases early, and to manage symptoms through less costly approaches. Patients themselves may demand behavioral interventions as a component of their care. The growing movement in complementary therapy, documented in the chapter by Wyatt, provides evidence that patients have created a demand for these services. Only recently have systematic trials been launched to document the effects of complementary therapies on patients receiving treatment for cancer.

However, behavioral interventions for the prevention, screening, early detection, and treatment of cancer, as well as the interventions' impact on one's quality of life, reach patients through traditional avenues where medical services are provided, and where patients receive treatment and care. Therefore, if behavioral interventions are to demonstrate their effects, they must be integrated into the treatment regimens that patients receive. As readers examine the chapters in this book, they may want to reflect upon how the interventions described recognize and integrate behavioral objectives into medical plans of care. More importantly, readers should consider how the testing of behavioral interventions among patients undergoing cancer treatment may unwittingly bias their outcomes by ignoring risk factors that may require greater doses to achieve the desired outcome.

Because we know that a physician's suggestions are among the most effective methods for enlisting patient compliance, we have to conclude that patients who have received regular advice from their physicians regarding health monitoring and health maintenance behaviors and have chosen not to follow it may be different from persons who have not had regular contact with their physicians and therefore, for possibly different reasons, they have chosen not to participate in such monitoring and maintenance behaviors. Research that does not incorporate these and related differences into their inclusion criteria or address different interventions to these groups will find their results greeted by skepticism in the healthcare community.

This book is an overview of the state-of-the-science evidence for selected behavioral interventions in cancer care. Each chapter summarizes the literature and the evidence for interventions designed to modify patient behaviors and reviews the impact of those behaviors on health-related outcomes. In addressing these issues, each of the authors has adopted a similar strategy for assessing the evidence. Each author has emphasized studies that employed clinical trials with control groups (most of which employed random assignment) when available, drew upon the theoretical frameworks that guided the design of the intervention, and identified health-related outcomes as endpoints of interest.

The goal of this introductory chapter is to suggest points of reference, with respect to how evidence is organized and accumulated, and to offer some guides as to essential elements of trials that allow for the creation of evidence. Although not all the studies reviewed conform to all these standards, this information provides some points of reference against which to evaluate the state of *our* science and the directions and rigor required if behavioral models of care are to be accepted as valid components in the treatment of patients with cancer. We have tried to identify issues regarding the elements of an intervention that lead to the specification of a therapeutic dose, the guiding theoretical framework, and the methodological issues readers may want to use to test the quality of the evidence provided. Readers can also assess the issues related to acknowledging how the medical plan of care may influence the delivery of behavioral interventions.

## REFERENCES

Benson, K., & Hartz, A. J. (2000). A comparison of observational studies and randomized, controlled trials. *New England Journal of Medicine, 342*, 1878–1886.

Concato, J., Shah, N., & Horwitz, R. I. (2000). Randomized, controlled trials, observational studies, and the hierarchy of research. *New England Journal of Medicine, 342*, 1887–1892.

Cox, D. R. (1958). *Planning of Experiments*. New York: Wiley.

Devine, E. C., & Westlake, S. (1995). Effects of psychoeducational care provided to adults with cancer: A meta-analysis of 116 studies. *Oncology Nursing Forum, 22,* 1369–1381.

Fawzy, F. I. (1999). Psychosocial interventions for patients with cancer: What works and what doesn't. *European Journal of Cancer, 35,* 1559–1564.

Fawzy, F. I., Cousins, N., Fawzy, N. W., Kemeny, M. E., Elashoff, R., & Morton, D. (1990). A structured psychiatric intervention for cancer patients. I. Changes over time in methods of coping and affective disturbance. *Archives of General Psychiatry, 47,* 720–725.

Fawzy, F. I., Fawzy, N. W., Arndt, L. A., & Pasnau, R. O. (1995). Critical review of psychosocial interventions in cancer care. *Archives of General Psychiatry, 52,* 100–113.

Fawzy, F. I., Kemeny, M. E., Fawzy, N. W., Elashoff, R., Morton, D., Cousins, N., & Fahey, J. L. (1990). A structured psychiatric intervention for cancer patients. II. Changes over time in immunological measures. *Archives of General Psychiatry, 47,* 729–735.

Friedman, L. M., Furberg, C. D., & DeMets, D. L. (1996). *Fundamentals of clinical trials.* London: Mosby.

Glanz, K. (1997). Behavioral research contributions and needs in cancer prevention and control: Dietary change. *Preventive Medicine, 26*(Suppl. 5), 43–55.

Guyatt, G., & Rennie, D. (Eds.). (2002). *Users' guide to the medical literature: A manual for Evidence-based clinical practice.* Chicago: American Medical Association.

Hadorn, D. C., Baker, D., Hodges, J. S., & Hicks, N. (1996). Rating the quality of evidence for clinical practice guidelines. *Journal of Clinical Epidemiology, 49,* 749–754.

Harbour, R., & Miller, J. (2001). A new system for grading recommendations in evidence based guidelines. *British Medical Journal, 323,* 334–336.

Holland, J. C. (Ed.) (1998). *Psycho-oncology.* New York: Oxford University Press.

Ioannidis, J. P., Haidich, A. B., Pappa, M., Pantazis, N., Kokori, S. I., Tektonidou, M. G., et al. (2001). Comparison of evidence of treatment effects in randomized and nonrandomized studies. *Journal of the American Medical Association, 286,* 821–830.

Kubler-Ross, E. (1975). On death and dying. *Bulletin of the American College of Surgeons, 60*(6), 15–17.

Last, J. (1995). Redefining the unacceptable. *Lancet, 346,* 1642–1643.

Lewis, F. M. (1997). Behavioral research to enhance adjustment and quality of life among adults with cancer. *Preventive Medicine, 26*(Suppl. 5), 19–29.

Meyer, T. J., & Mark, M. M. (1995). Effects of psychosocial interventions with adult cancer patients: A meta-analysis of randomized experiments. *Health Psychology, 14,* 101–108.

National Cancer Institute. (1986). Cancer control objectives for the nation: 1985–2000. DHHS publication no. (NIH) 86-2880. Bethesda, Maryland: U.S. Department of Health and Human Services, Public Health Service.

Piantadosi, S. (1997). *Clinical trials: A methodologic perspective.* New York: John Wiley & Sons.

Pocock, S. J. (1983). *Clinical trials: A practical approach.* New York: John Wiley & Sons.

Redd, W. H., Montgomery, G. H., & DuHamel, K. N. (2001). Behavioral intervention for cancer treatment side effects. *Journal of the National Cancer Institute, 93,* 810–823.

Sacket, D. L., Haynes, R. B., Guyatt, G. H., & Tugwell, P. (1991). *Clinical epidemiology: A basic science for clinical medicine* (2nd ed.). Boston: Little, Brown & Co.

Wilson, E. O. (1992). *The diversity of life.* Cambridge, MA: Harvard University Press.

# 2

# Behavioral Interventions for Cancer Prevention: Dietary Intake and Physical Activity

**Debra Haire-Joshu**
**Marilyn S. Nanney**

Substantial evidence exists that lifestyle factors (dietary intake and physical activity are identified in this chapter) are associated with cancer risk (Paffenbarger et al., 1993). In many cases, diet and activity are considered alone with regard to cancer risk (e.g., diet alone). However, that risk is enhanced in the combined presence of both poor diet and sedentary activity, as seen through the association of obesity with cancer incidence (McTiernan, 2000). These two health behaviors are the focus of the cancer prevention guidelines supported by the American Cancer Society and others, as described in Table 2.1 (American Cancer Society Advisory Committee on Diet Nutrition, 1996).

This chapter reviews current evidence for the effectiveness of behavioral and educational interventions in cancer prevention, targeting dietary intake and physical activity. The following paragraphs describe the systematic approach used to conduct this review, which addresses methods, the selection of outcomes for review, the selection of interventions for review, and search strategy.

A behavioral epidemiological approach was used to organize phases of research on lifestyle factors and cancer (Sallis, Owen, & Fotheringham, 2000). Phase I addresses the link between diet, physical activity, and cancer

**TABLE 2.1   Recommended Diet and Physical Activity Guidelines for Cancer Prevention**

Persons over the age of 2 years should follow the following cancer-prevention guidelines:

1. Choose most foods from plant sources:
   - At least 2 daily servings of fruits
   - At least 3 daily servings of vegetables with at least one-third being dark green or orange vegetables
   - Eat other foods from plant sources, such as breads, cereals, grains, pasta, or beans several times each day

2. Limit intake of high-fat foods with total fat no more than 30% of total caloric intake and saturated fat no more than 10%. Limit consumption of meats, especially high-fat meats.

3. Be physically active, and achieve and maintain a healthy body weight. Be at least moderately active for 30 minutes or more most days of the week.

4. Limit consumption of alcoholic beverages.

(American Cancer Society [American Cancer Society Advisory Committee on Diet Nutrition 1996; American Institute for Cancer Research World Cancer Research Fund and American Institute for Cancer Research 1997])

incidence. Phase II addresses issues of measurement regarding these target behaviors. Phase III describes determinants of diet and physical activity behaviors, including sociodemographic factors and psychosocial variables as incorporated within theoretical perspectives. Phase IV reviews interventions designed to improve diet and physical activity, based upon an ecological model.

Studies were selected for review if the target was diet alone or physical activity alone. Studies that targeted changes in multiple risk factors (e.g., diet, activity, and smoking) were classified based on the primary outcome. An ecological approach was used to first evaluate dietary interventions, and then to evaluate physical activity interventions. Based on this conceptual model, interventions are reviewed that address three levels: individual, organizational, and community. *Individual* interventions are defined as those conducted in healthcare settings. Worksite studies comprise interventions conducted at the *organizational* level. Studies conducted within the *community* environment are defined as mass media interventions and/or intervention components targeting policies.

The reviews of interventions to improve dietary intake and increase physical activity reflect systematic searches of multiple databases as well as reviews of reference lists and consultations with experts in the field. In general, studies were published within the past 15 years; however, studies considered classic are cited when relevant. Studies citing randomized control designs were included. This chapter draws from several major national reviews and guideline development reports in the field (Ammerman et al., in press; Willett, 1999).

Dietary studies with a stated focus on cancer prevention are identified; those primarily addressing cardiovascular, diabetes, or other related risks are not included. Dietary studies citing purposes of general risk reduction were also included if the results were consistent with those noted for cancer prevention (e.g., increased fruit and vegetable consumption).

In contrast, cancer prevention interventions targeting physical activity have not been conducted. Physical activity interventions have instead focused on the prevention of other chronic diseases (e.g., cardiovascular). Therefore, the section on physical activity interventions is inclusive of behavioral studies focused on meeting recommended guidelines and reducing general risk, extrapolating that these findings are relevant to cancer prevention.

# PHASE I: EPIDEMIOLOGICAL EVIDENCE FOR DIET, PHYSICAL ACTIVITY, AND CANCER

## Dietary Intake and Cancer

About one-third of the 500,000 cancer deaths that occur in the United States each year are due to dietary factors (Willett, 1995; World Cancer Research Fund and American Institute for Cancer Research, 1997). High-risk dietary patterns have been cited as risk factors for a variety of cancers (Hunter et al., 1996; Potter, 1996; Williamson et al., 1995). These patterns reflect the intake of a variety of dietary constituents, with the majority of evidence addressing fat and cholesterol intake, and fruit and vegetable consumption. Additional evidence related to energy factors, carbohydrates, alcohol, and vitamins also exists (World Cancer Research Fund and American Institute for Cancer Research, 1997). This review focuses on fruit and vegetable consumption, fat intake, and other constituents as related to the incidence of specific cancers.

FRUIT AND VEGETABLE CONSUMPTION AND CANCER

Diets containing a substantial variety of fruits and vegetables will prevent 20% or more of all cancer cases (World Cancer Research Fund and American Institute for Cancer Research, 1997). Inverse relationships with fruit and vegetable intake have been reported in more than 200 case-control and prospective cohort studies. In addition, several studies cite biochemical indicators of fruit and vegetable consumption—such as serum carotenoid levels—as associated with reduced risks (Block, Patterson, & Subar, 1992; Steinmetz & Potter, 1996). Numerous studies have consistently found inverse associations between fruit and vegetable consumption and cancers of the lung (Ziegler, Mayne, & Swanson, 1996) and stomach (Kono & Hirohata, 1996). Fewer studies have suggested inverse associations for cancers of the oral cavity, larynx, esophagus, endometrium, cervix, bladder, kidney, and breast (Willett & Trichopoulos, 1996). More work is needed to identify which constituents of fruits and vegetables contribute to cancer-protective relationships (e.g., carotenoids, folic acid,vitamin C).

FAT INTAKE AND CANCER

In an analysis study of more than 200 cases of breast cancer, no overall association was seen for total fat intake ranging from 15% to greater than 45% of energy from fat (Hunter et al., 1996). In contrast, national rates of colon cancer are strongly associated with per capita consumption of animal fat and meat (Giovannucci et al., 1994). In a recent meta-analysis of 13 case-control studies, a significant association between total energy intake and colon cancer was observed, but saturated, monounsaturated, and polyunsaturated fat were not related to colon cancer risk after adjustment for total energy (Howe et al., 1997). For prostate cancer, the available evidence supports an association between animal fat products and risk (Willett, 1998; World Cancer Research Fund and American Institute for Cancer Research, 1997). Consistent findings across multiple studies support an association between the consumption of fat-containing animal products and prostate cancer incidence, but they do not support a relationship with vegetable fat intake (Giovannucci et al., 1993; Whittemore et al., 1995; Willett, 1999). Limited evidence exists to support a relationship between fat intake and the incidence of other cancers, such as ovarian, skin, and lung. In summary, the relationship between dietary fat intake and cancer incidence appears to be correlated with the intake of animal rather than vegetable fat, and appears to be primarily related to colon cancer risk (Willett, 1999).

OTHER DIETARY CONSTITUENTS

Some epidemiological evidence exists regarding cancer risk and dietary fiber, alcohol, and vitamin intake. In several large prospective studies, even after adjustments for other risk factors, overall fiber intake was not significantly associated with a lower risk of colon cancer incidence (Fuchs et al., 1999; Giovannucci et al., 1994; Goldbohm et al., 1994). In prospective studies, little or no relationship has been observed between fiber intake and the risk of breast cancer (Verhoeven et al., 1997). The high consumption of alcohol is associated with cancer of the oral cavity, larynx, esophagus, and liver (Willett, 1999). The data on vitamin intake are less clear. High doses of vitamins C and E are not associated with reduced breast cancer risk; vitamin E is not associated with the risk of prostate cancer. Beta carotene, as a supplement, actually increased the risk of lung cancer in two studies (Kushi, Fee, Sellers, Zheng, & Folsom, 1996; Rohan, Howe, Friedenreich, Jain, & Miller, 1993; Verhoeven et al., 1997; Willett, 1999).

## Physical Activity and Cancer

A large body of research has established that regular physical activity reduces the risk of premature death and disability from a variety of health conditions, including cancer (Eyler & Brownson, in press). In the United States, the annual number of lives lost through physical inactivity is estimated at more than 250,000, and relatively small increases in physical activity at the population level could avert 30,000 to 35,000 deaths per year (Powell & Blair, 1994). Only 25% of adults in the United States report engaging in moderate-intensity physical activity (30 minutes, 5 or more days per week). Forty percent report no leisure-time regular physical activity, and only 27% of students (grades 9 through 12) engage in moderate-intensity physical activity (U.S. Department of Health and Human Services, 2000).

Physical activity may have protective effects against cancer, based on early observations that activity on the job influences cancer risk (Powell & Blair, 1994). The strongest evidence for physical activity reducing cancer risk is found through the association with colon cancer. Numerous case-control and cohort studies representing over 13,000 colon cancer cases have found an inverse association between physical activity and the risk of colon cancer (Batty, 2000; Giovannucci et al., 1995; McTiernan, Ulrich, Slate, & Potter, 1998). Powell and Blair (1994) estimated, based on findings from 30 studies on colon cancer, that *inactivity* increases colon cancer risk by 32%. Marrett, Theis, and Ashbury, working with an expert panel (2000), cited convincing evidence from 42 of 48 studies of a 70% overall reduction in colon cancer risk related to physical activity.

McTiernan (1998) reported that 17 of 22 studies found an inverse association between physical activity and the risk of breast cancer, ranging from a relative risk of .20 to .89 for participation in the highest level of activity as compared with a sedentary lifestyle. Marrett et al. (2000) reported 22 of 33 studies citing a relationship between breast cancer risk and physical activity. In the largest published study of over 25,000 Norwegian women, an observed trend was that increased leisure and work-related physical activity decreased the risk of breast cancer. Women who exercised regularly had a 37% reduction in breast cancer risk, even after adjusting for parity and body mass index (Ainsworth, Steinfeld, Slattery, Daguise, & Zahn, 1998). Occupational and recreational activity were of equal importance in decreasing risk, suggesting that the type of activity may not be critical to a beneficial effect (Freindenreich, Thune, Brinton, & Albanes, 1998). Mechanisms that explain these findings include a reduction in fat stores from which estrogen is produced, protection against insulin resistance, which is a contributor to breast cancer, and bolstering of the immune system. However, definitive evidence is lacking, as the Norwegian study did not account for smoking, alcohol, or dietary intake (Chen, White, Malone, & Daling, 1996; Rockhill et al., 1998).

Evidence of the relationship between various cancers and activity is less convincing. For prostate cancer, Marrett and others cite that 14 of 23 studies identified a 50% reduction in risk, suggesting a possible relationship (Marrett et al., 2000; Thune, 1996; Thune & Lund, 1994). Also, data from three case-control studies indicate a negative association between physical activity and endometrial cancer risk (McTiernan et al., 1998). Few and inconsistent findings have also been reported for testicular, ovarian, and lung cancer (Marrett et al., 2000; World Cancer Research Fund and American Institute for Cancer Research, 1997).

It is unclear whether the type, intensity, or frequency of physical activity at different stages of life decreases risk for any of the cancer types (Wood, 2000). It appears that physical activity affects several physiologic and metabolic mechanisms that may influence cancer risk, including cardiovascular and pulmonary capacity, bowel motility, endogenous hormones, energy balance and reduced obesity, enhanced immune function, antioxidant defense, and DNA repair (Batty, 2000). Table 2.2 summarizes the evidence to date suggesting the relationship of cancer incidence with dietary intake and physical activity.

**TABLE 2.2   Summary of the Biologic Evidence of Cancer Risk Related to Dietary Intake and Physical Activity**

| *Evidence | Fruit and vegetable intake | Fat intake (total and saturated) | Other dietary constituents (fiber, alcohol, vitamin) intake | Physical activity |
|---|---|---|---|---|
| Convincing | ↓Mouth, pharynx, esophagus, lung, stomach, colon, rectum | | | ↓Colon |
| Probable | ↓Larynx, pancreas, breast, bladder | | *Carotenoids* ↓Lung *Vitamin C* ↓Stomach | ↓Breast |
| Possible | ↓Cervical, ovary, endometrium, thyroid, liver, prostate, kidney | —Breast ↑Lung, colon, rectum, breast, prostate | *Carotenoids* ↓Esophagus, stomach, colon, rectum, breast, cervix —prostate | ↓Prostate, lung |
| Insufficient | | ↑Ovary, endometrium, bladder | *Carotenoids* ↓Larynx, ovary, endometrium, bladder *Vitamin C* ↓Larynx, colon, rectum, breast, bladder | ↑Ovary, endometrium |

Level of risk
(↓)          Decreases risk
(↑)          Increases risk
(—)          No relationship

*Strength of the evidence

Convincing: Epidemiological studies show consistent associations, with little or no evidence to the contrary. A substantial number of acceptable studies (more than 20), preferably including prospective designs, should be conducted in different population groups and controlled for possible confounding factors. Exposure data should refer to the time preceding the occurrence of cancer. Dose-response relationships should be supportive of a causal relationship. Associations should be biologically plausible. Laboratory evidence is usually supportive.

Probable: Epidemiological studies showing associations are either not so consistent, with a number of studies not supporting the association, or the number or type of studies is not extensive enough to make a more definite judgment. Mechanistic and laboratory evidence is usually supportive.

Possible: Epidemiological studies are generally supportive but are limited in quantity, quality, or consistency. There may or may not be supportive mechanistic or laboratory evidence. Alternatively, few or no epidemiological data exist, but strongly supportive evidence from other disciplines can be found.

Insufficient: Only a few studies have been done, which are generally consistent but really do no more than hint at a possible relationship. Well-designed research is needed.

## PHASE II: ISSUES OF MEASUREMENT

### Dietary Assessment

The construct of diet is very complex, comprised of multiple behaviors and constituents that change daily as well as over the course of one's lifespan. Methods for capturing intake often focus on biomarkers, observation, or self-report; each has limitations that influence study interpretation. Biochemical indicators are potentially useful but do not exist for many dietary nutrients, they are expensive, and they are affected by genetic and lifestyle factors. Observation methods of food intake have been used but are expensive, require trained interviewers, and are limited to intake in specified settings in limited time frames (Briefel, 1994; Kristal, Beresford, & Lazovich, 1994; Thompson, Byers, & Kohlmeier, 1994).

Other methods rely on short-term self-report. The food diary method consists of a detailed listing of all foods consumed by an individual, typically for 3 to 7 days. This method is especially burdensome to the respondents, requiring a high level of subject motivation and literacy. The 24-hour dietary recall method solicits detailed information about everything the individual had to eat and drink over the past 24 hours. This method does not address variability in day-to-day eating habits, relies on memory, and requires a highly trained interviewer (Willett, 1998). These short-term recall methods may be unrepresentative of usual intake and are inappropriate for an assessment of past diet (Kristal, Andrilla, Koepsell, Diehr, & Cheadle, 1998; Rockett, Wolf, & Colditz, 1995).

Food-frequency questionnaires are commonly used to assess average intake over an extended period of time (past month or year). These questionnaires are easy to self-administer. However, questionnaires often vary by study, population, and time frames assessed, limiting comparisons of results across studies (Coates & Monteilh, 1997; World Cancer Research Fund and American Institute for Cancer Research, 1997).

In general, multiple weeks of diet records provide the best available comparison method with the least correlated error, albeit being a costly process (Willett, 1998). The use of multiple methods per subject with statistical correlation for within-person variation provides an alternative approach to validation.

## Physical Activity Assessment

The assessment of physical activity behavior is difficult to characterize because it is based on individual habits and practices that vary from day to day (Freedson & Miller, 2000). In a review by Sallis and Saelens (2000), five key points in assuring the accurate assessment of physical activity were identified: (a) the frequency, intensity, duration, type, and context of physical activity should be considered when evaluating the content and concurrent validity of instruments, (b) inaccurate reporting by respondents is likely and therefore test developers should consider the cognitive demands, (c) tests required for different populations should be calibrated, (d) test/ retest reliability studies should cover the same time period as the initial recall period and employ intraclass reliability coefficients, and (e) developers should assess the validity of measures.

Despite numerous limitations, self-report instruments are the most widely used type of physical activity measure (Sallis & Saelens, 2000). With the current public health emphasis on exposure, more objective methods such as motion sensors and heart rate monitors are suggested for quantifying physical activity (Freedson & Miller, 2000). However, these devices are relatively expensive and prone to instrument malfunction; further, they do not distinguish among types of activities and are difficult to interpret (Wood, 2000). The use of combined instruments in studies is recommended, such as an accelerometer plus a questionnaire (Bassett, 2000).

## PHASE III: DETERMINANTS OF DIET AND PHYSICAL ACTIVITY BEHAVIORS

### Sociodemographic Determinants

Income, age, and ethnicity of study participants influence the performance of lifestyle behaviors. Poor dietary intake is most likely among low-income adults, those with little education, and ethnic minorities. Several studies suggest that poverty and environmental inadequacies found in rural settings place individuals at increased risk for poor dietary intake (Kumanyika, 1993; McGinnis, 1991). Issues of access and availability to healthy foods in the environment have been a substantial predictor of intake (Hearn et al.,

1998). Low educational attainment and limited literacy skills found in rural communities may result in limited exposure and receptivity to health messages designed for better educated, urban groups.

Poorer dietary patterns are also notable among various ethnic groups. Among African-Americans, dietary patterns linked to cancer include over-consumption of calories and fat, excess intake of sodium or salt-cured foods (associated with stomach cancer), and inadequate consumption of fruits and vegetables that may protect against cancer (Kumanyika, 1990). Surveys of African-Americans have found barriers to achieving nutritious eating styles, including fear of giving up food (37%), belief that eating well is too time consuming (29%), and confusion over nutrition reports (29%; Harnack, Block, Subar, Lane, & Brand, 1997). In addition, African-American women are less concerned about weight (Jeffery, 1991). This may explain, in part, the higher rates of specific kinds of obesity-related cancers in this population.

Sociodemographic factors affecting diet are also mirrored in physical activity. Women are more likely to be inactive than men, physical inactivity increases with age, and inactivity decreases as education and income increase (Department of Health and Human Services, 1999). Low-income persons, those with disabilities, and racial and ethnic minority groups are more likely to be sedentary than the general population (Brownson et al., 1999). Because the prevalence of physical inactivity ranges as high as 43% in these population groups (Department of Health and Human Services, 1999), they are more likely to develop inactivity-related diseases. King et al. (2000) described determinants associated with physical activity common for both younger and older adults, including educational level, smoking status, weight, social support, exercise-related self-efficacy, and motives to improve physical fitness and appearance.

## Psychosocial Factors and Theoretical Perspectives

A variety of theories have been employed to understand psychosocial factors that influence lifestyle behavior changes. Such theories guide the development of interventions designed to target behaviors that mediate change. For this chapter, several theoretical perspectives and the psychosocial constructs that comprise these perspectives, which are consistently cited as influencing behaviors of both dietary intake and physical activity are reviewed.

## THEORY OF REASONED ACTION (TRA) OR THEORY OF PLANNED BEHAVIOR (TPB)

The Theory of Reasoned Action (TRA) or the Theory of Planned Behavior (TPB) has guided much of the research on health-related behaviors (Montano, Kasprzyk, & Taplin, 1997). TRA suggests that intention is the primary determinant of behaviors under personal control. The addition of perceived behavioral control is an effort to account for factors outside an individual's control that may affect intention and behavior. Among dietary studies based on this model, prediction is improved when specific behaviors are targeted for change (e.g., drinking low-fat milk versus eating low-fat foods; Baranowski, Cullen, & Baranowski, 1999). A review conducted by Baranowski et al. (1999) found the use of TRA to design fat-intake interventions among adults yielded $R^2$ values of less than .30. A review of the use of TRA in exercise interventions revealed that across 12 studies, the correlation of intention with exercise varied from $r = .19$ to .82, with a mean of $r = .55$. Variations in measures of intention, timing, and type of intervention may account for differences in results.

## TRANSTHEORETICAL MODEL (TTM)

The Transtheoretical Model (TTM), developed by Prochaska (1994), views change as a process involving progress through a series of stages, including precontemplation (no intention to change), contemplation (seriously considering change), preparation (making small changes), action (actively engaging in changing behavior), and maintenance (continuing successful change efforts). Several dietary studies have assessed TTM to guide intervention development or to evaluate progress (Campbell et al., 1998; Curry, Kristal, & Bown, 1992; Glanz et al., 1994; Greene & Rossi, 1998; Haire-Joshu, Auslander, Houston, & William, 1999). Auslander, Haire-Joshu, Williams, Houston, and Krebill (2000) used TTM to individually tailor information to dietary change among African-American women, achieving significantly positive results. TTM has also been used to develop physical activity interventions in worksites, primary care, and other settings (Cowan, Britton, Logue, Smucker, & Milo, 1995; Marcus, Selby, Niaura, & Rossi, 1992).

## SOCIAL COGNITIVE THEORY (SCT)

Social Cognitive Theory (SCT), developed by Bandura (1986), is a broad model that highlights the interactions among intrapersonal, social, and physical factors. SCT and related constructs have also been used extensively to encourage dietary change (Nestle et al., 1998; Resnicow et al., 1997). One SCT construct is self-efficacy, the strongest correlate of physical activity in virtually every study in which it is included—evident despite variations in the definition of the construct and its measurement. Other constructs of SCT, including self-monitoring and goal setting, have also been consistently noted as successful for diet and activity studies (Sorensen et al., 1992; Strychar et al., 1998; Tilley et al., 1999). Similarly, virtually every study that has included a measure of social influence on physical activity has found a significant association (Eyler et al., 1999). Social support can be direct (watching children or doing chores for the exerciser) indirect (encouraging or talking about activity) or modeled (Baron, Cutrona, Russell, Hicklin, & Lubaroff, 1990). In analyses of different subgroups of a community sample of adults, either social support or the presence of an exercise model was related to exercise habits in young men and women, older men and women, Latinos, and the obese (Department of Health and Human Services, 1999).

## ECOLOGICAL MODELS

Ecological models suggest that behaviors are influenced by interpersonal, social, and physical environmental variables; that these variables interact; and that an understanding of the multiple levels of the sociocultural environment is relevant for changing health behaviors (Sallis & Owen, 1997). McLeroy, Bibeau, and Steckler (1988) described the following five levels of intervention targeting: intrapersonal (toward characteristics of the individual), interpersonal (family-focused interventions), organizational (worksite), community, and public policy (regulatory procedures; McLeroy et al., 1988; McLeroy et al., 1995). Ecological models consider the connections between people and their environment, and address both individual behavior change and community-wide change. To date, this model has been used as an organizing framework to assure that interventions target multiple levels (Brownson et al., 1996; Campbell, Demark-Wahnefried, et al., 1999). For example, a coalition to reduce cardiovascular disease risk factors in rural Missouri implemented strategies that included screening individuals for high blood pressure, serving heart-healthy church dinners, and constructing a walking fitness path (Brownson, Dean, Dabney, & Brownson, 1998). Strategies aimed at creating a fuller health-promoting environment may be important in improving intervention effectiveness. An analysis of the interaction of interventions across levels has not been conducted.

## PHASE IV: EVALUATING INTERVENTIONS DESIGNED TO PREVENT CANCER

This section reviews intervention studies that addressed dietary intake and physical activity as the primary outcome. These studies are organized around an ecologic model. Dietary intervention studies are addressed first, across individual, organizational, and community levels. This is followed by physical activity intervention studies.

### Dietary Interventions

DIETARY INTERVENTIONS: INDIVIDUAL LEVEL

Healthcare settings are appropriate environments for targeting populations at risk for, or interested in, health-related concerns. Ammerman et al. (in press) reviewed 45 dietary change interventions conducted in healthcare settings, with 11 of those specifically citing participants at risk for cancer. Ten studies focused on fat as the primary result of interest, while one also included fruit and vegetable intake (Insull et al., 1990). In general, studies in these settings allowed for additional biochemical measures and more intensive dietary measures (e.g., 3-day food records) not as frequently attainable as in other settings. Eight of the interventions were delivered by dietitians, with one study using community volunteers, 40% of whom were dietitians (Kristal et al., 1997). In addition, as noted in Table 2.3, 9 of the 10 studies reviewed here recruited women at risk for or diagnosed with cancer. The most frequently tested interventions were individualized counseling, including self-monitoring, goal-setting, and problem-solving (Boyd et al., 1997; Chlebowski et al., 1993; McKeown-Eyssen et al., 1994; Simon et al., 1997); interactive recipe preparations (Boyd et al. 1996); and/or group sessions (Kristal et al., 1992; Nordevang et al., 1990; White et al., 1992). Follow-up contacts ranged from 12 months to 7 to 8 years. Significant reductions in self-reported measures of fat intake were noted in all studies.

DIETARY INTERVENTIONS: ORGANIZATIONAL LEVEL

In a recent review of dietary interventions (Ammerman et al., in press), six studies cited cancer prevention—or general risk reduction meeting cancer prevention dietary guidelines—as their purposes (see Table 2.4). Fat-related and fruit and vegetable intake were the combined primary result of four studies (Reynolds et al., 1997; Sorensen et al., 1996; Strychar et al., 1998; Tilley et al., 1999), with one citing fat intake only (Sorensen et al., 1992),

**TABLE 2.3  Dietary Interventions at the Individual Level: Health Care Settings**

| | Theoretical/ conceptual framework | Design | Sample | Measures | Results |
|---|---|---|---|---|---|
| Boyd, Lockwood, Greenberg, Martin, & Tritchler (1997) | None reported | RCT; dietary counseling with written guide delivered by RD; monthly for 12 months, quarterly for 12 months | N = 216, women healthcare workers aged 30–65 years screened for cancer risk | 3-day food record, follow-up at 2 years | Significant reduction in total fat (%), saturated fat |
| Boyd, Martin, Beaton, Cousins, & Kriukov (1996) | None reported | RCT; individualized dietary counseling, self-help materials, low-fat recipe testing; monthly for 12 months | N = 157, women aged 30–65 years at risk for cancer | Food frequency questionnaire, cholesterol, follow-up at 7–8 years | Significant reduction in total fat (%), total fat (grams), saturated fat, improved cholesterol |
| Chlebowski et al. (1993) | Social Learning Theory | RCT; individualized instruction, fat goal-setting, self-monitoring; biweekly sessions (4), monthly (8), bimonthly through 12 months, quarterly through 24 months | N = 196, women aged more than 50 years at risk for cancer | Food record, cholesterol | Significant reduction in total fat (%), total fat (grams), saturated fat |

| | Theoretical/ conceptual framework | Design | Sample | Measures | Results |
|---|---|---|---|---|---|
| Insull et al. (1990) | None reported | RCT; group and individualized counseling sessions plus self-help materials; small group for 8 sessions, biweekly for 4 sessions, and individual counseling at 12 weeks, 12 months, and 24 months | $N = 292$, women aged 45–69 years, at risk for cancer | 4-day food record, follow-up at 6, 12, and 24 months | Significant reduction in total fat (%), total fat (grams), saturated fat, total cholesterol |
| Kristal et al. (1992) | None reported | RCT; group session, conducted by RD over 18 months | $N = 904$, women aged 45–69 years, at risk for cancer | Food frequency questionnaire, diet-related habits, follow-up at 12 months | Significant reduction in total fat (grams) and change in diet-related habits (i.e., avoiding fat as flavoring) |

*(continued)*

31

**TABLE 2.3  Dietary Interventions at the Individual Level: Health Care Settings** (*continued*)

| | Theoretical/ conceptual framework | Design | Sample | Measures | Results |
|---|---|---|---|---|---|
| Kristal, Shattuck, Bowen, Sponzo, & Nixon (1997) | Social Learning Theory, Cognitive Behavior Therapy, Self-Control Theory | RCT; individual and group session interactive activities, self-assessment, and cancer treatment; delivered by community volunteers; 7 weekly and 10 group sessions for 12 months | $N = 144$, women aged less than 75 years and postmenopausal, previously treated for cancer | 4-day food records, follow-up at 3, 6, and 12 months | Significant improvements in reduction of total fat (%), total fat (grams) |
| McKeown-Eyssen et al. (1994) | None reported | RCT; dietary counseling by RD and prepackaged fiber snacks; monthly counseling for 12 months | $N = 122$, both genders, aged less than 85 years at risk for cancer | 4-day food record, follow-up at 12 and 24 months | Significant reduction in dietary fat (%) and total fat (grams) for women, dietary fat (%) for men |

| Theoretical/conceptual framework | Design | Sample | Measures | Results |
|---|---|---|---|---|
| Nordevang, Ikkala, Callmer, Hallstrom, & Holm (1990) | None reported | RCT; individualized counseling, group meetings, low-fat cooking classes, RD delivered, regular cancer treatment; counseling 4–6 times for 2 months, then every third month, and group meetings every 6–8 weeks over 24 months | N = 169, women aged 50–65 years, at risk for cancer | Diet history interview, follow-up at 24 months |
| White et al. (1992) | None reported | RCT; small-group education and counseling, goal setting, fat counter; weekly, monthly, and bimonthly sessions over 3 years | N = 908 women aged 45–69 years, at risk for cancer | Food frequency questionnaire; follow-up at 12 months |
| | | | | Significant intervention effects for all (total fat, saturated fat, fiber, calcium, cereals, bread, milk, and beef); no significant effects for pasta or rice |

**Table 2.4   Dietary Interventions at the Organizational Level: Worksite Settings**

| | Theoretical/conceptual framework | Design | Sample | Measures | Results |
|---|---|---|---|---|---|
| Buller et al. (1999) | Theory to use paraprofessionals | RCT; five-a-day plus environmental/cafeteria promotions, peer-education program, printed materials: newsletters for 18 months | 10 public employers | 24-hour recall and food frequency questionnaire, follow-up at 18 and 24 months | Significant effect on fruit and vegetable intake by recall and by food frequency questionnaire at follow-up 1 |
| Sorensen et al. (1992) | Community organization, social learning, diffusion of innovation, adult learning theories | RCT; advisory board, direct and environmental interventions including cholesterol screenings, counseling, and referrals; BBQ parties; classes with skill building; goal-setting and self-monitoring; modified food service, cafeteria environment for 15 months | 16 worksites | Food frequency questionnaire, follow-up at 15 months | Significant reduction in total fat (%) |

| | Theoretical/ conceptual framework | Design | Sample | Measures | Results |
|---|---|---|---|---|---|
| Sorensen et al. (1996) | Stages of change, community activation | RCT, matched-pair design; interactive activities, posters, self-assessment, contests, smoking cessation, food environment alterations for 24 months | 111 worksites | Food frequency questionnaire, follow-up at 30 months | Significant decrease in fat (%) consumption, significant increase in fruit and vegetable intake |
| Strychar et al. (1998) | Social Learning Theory | RCT; nutrition education, assessment of eating habits, contracts, information on cholesterol level pregroup 1 or at follow-up for group 2; 1 session and mailing | 6 hospital worksites | 24-hour recall, follow-up at 16 and 20 weeks | Significant decrease in total fat group 1, not significant for group 2; decrease in saturated fat for groups 1 and 2; significant cholesterol change for both intervention groups |

*(continued)*

**Table 2.4  Dietary Interventions at the Organizational Level: Worksite Settings** (*continued*)

| | Theoretical/ conceptual framework | Design | Sample | Measures | Results |
|---|---|---|---|---|---|
| Tilley et al. (1999) | Health Belief Model, Social Learning Theory, stages of change, Social Support Theory | RCT; nutrition classes, skill development, goal setting, self-help materials, personalized dietary feedback, family component and support; classes year 1, mailed information year 2 | 28 worksites | Food frequency questionnaire, health habits questionnaire, follow-up at 1 and 2 years | Significant effects in fruit, vegetable, and fiber consumption; decrease in fat intake |

and one citing fruit and vegetable intake only (Buller et al., 1999). Intervention delivery was diverse. Five of the studies cited multiple theoretical approaches to intervention development, including community-based theories (Sorensen et al., 1992; Sorensen et al., 1996), social learning theory (Sorensen et al., 1992; Strychar et al., 1998; Tilley et al., 1999), and stages of change theory (Buller et al., 1999). Employees were actively involved in the development of several studies, while family components were included in at least two studies (Sorensen et al., 1992; Strychar et al., 1998; Tilley et al., 1999). Environmental changes altering food access were also reported (Kristal, Glanz, Tilley, & Li, 2000; Sorensen et al., 1992; Sorensen et al., 1996; Tilley et al., 1999). Significant improvements were noted in dietary results across all studies.

DIETARY INTERVENTIONS: COMMUNITY LEVEL

Ammerman et al. (in press) identified 15 studies addressing cancer-specified or related dietary behavior change at the community level (see Table 2.5). Of these, three addressed fat intake alone as the primary outcome (Baranowski et al., 1990; Campbell, Honess-Morreale, Farrell, Carbone, & Brasure, 1999; Stolley & Fitzgibbon. 1997), five addressed fruit and vegetable consumption alone (Campbell, Demark-Wahnefried, et al., 1999; Havas et al., 1998; Lutz et al., 1999; Marcus, Heimendinger, et al., 1998; Marcus, Morra, et al., 1998), and seven addressed combined intake (Brug, Glanz, van Assema, Kok, & van Breukelen, 1998; Brug, Steenhuis, van Assema, & de Vries, 1996; Brug, Steenhuis, van Assema, Glanz, & De Vries, 1999; Fitzgibbon, Stolley, Avellone, Sugerman, & Chavez, 1996; Hartman, McCarthy, Park, Schuster, & Kushi, 1997; Pierce et al., 1997; Rodgers et al., 1994). Nine studies cited use of theory in intervention development, with SCT, TTM, and the Health Belief Model most frequently used.

Several studies targeted fruit and vegetable consumption-related results along with individual change strategies (e.g., goal setting) and the inclusion of family components (Baranowski et al., 1990; Fitzgibbon et al., 1996; Stolley & Fitzgibbon, 1997). Marcus et al. (1998) delivered telephone messages and mailings based on participant stage of change, yielding significant improvements in meeting five-a-day guidelines ($p<.01$) (Marcus, Heimendinger, et al., 1998; Marcus, Morra, et al. 1998). Several studies achieved significant effects in both fruit and vegetable consumption and fat intake through intensive interventions using home visits or classes

**TABLE 2.5  Dietary Interventions at the Community Level**

| | Theoretical/ conceptual framework | Design | Sample | Measures | Results |
|---|---|---|---|---|---|
| Baranowski et al. (1990) | Social Cognitive Theory, Social Support Theory, Adult Education Theory | RCT; culturally appropriate materials; group and family counseling; aerobic activity; delivered by RD, educator, aerobics instructor | N = 198, African-American families of 5th to 7th graders | Food frequency questionnaire, follow-up at 14 weeks | Significant improvement in high total fat and saturated fat intake for mothers and children, dose-response relationship noted |
| Brug, Steenhuis, van Assema, Glanz, and De Vries (1999) | None reported | RCT; computer-tailored dietary letters; one letter | N = 347, home computer participants, aged 19–59 years | Food frequency questionnaire, follow-up at 4 weeks | Significant improvement in vegetable intake, not significant for fruit intake |
| Campbell, Honess-Morreale, Farrell, Carbone, and Brasure (1999) | Social Cognitive Theory, stages of change, Transtheoretical Model | RCT; videos and individually tailored media; one 30-minute session | N = 377, Low-income women, at least 18 years old | Food frequency questionnaire, follow-up at 1 and 3 months | Significant reduction in fat intake |

| | Theoretical/ conceptual framework | Design | Sample | Measures | Results |
|---|---|---|---|---|---|
| Campbell et al. (1999) | Social Cognitive Theory, stages of change, social support, Precede-Proceed Models | RCT; lay health advisors with Five-a-Day sessions, cookbooks, recipe tasting, tailored church bulletins, grocery involvement, pastor support and nutrition-action teams | 49 black, rural churches | Food frequency questionnaire, follow-up at 24 months | Significant increase in fruit and vegetable consumption |
| Lutz et al. (1999) | Health Belief Model, Social Cognitive Theory, stages of change, goal setting | RCT; newsletters, nontailored; newsletters tailored with goal setting; newsletters tailored without goal setting; 4 monthly newsletters | $N = 573$, home HMO population randomized to one of three intervention or control groups | Fruit and vegetable servings and variety; follow-up at 6 months | Significant increase in fruit and vegetable intake and variety for all intervention and control groups |

*(continued)*

39

**TABLE 2.5  Dietary Interventions at the Community Level (continued)**

| | Theoretical/ conceptual framework | Design | Sample | Measures | Results |
|---|---|---|---|---|---|
| Marcus, Heimendinger, et al. (1998) | Reasoned action, Health Belief Model, Social Cognitive Theory, stages of change | RCT; staged phone messages and interactive counseling, behavioral strategies, follow-up mailings; one call and mailings | N = 1,286 Cancer Information Service | Single-item and food frequency questionnaires; follow-up at 4 weeks and at 4 months | Significant increase in fruit and vegetable consumption |
| Marcus, Morra et al. (1998) | Health Belief Model, Social Cognitive Theory, stages of change | RCT; telephone message based on stage of change; one call, two mailings | N = 277 Cancer Information Service participants older than 18 years | Food frequency questionnaire, follow-up at 4 weeks | Significant increase in fruit and vegetable consumption<br><br>Rodgers et al. (1994) |
| None reported | Matched pair quasi-experimental design, altered shelf labels, food guide signs, and advertising | N = 60, store pairs supermarket shoppers aged 21–75 years | Food frequency questionnaire, health habits questionnaire, follow-up at 2 years | Significant reduction in reported fat intake, not significant differences in fruit and vegetable, fats, and oil intake | |

(Fitzgibbon et al., 1996; Hartman et al., 1997), and using minimal interventions, such as computer-tailored letters (Brug et al., 1996; Brug et al., 1998; Brug et al., 1999).

DIETARY INTERVENTIONS: SPECIAL POPULATIONS

Interventions addressing sociodemographic factors and special needs of various ethnic groups frequently involve participants in intervention development while institutionalizing the intervention within the community. Havas et al. (1998) trained peer educators to work with low-income USDA Women, Infants, and Children (WIC) participants, resulting in a significant increase in fruit and vegetable intake by intervention participants (.56 versus .13, $p<.002$). Stolley and Fitzgibbon (1997) intervened with low-income mothers and daughters participating in a tutoring program and were able to achieve significant reductions in dietary fat. Campbell, Demark-Wahnefried, et al. (1999) worked with African-American churches to implement a fruit and vegetable intervention using tailored bulletins and other print materials, as well as group activities such as gardening, including lay health advisors, pastor support, and the distribution of materials through local grocers. The result was a statistically significant difference between the intervention and delayed treatment counties of 0.85 servings per day of fruits and vegetables.

## Physical Activity Interventions

PHYSICAL ACTIVITY INTERVENTIONS: INDIVIDUAL LEVEL

A comprehensive review by Simons-Morton (1998) evaluated physical activity education or counseling primary prevention methods. Seven randomized clinical trials addressed primary prevention through physical activity counseling (see Table 2.6). Five reported significant increases in physical activity at one or more follow-up measures. All the studies used moderate-intensity aerobic activity as the chief behavioral target, with SCT and the TTM cited as the basis for six interventions. The majority of the physical activity interventions were delivered by physicians, with two delivered by nurses and two by allied health specialists. Intervention components were categorized as advice and/or instruction, behavioral approaches (feedback, reinforcement, and goal setting), the provision of equipment, and supervised training. Several reviews concluded that long-term intervention and multiple contacts are needed, and supervised exercise, the

**TABLE 2.6 Physical Activity Interventions at the Individual Level: Healthcare Settings**

| | Theoretical/ conceptual framework | Design | Sample | Measures | Results |
|---|---|---|---|---|---|
| Bull, Jamrozik, & Blacksby (1999) | Transtheoretical Model | RCT; verbal advice on exercise and follow-up pamphlet mailed within 2 days of visit | N = 534, sedentary patients aged 18–60+ with appointments to see general practice | Self-report of more than 1 episode of physical activity in past 2 weeks, follow up at 1, 6, and 12 months | Significant improvement in physical activity at 1 and 6 months, not significant at 12 months |
| Burton, Paglia, German, Shapiro, & Damiano (1995) | None reported | RCT; two multiple risk factor visits 1 year apart with optional follow-up visit | N = 3,097, Medicare patients aged 65–85 | Self-report of sedentary lifestyle, follow-up at 2 years | Not significant difference percentage, sedentary at 2 years |
| Calfas et al. (1996) | Social Cognitive Theory, stages of change | RCT; assessment and 2–5 minute provider counseling, 5–10 minute call with health educator, follow-up 2 weeks later | N = 225, sedentary patients, M age = 39 | Report of total walking, weekly minutes walking for exercise, and Caltrac motion sensor, with follow-up at 4–6 weeks | Significant improvement in minutes of walking, total walking, Caltrac counts at 4–6 weeks |

| | Theoretical/ conceptual framework | Design | Sample | Measures | Results |
|---|---|---|---|---|---|
| Graham-Clarke & Oldenburg (1994) | Stages of change, cognitive behavioral | RCT; risk assessment and video or risk assessment, video, plus self-help booklets | N = 382, patients aged 18–69 with one or more cardiovascular disease risk factors | Self-report frequency for the duration of vigorous, moderate physical activity and walking, with follow-up at 4 and 12 months | No significant difference between groups in type, frequency, duration, and energy expenditure at follow-up |
| Imperial Cancer Research Fund OXCHECK Study Group (1994) | None reported | RCT; annual 45–60-minute, multiple-factor consultation; goal-setting and health education | N = 6124, general practice patients aged 35–64 | Self-report of sedentary lifestyle, follow-up at 1 year | Significant decrease in percentage sedentary at follow-up |
| Marcus et al. (1997) | Stages of change, Social Cognitive Theory | RCT; counseling sessions by physicians on physical activity during visit, plus 1-month follow-up | N = 44, middle/older-age sedentary adults, M age = 67 | Completion of physical activity scale for the elderly (PASE), follow-up at 6 weeks | Not significant increase in physical activity among both groups, but greater in patients who received more counseling messages |

*(continued)*

43

**TABLE 2.6  Physical Activity Interventions at the Individual Level: Healthcare Settings** *(continued)*

| | Theoretical/ conceptual framework | Design | Sample | Measures | Results |
|---|---|---|---|---|---|
| McTiernan, Ulrich, Slate, & Potter (1998) | None reported | Feasibility study, convenience sample; aerobic exercise sessions and a low-fat (20% of calories from fat) diet for 2 weeks | N = 9, stage 1 or 2 breast cancer patients aged 40–74 years | Measurement of outcomes in weight, waist/hip circumference, body fat, and lean mass | Lost 2.6 pounds, 3.4 cm in waist circumference, 4.6 cm in hip circumference, 2.3% body fat, and gained 2.3% lean mass |
| Schultz (1993) | Education principles | RCT; 20–30-minute education session plus behavioral skills counseling; a phone follow-up at 2, 4, and 6 weeks | N = 54, sedentary patients aged 36–65 | Self-report frequency for duration of leisure versus vigorous physical activity in past week, with follow-up at 6 and 12 weeks | Significant increase in physical activity frequency at 6 weeks, not significant physical activity frequency at 12 weeks, not significant change in duration of physical activity |
| Winburn, Walter, Arroll, Milyard, & Russell (1998) | None reported | RCT; brief goal-oriented verbal advice and written prescription given by general practice | N = 456, sedentary patients, M age = 49 | Self-report time in physical activity during past 2 weeks, with follow-up at 6 weeks | Significant increase in any physical activity and percentage increasing physical activity at 6 weeks, not significant physical activity duration change |

provision of equipment, and behavioral approaches seem to improve success (Eyler & Brownson, in press; Fisher, Brownson, Eyler, Haire-Joshu, & Schootman, 2001; Simons-Morton, 1998).

PHYSICAL ACTIVITY INTERVENTIONS: ORGANIZATIONAL LEVEL

In a recent review of worksite physical activity interventions, Dishman, Oldenburg, O'Neal, and Shephard (1998) evaluated 26 studies involving nearly 9,000 subjects as yielding a small but nonsignificant positive effect equivalent to increasing physical activity among 6 people per 100. Effects were larger in studies employing a nonrandomized quasi-experimental design and intervention incentives, and smaller in studies employing a randomized experimental design using a health education/risk appraisal intervention. The follow-up results from eight studies yielded a mean effect of 0.12 (95% CI, $-0.08$, 0.32). Among the moderating variables, the intervention type ($r = 0.47$, $p = 0.013$), especially those using exercise prescriptions, yielded larger effects (see Table 2.7).

Other reviews suggest that design and issues involving the conduct of worksite studies influence enthusiasm for results (Shephard, 1996; Shephard & Shek, 1998). Although most reported interventions yield small but favorable changes in body mass, skinfold, aerobic power, muscle strength, and flexibility, studies are limited by low participation rates and attrition. In contrast, the Johnson and Johnson worksite program is an example of a well-conducted, comprehensive, quasi-experimental study with a large study population. This program reported significant increases in the intervention group with regard to cardiorespiratory fitness as measured by $VO_2$ max or maximal oxygen intake (Breslow, Fielding, Herrman, & Wilbur, 1990). Worksite programs hold promise due to their ability to reach a variety of racial, ethnic, and economic groups (Briss et al., 2000; Eyler & Brownson, in press).

PHYSICAL ACTIVITY INTERVENTIONS: COMMUNITY LEVEL

The majority of community-based studies targeting physical activity has targeted the prevention of cardiovascular disease, not cancer. This is likely due to the recent recognition of physical activity as a valuable tool in preventing cancer through weight maintenance and other mechanisms, and the limited ability to measure cancer prevention in the absence of long-term studies. However, the extensive research on physical activity across chronic

**TABLE 2.7  Physical Activity Interventions at the Organizational Level: Worksite Settings**

| | Theoretical/ conceptual framework | Design | Sample | Measures | Results |
|---|---|---|---|---|---|
| Blair, Piserchia, Wilbur, & Crowder (1986) | Public Health Intervention Model | Nonrandomized control trial; health promotion program, health education focused on energy expenditure and vigorous exercise; follow-up at 2 years | $N = 992$, volunteer employees at 4 worksites | Validated self-report of energy expenditure in vigorous physical activity, estimates of maximal oxygen uptake | 104% increase of daily energy expenditure in vigorous activity |
| Gomel, Oldenburg, Simpson, & Owen (1993) | Transtheoretical Model, stages of change | RCT; allocation to health risk assessment, risk-factor education, behavioral counseling, or behavioral counseling plus incentives; follow-up at 3, 6, and 12 months | $N = 431$, employees at 28 sites, $M$ age $= 32$ | Aerobic capacity determined by heart rate response to fitness test | Short-term increase in aerobic capacity |
| Heirich, Foote, Erfut, & Konopka (1993) | None reported | RCT; staffed fitness facility, counseling with at-risk employees, peer support at work; 3-year post-test | $N = 1880$, employees at 4 worksites | Self-report health screen, participation in physical activities | Significant increases in frequency of physical activity |

diseases is relevant, given the etiologic evidence suggesting a relationship between cancer and physical activity (Eyler & Brownson, in press; McTiernan, 1998a; McTiernan, Stanford, Weiss, Daling, & Voigt, 1996).

Three comprehensive, large-scale, community-based heart disease prevention trials were conducted. The Stanford Five-City Project, the Minnesota Heart Health Program (MHHP), and the Pawtucket Heart Health Program involved 12 cities; 6 received a 5- to 8-year multifactorial risk-reduction program (Carleton, et al. 1995; Farquhar, et al. 1984; Jacobs, et al., 1986; see Table 2.8). All three community trials targeted changes in biological risk factors (e.g., blood pressure and blood cholesterol) and also reported physical activity results.

Young and Lee (1998) used cross-sectional data to report modest but statistically significant changes in physical activity in the intervention communities. The MHHP had less of a focus on media education and concentrated more on promoting physical activity through local health professions and community organizations. Luepker et al. (1994) reported MHHP cross-sectional physical activity outcome data as having small but significant effects over the first 3 years of the program. In the Pawtucket Heart Health Program, no differences were reported in self-reported knowledge of the benefits of physical activity, attempts to increase exercise, or the prevalence of physical inactivity between Pawtucket and the comparison community (Carleton et al., 1995). These findings suggest that community-wide interventions for increased physical activity are feasible, acceptable to community residents, and potentially effective in bringing about change in at least some aspects of physical activity and fitness (Fisher et al., 2001).

PHYSICAL ACTIVITY INTERVENTIONS: SPECIAL POPULATIONS

In a review by Taylor et al. (1998), 10 studies were found concerning physical activity interventions among ethnic minority groups. Six studies were among African-Americans, one study among Mexican-Americans, and three studies included multiethnic populations. Most interventions were designed using information from the target group (e.g., instructions in Spanish and convenient locations), were flexible in response to participant concerns, and were focused on involving community members in advisory panels and/or delivering the intervention (Avila & Hovell, 1994). Only two interventions reported consistent and positive changes; both of these were weight-loss programs for women.

**TABLE 2.8  Physical Activity Interventions at the Community Level**

| | Theoretical/ conceptual framework | Design | Sample | Measures | Results |
|---|---|---|---|---|---|
| Andersen, Franckowiak, Snyder, Bartlett, & Fontaine (1998) | None reported | Convenience sample of shopping center shoppers; signs promoting the health and weight-control benefits of taking the stairs were placed beside escalators | Convenience sample of shopping center shoppers | Direct observation of sex, age, race, weight classification, and use of stairs | Stair use increased for all demographics observed |
| Avila & Hovell (1994) | Constructs from Social Cognitive Theory | RCT; instruction for diet modification and walking for exercise (20 minutes each session); 1 session per week for 8 weeks | $N = 44$, obese Mexican-American women | Measurement of moderate exercise with five questions for an index of moderate intensity lifestyle activity | Significant increases for fitness, exercise rate and frequency, and diet/exercise knowledge; significant decreases for BMI, waist-to-hip ratio, and serum cholesterol |

| | Theoretical/conceptual framework | Design | Sample | Measures | Results |
|---|---|---|---|---|---|
| Blamey, Mutrie, & Aitchison (1995) | None reported | Convenience sample of underground station pedestrians; signs encouraging use of stairs placed where stairs and escalators were adjacent | Convenience sample of underground station pedestrians | Observations of stair usage; follow-up at 2, 4, 12 and weeks | Significant higher usage of stairs during posting of signs |
| Eaton et al. (1999) | None reported | RCT; community-based physical activity programs | $N = 15{,}261$ community residents | Delivery of cross-sectional surveys at 2-year intervals for 7 years | Not significant differences in self-reported knowledge of the benefits of physical activity, attempts to increase physical activity, or prevalence of physical inactivity between groups |

*(continued)*

**TABLE 2.8   Physical Activity Interventions at the Community Level** *(continued)*

| | Theoretical/ conceptual framework | Design | Sample | Measures | Results |
|---|---|---|---|---|---|
| Haskell et al. (1994) | None reported | RCT; community-wide health education programs on knowledge, attitudes, self-efficacy, and behavior regarding physical activity | Four central California cities | Examination of physical activity knowledge, attitudes, self-efficacy, and behavior; follow-up every 2 years | Significant effect in men for energy expenditure and participation in vigorous activities; significant effect in women for participation in moderate activities |
| Kanders et al. (1994) | None reported | RCT; interactive group sessions with handouts on nutrition, exercise, and behavior modification; 1 hour per week for 10 weeks | $N = 67$, obese African-American women | Examination of self-reported time exercising (minutes per week) | Significant increase in time spent exercising |
| Lewis et al. (1993) | None reported | RCT; community-based group exercise classes and literature, competitions, social support, motivation, and barrier reduction | African-American residents of 8 communities | Examination of class attendance, self-report, total physical activity score, and participation in 13 specific activities | Significant differences in average attendance by community at group exercise sessions |

## CONCLUSIONS AND IMPLICATIONS
## FOR FUTURE RESEARCH

The first conclusion is that the evidence of dietary protection against cancer is strongest and most consistent for diets high in fruits and vegetables. Evidence that physical activity protects against colon cancer is convincing. Evidence that alcohol increases risk for a variety of cancers and that obesity is associated with cancer is also convincing. Implications for further research in this area are related to specific constituents (e.g., vitamins and types of activity), timing (patterns of intake and activity over the lifespan), and dose (amount needed for protection).

This review also suggests that a consistent positive improvement exists among studies across all settings addressing fruit and vegetable intake. For fat intake, in general, the median difference between intervention and control groups has been cited for total fat as −15.5 percentage points and for saturated fat as −14.5 (Ammerman et al., in press). In addition, the consistent effectiveness of physical activity interventions is documented (Eyler & Brownson, in press).

Third, the way diet and physical activity are measured has an effect on intervention results. For example, in this review, studies defined dietary results as fat intake (percentage and/or grams of total and/or saturated fat) and fruit and vegetable intake. Studies defined physical activity as vigorous and moderate physical activity, or lifestyle physical activity. Results were measured by self-report, biomarkers, observation, or technological monitoring. All these variations make interpretation complex. Consensus measurement standards for dietary and physical activity intake are needed to allow comparisons across studies.

Further, common determinants are associated with both high-risk diet and activity behaviors, including being poor, female, and less educated. Studies that examine the cumulative effect of these variables over one's lifespan (e.g., long-term versus short-term poverty) and in combination (e.g., poverty alone or poverty plus gender) may allow for further interpretation of the impact of poverty-related lifestyle patterns on cancer risk.

Fifth, theoretical models have been used consistently to understand psychosocial and mediating factors that result in individual diet and activity behavior changes. Additional research is needed that allows for understanding which aspects of the theory are most effective to specific aspects of behavior change, and how these approaches can inform additional theoretical development. Theories that address factors that mediate changes in *both* combined diet and activity behavior changes are needed.

Sixth, certain factors enhance effectiveness across interventions. The determination of behavior change is influenced by diverse factors, including individual characteristics (self-efficacy) and environmental characteristics (e.g., access; Sherwood, 2000). Longer interventions, interventions that use a variety of methods to reach the population, and interventions that pay specific attention to methods of behavior change seem to be the most effective. However, it is difficult to isolate the effects of the intervention components or generalize findings. Studies need to be conducted that allow for identifying determinants and intervention components most effective in altering diet and activity behaviors.

In addition, no one setting or approach will work universally to improve diet and activity behaviors. Variations will take place among people in different settings who will change behavior for multiple reasons. Research is needed to identify characteristics where interventions can be better tailored to meet the needs of specific persons or groups. Finally, issues of intervention maintenance have been minimally addressed by diet or activity studies; whether or not patients continue to engage in positive behaviors after the interventions is not known. If and when decay in intervention effects begins needs to be determined, and designs that allow for measuring the impact over time are also needed.

## ACKNOWLEDGMENT

The authors would like to acknowledge the research conducted by two research assistants: Julie M. Bender and Cynthia D. Linneman.

## REFERENCES

Ainsworth, B. E., Steinfeld, B., Slattery, M. L., Daguise, V., & Zahn, S. H. (1998). Physical activity and breast cancer. *Cancer, 83*, 611–620.

American Cancer Society's 1996 Advisory Committee on Diet Nutrition. (1996). Guidelines on diet, nutrition, and cancer prevention: Reducing the risk of cancer with healthy food choices and physical activity. *CA-A Cancer Journal for Clinicians, 25*, 325–341.

Ammerman, A., Lindquist, C., Hersey, J., Jackman, A. M., Gavin, N. I., Carces, C., et al. (in press). Evidence report on the efficacy of intervention to modify dietary behavior related to cancer risk: Final evidence report (Contract No. 290-97-0011, No. 5). Research Triangle Institute, NC: Agency for Healthcare Research and Quality.

Andersen, R., Franckowiak, S., Snyder, J., Bartlett, S., & Fontaine, K. (1998). Can inexpensive signs encourage the use of stairs? Results from a community intervention. *Annals of Internal Medicine, 129*, 363–369.

Auslander, W. F., Haire-Joshu, D., Williams, J. H., Houston, C., & Krebill, H. (2000). The short-term impact of a health promotion program for African-American women. *Research on Social Work Practice, 10*, 56–77.

Avila, P., & Hovell, M. (1994). Physical activity training for weight loss in Latinas: A controlled trial. *International Journal of Obesity, 18*, 476–482.

Bandura, A. (1986). *Social Foundations of Thought and Action. A Social Cognitive Theory*. Englewood Cliffs, NJ: Prentice Hall.

Baranowski, T., Cullen, K. W., & Baranowski, J. (1999). Psychosocial correlates of dietary intake: Advancing dietary intervention. *Annual Review of Nutrition, 19*, 17–40.

Baranowski, T., Simons-Morton, B., Hooks, P., Henske, J., Tiernan, K., et al. (1990). A center-based program for exercise change among black-American families. *Health Education Quarterly, 17*, 179–196.

Baron, R. S., Cutrona, C. E., Russell, D. W., Hicklin, D., & Lubaroff, D. M. (1990). Social support and immune function among spouses of cancer patients. *Journal of Personality and Social Psychology, 59*, 344–352.

Bassett, D. R. (2000). Validity and reliability issues in objective monitoring of physical activity. *Research Quarterly for Exercise & Sport, S-71*(12), 30–33.

Batty, D. (2000). Does physical activity prevent cancer? *British Medical Journal, 321*, 1424–1425.

Blair, S., Piserchia, P., Wilbur, C., & Crowder, J. (1986). A public health intervention model for worksite health promotion. *Journal of the American Medical Association, 255*, 921–926.

Blamey, A., Mutrie, N., & Aitchison, T. (1995). Health promotion by encouraged use of stairs. *British Medical Journal, 311*, 289–291.

Block, G., Patterson, B., & Subar,A. (1992). Fruit, vegetables, and cancer prevention: A review of the epidemiological evidence. *Nutrition and Cancer, 18*, 1–29.

Boyd, N. F., Lockwood, G. A., Greenberg, C. V., Martin, L. J., & Tritchler, D. L. (1997). Effects of a low-fat high-carbohydrate diet on plasma sex hormones in premenopausal women: Results from a randomized controlled trial. *British Journal of Cancer, 76*, 127–135.

Boyd, N. F., Martin, L. J., Beaton, M., Cousins, M., & Kriukov, V. (1996). Long-term effects of participation in a randomized trial of a low-fat, high-carbohydrate diet. *Cancer Epidemiology, Biomarkers and Prevention, 5*, 217–222.

Breslow, L., Fielding, J., Herrman, A. A., & Wilbur, C. S. (1990). Worksite health promotion: Its evolution and the Johnson & Johnson experience. *Preventive Medicine, 19*, 13–21.

Briefel, R. R. (1994). Assessment of the US diet in national nutrition surveys: National collaborative efforts and NHANES. *American Journal of Clinical Nutrition, 59* (Suppl.), 164–167.

Briss, P., Zaza, S., Pappaioanou, M., Fielding, J., Wright-De Aguero, L., Truman, B., et al. (2000). Developing an evidence-based Guide to Community Preventive Services methods. The Task Force on Community Preventive Services. *American Journal of Preventive Medicine, 18*(Suppl. 1), 35–43.

Brownson, C. A., Dean, C., Dabney, S., & Brownson, R. C. (1998). Cardiovascular risk reduction in rural minority communities: The Bootheel Heart Health Project. *Journal of Health Education, 29,* 158–165.

Brownson, R. C., Eyler, A. A., King, A. C., Shyu, Y., Brown, D. R., & Homan, S. M. (1999). Reliability of information on physical activity and other chronic disease risk factors among US women aged 40 years or older. *American Journal of Epidemiology, 149,* 379–391.

Brownson, R. C., Smith, C., Pratt, M., Mack, N., Jackson-Thompson, J., Dean, C., et al. (1996). Preventing cardiovascular disease through community-based risk reduction: The Bootheel Heart Health Project. *American Journal of Public Health, 86,* 206–213.

Brug, J., Glanz, K., van Assema, P., Kok, G., & van Breukelen, G. J. (1998). The impact of computer-tailored feedback and iterative feedback on fat, fruit, and vegetable intake. *Health Education and Behavior, 25,* 517–531.

Brug, J., Steenhuis, I., van Assema, P., & de Vries, H. (1996). The impact of a computer-tailored nutrition intervention. *Preventive Medicine, 25,* 236–242.

Brug, J., Steenhuis, I., van Assema, P., Glanz, K., & de Vries, H. (1999). Computer-tailored nutrition education: differences between two interventions. *Health Education Research, 14,* 249–256.

Bull, F. C., Jamrozik, K., & Blacksby, B. A. (1999). Tailored advice on exercise—does it make a difference? *American Journal of Preventive Medicine, 16,* 230–239.

Buller, D. B., Morrill, C., Taren, D., Aickin, M., Sennott-Miller, L., Buller, M. K., et al. (1999). Randomized trial testing the effect of peer education at increasing fruit and vegetable intake. *Journal of the National Cancer Institute, 91,* 1491–1500.

Burton, L., Paglia, M., German, P., Shapiro, S., & Damiano, A. (1995). The effect among older persons of a general preventive visit of three health behaviors: Smoking, excessive alcohol drinking, and sedentary lifestyle. *Preventive Medicine, 24,* 492–497.

Calfas, K., Long, B., Sallis, J., Wooten, W., Pratt, M., & Patrick, K. (1996). A controlled trial of physician counseling to promote the adoption of physical activity. *Preventive Medicine, 25,* 225–233.

Campbell, M., Symons, M., Demark-Wahnefried, W., Polhamus, B., Bernhardt, J., McClelland, J. W., et al. (1998). Stages of change and psychosocial correlates of fruit and vegetable consumption among rural African-American church members. *American Journal of Health Promotion, 12,* 185–191.

Campbell, M. K., Demark-Wahnefried, W., Symons, M., Kalsbeek, W. D., Dodds, J., Cowan, A., et al. (1999). Fruit and vegetable consumption and prevention of cancer: The Black Churches United for Better Health project. *American Journal of Public Health, 89,* 1390–1396.

Campbell, M. K., Honess-Morreale, L., Farrell, D., Carbone, E., & Brasure, M. (1999). A tailored multimedia nutrition education pilot program for low-income women receiving food assistance. *Health Education Research, 14,* 257–267.

Carleton, R. A., Lasater, T. M., Assaf, A. R., Feldman, H. A., McKinlay, S., & Pawtucket Heart Health Program Writing Group. (1995). The Pawtucket Heart Health

Program: Community changes in cardiovascular risk factors and projected disease risk. *American Journal of Public Health, 85*, 777–785.

Chen, C. L., White, E., Malone, K., & Daling, J. (1996). Leisure-time physical activity in relation to breast cancer among young women. *Cancer Causes & Control, 8*, 77–84.

Chlebowski, R. T., Blackburn, G. L., Buzzard, I. M., Rose, D. P., Martino, S., Khandekar, J. D., et al. (1993). Adherence to a dietary fat intake reduction program in postmenopausal women receiving therapy for early breast cancer. The Women's Intervention Nutrition Study. *Journal of Clinical Oncology, 11*, 2072–2080.

Coates, R. J., & Monteilh, C. P. (1997). Assessments of food-frequency questionnaires in minority populations. *American Journal of Clinical Nutrition, 65*(Suppl.), 1108–1115.

Cowan, R., Britton, P. J., Logue, E., Smucker, W., & Milo, L. (1995). The relationship among the transtheoretical model of behavioral change, psychological distress, and diet attitudes in obesity: Implications for primary care intervention. *Journal of Clinical and Psychological Medical Settings, 2*, 249–267.

Cox, R. H., Parker, G. G., Watson, A. C., Robinson, S. H., Simonson, S. H., Elledge, C. J., Diggs, J. C., & Smith, E. (1995). Dietary cancer risk of low-income women and change with intervention. *Journal of the American Dietetic Association, 95*, 1031–1034.

Curry, S. J, Kristal, A. R., & Bown, D. J. (1992). An application of the stage model of behavior change to dietary fat reduction. *Health Education and Research, 7*, 97–105.

Department of Health and Human Services. (1999). *Physical activity and health: A report of the surgeon general.* Atlanta, GA: U.S. Department of Health and Human Services, Centers for Disease Control and Prevention, National Center for Chronic Disease Prevention and Health Promotion.

Dishman, R. K., Oldenburg, B., O'Neal, H., & Shephard, R. J. (1998). Worksite physical activity interventions. *American Journal of Preventative Medicine, 15*, 344–361.

Eaton, C., Lapane, K., Garber, C., Gans, K., Lasater, T., & Carleton, R. (1999). Effects of a community-based intervention on physical activity: The Pawtucket Heart Health Program. *American Journal of Public Health, 89*, 1741–1744.

Eyler, A., & Brownson, R. (in press). Effectiveness of interventions for cancer prevention and early detection: Promoting physical activity. *Preventive Medicine.*

Eyler, A., Brownson, R., Donatelli, R. J., King, A. C., Brown, D., & Sallis, J. F. (1999). Physical activity social support and middle- and older-aged minority women: Results from a US survey. *Social Science & Medicine, 49*, 781–789.

Farquhar, J. W., Fortmann, S. P., Maccoby, N., Woods, P. D., Haskell, W. L., Taylor, C. B., et al. (1984). The Stanford Five City Project: An overview. In J. D. Matarazzo, S. M. Weiss, J. A. Herd, N. E. Miller, & S. M .Weiss (Eds.), *Behavioral health: A handbook of health enhancement and disease prevention.* New York: Wiley.

Fisher, E. B., Brownson, R. C., Eyler, A. A., Haire-Joshu, D. L., & Schootman, M. (2001). *Effectiveness of interventions to promote cancer prevention and early detection.* Paper presented at the National Cancer Policy Board, Washington, D.C.

Fitzgibbon, M. L., Stolley, M. R., Avellone, M. E., Sugerman, S., & Chavez, N. (1996). Involving parents in cancer risk reduction: A program for Hispanic American families. *Health Psychology, 15,* 413–422.

Freedson, P. S., & Miller, K. (2000). Objective monitoring of physical activity using motion sensors and heart rate. *Research Quarterly for Exercise & Sport, S-71* (Suppl. 2), 21–29.

Freindenreich, C. M., Thune, I., Brinton, L. A., & Albanes, D. (1998). Epidemiologic issues related to the association between physical activity and breast cancer. *American Cancer Society, 83,* 600–610.

Fuchs, C. S., Giovannucci, E. L., Colditz, G. A., Hunter, D. J., Stampfer, M. J., Rosner, B., Speizer, F. E., & Willett, W. C. (1999). Dietary fiber and the risk of colorectal cancer and adenoma in women. *New England Journal of Medicine, 340,* 169–176.

Giovannucci, E., Ascherio, A., Rimm, E. B., Colditz, G. A., Stampfer, M. J., & Willett, W. C. (1995). Physical activity, obesity and risk for colon cancer and adenoma in men. *Annals of Internal Medicine, 122,* 327–334.

Giovannucci, E., Rimm, E. B., Colditz, G. A., Stampfer, M. J., Ascherio, A., Chute, C. C., et al. (1993). A prospective study of dietary fat and risk of prostate cancer. *Journal of the National Cancer Institute, 85,* 1571–1579.

Giovannucci, E., Rimm, E. B., Stampfer, M. J., Colditz, G. A., Ascherio, A., & Willett, W. C. (1994). Intake of fat, meat, and fiber in relation to risk of colon cancer in men. *Cancer Research, 54,* 2390–2397.

Glanz, K., Patterson, R. E., Kristal, A. R., DiClemente, C. C., Heimendinger, J., Linnan, L., et al. (1994). Stages of change in adopting healthy diets: Fat, fiber, and correlates of nutrient intake. *Health Education Quarterly, 21,* 499–519.

Goldbohm, R. A., van den Brandt, P. A., van Veer, P., Brants, H. A., Dorant, E., Sturmans, F., et al. (1994). A prospective cohort study on the relation between meat consumption and the risk of colon cancer. *Cancer Research, 54,* 718–723.

Gomel, M., Oldenburg, B., Simpson, J., & Owen, N. (1993). Worksite cardiovascular risk reduction: A randomized trial of health risk assessment, education, counseling, and incentives. *American Journal of Public Health, 83,* 1231–1238.

Graham-Clarke, P., & Oldenburg, B. (1994). The effectiveness of general practice-based physical activity intervention on patient physical activity status. *Behavior Change, 11,* 132–144.

Greene, G. W., & Rossi, S. R. (1998). Stages of change for reducing dietary fat intake over 18 months. *Journal of the American Dietetic Association, 98,* 529–534.

Haire-Joshu, D., Auslander, W., Houston, C., & William, J. H. (1999). Staging of dietary patterns in African-American women. *Health Education and Behavior, 26,* 90–102.

Harnack, L., Block, G., Subar, A., Lane, S., & Brand, R. (1997). Association of cancer prevention-related nutrition knowledge, beliefs, and attitudes to cancer prevention dietary behavior. *Journal of the American Dietetic Association, 97,* 957–965.

Hartman, T. J, McCarthy, P. R., Park, R. J., Schuster, E., & Kushi, L. H. (1997). Results of a community-based low-literacy nutrition education program. *Journal of Community Health, 22,* 325–341.

Haskell, W. L., Alderman, E. L., Fair, J. M., Maron, D. J., Mackey, S. F., Superko, H. R., et al. (1994). Effects of intensive multiple risk factor reduction on coronary arteriosclerosis and clinical cardiac events in men and women with coronary artery disease. The Stanford Coronary Risk Intervention Project (SCRIP). *Circulation, 89*, 975–990.

Havas, S., Anliker, J., Damron, D., Langenberg, P., Ballesteros, M., & Feldman, R. (1998). Final results of the Maryland WIC Five-a-Day Promotion Program. *American Journal of Public Health, 88*, 1161–1167.

Hearn, M. D., Baranowski, J., Doyle, C., Smith, M., Lin, L. S., & Resnicow, K. (1998). Environmental influences on dietary behavior among children: Availability and accessibility of fruits and vegetables enable consumption. *Journal of Health Education, 29*, 26–32.

Heirich, M., Foote, A., Erfut, J., & Konopka, B. (1993). Worksite physical fitness programs: Comparing the impact of different programs designs on cardiovascular risks. *Journal of Occupational Medicine, 5*, 510–517.

Howe, G. R., Aronson, K. J., Benito, E., Castelleto, R., Cornee, J., Duffy, S., et al. (1997). The relationship between dietary fat intake and risk of colorectal cancer: Evidence from the combined analysis of 13 case-control studies. *Cancer Causes and Control, 8*, 215–228.

Hunter, D. J., Spiegelman, D., Adami, H. O., Beeson, L., van den Brandt, P. A., Folsom, A. R., et al. (1996). Cohort studies of fat intake and the risk of breast cancer —A pooled analysis. *New England Journal of Medicine, 334*, 356–361.

Imperial Cancer Research Fund OXCHECK Study Group. (1994). Effectiveness of health checks conducted by nurses in primary care: Results of OXCHECK study after one year. *British Medical Journal, 308*, 308–312.

Insull, W., Henderson, M. M., Prentice, R. L., Thompson, D. J., Clifford, C., Goldman, S., et al. (1990). Results of a randomized feasibility study of a low-fat diet. *Archives of Internal Medicine, 150*, 421–427.

Jacobs, D. R., Luepker, R. V., Mittlemark, M. B., Folsom, A. R., Pirie, P. L., Mascioili, S. R., et al. (1986). Community-wide prevention strategies: Evaluation design of the Minnesota Heart Health Program. *Journal of Chronic Disease, 39*, 775–787.

Jeffery, R. W. (1991). Population perspectives on the prevention and treatment of obesity in minority populations. *American Journal of Clinical Nutrition, 53*(Suppl.), 1621–1624.

Kanders, B. S., Ullmann-Joy, P., Foreyt, J. P., Heymsfield, S. B., Heber, D., Elashoff, R., et al. (1994). The black American lifestyle intervention (BALI): The design of a weight loss program for working-class African-American women. *Journal of the American Dietetic Association, 94*, 310–312.

King, A., Castro, C., Wilcox, S., Eyler, A., Sallis, J., & Brownson, R. (2000). Personal and environmental factors associated with physical inactivity among different racial-ethnic groups of U.S. middle-aged and older-aged women. *Health Psychology, 19*, 354–364.

Kono, S., & Hirohata, T. (1996). Nutrition and stomach cancer. *Cancer Causes and Control, 7*, 41–55.

Kristal, A. R., Andrilla, C. H., Koepsell, T. D., Diehr, P. H., & Cheadle, A. (1998). Dietary assessment instruments are susceptible to intervention-associated response set bias. *Journal of the American Dietetic Association, 98*, 40–43.

Kristal, A. R., Beresford, S. A., & Lazovich, D. (1994). Assessing change in diet-intervention research. *American Journal of Clinical Nutrition, 59*(Suppl.), 185–189.

Kristal, A. R., Glanz, K., Tilley, B. C., & Li, S. (2000). Mediating factors in dietary change: Understanding the impact of a worksite nutrition intervention. *Health Education Behavior, 27*, 112–125.

Kristal, A. R., Shattuck, A. L., Bowen, D. J., Sponzo, R. W., & Nixon, D. W. (1997). Feasibility of using volunteer research staff to deliver and evaluate a low-fat dietary intervention: The American Cancer Society Breast Cancer Dietary Intervention Project. *Cancer Epidemiology, Biomarkers & Prevention, 6*, 459–467.

Kristal, A. R., White, E., Shattuck, A. L., Curry, S., Anderson, G. L., Fowler, A., et al. (1992). Long-term maintenance of a low-fat diet: Durability of fat-related dietary habits in the Women's Health Trial. *Journal of the American Dietetic Association, 92*, 553–559.

Kumanyika, S. (1990). Diet and chronic disease issues for minority populations. *Journal Nutritional Education, 22*, 89–96.

Kumanyika, S. (1993). Special issues regarding obesity in minority populations. *Annals of Internal Medicine, 119*, 650–654.

Kushi, L. H., Fee, R. M., Sellers, T. A., Zheng, W., & Folsom, A. R. (1996). Intake of vitamins A, C, and E and postmenopausal breast cancer. *American Journal of Epidemiology, 144*, 165–174.

Lewis, C., Raczynski, J., Heath, B., Levinson, R., Hilyer, J., & Cutter, G. (1993). Promoting physical activity in low-income African-American communities: The PARR project. *Ethnicity and Disease, 3*, 106–118.

Luepker, R. V., Murray, D. M., Jacobs, D. R., Jr., Mittelmark, M. B., Bracht, N., Carlaw, R., et al. (1994). Community education for cardiovascular disease prevention: Risk factor changes in the Minnesota Heart Health Program. *American Journal of Public Health, 84*, 1383–1393.

Lutz, S. F., Ammerman, A. S., Atwood, J. R., Campbell, M. K., De Vellis, R. F., & Rosamond, W. D. (1999). Innovative newsletter interventions improve fruit and vegetable consumption in healthy adults. *Journal of the American Dietetic Association, 99*, 705–709.

Marcus, A. C., Heimendinger, J., Wolfe, P., Rimer, B. K., Morra, M., Cox, D., et al. (1998). Increasing fruit and vegetable consumption among callers to the CIS: Results from a randomized trial. *Preventative Medicine, 5*(Suppl. 2), 16–28.

Marcus, A. C., Morra, M., Rimer, B. K., Stricker, M., Heimendinger, J., Wolfe, P., et al. (1998). A feasibility test of a brief educational intervention to increase fruit and vegetable consumption among callers to the Cancer Information Service. *Preventative Medicine, 27*, 250–261.

Marcus, B. H., Goldstein, M. G., Jette, A., Simkin-Silverman, L., Pinto, B. M., Milan, F., et al. (1997). Training physicians to conduct physical activity counseling. *Preventative Medicine, 26*, 382–388.

Marcus, B. H., Selby, V. C., Niaura, R. S., & Rossi, J. S. (1992). Self-efficacy and the stages of exercise behavior change. *Research Quarterly for Exercise & Sports, 63,* 60–66.

Marrett, L. D., Theis, B., Ashbury, F. D., & Expert Panel. (2000). Chronic Diseases in Canada Workshop report: Physical activity and cancer prevention. *CDIC, 21*(4).

McGinnis, J. M. (1991). Obesity in minority populations: Policy implications. *American Journal of Clinical Nutrition, 53*(Suppl.), 1512–1514.

McKeown-Eyssen, G. E., Bright-See, E., Bruce, W. R., Jazmaji, V., Cohen, L. B., Pappas, S. C., et al. (1994). A randomized trial of a low fat high fiber diet in the recurrence of colorectal polyps. *Journal of Clinical Epidemiology, 47,* 525–536.

McLeroy, K., Bibeau, D., & Steckler, A. (1988). An ecological perspective on health promotion programs. *Health Education Quarterly, 15,* 351–377.

McLeroy, K. R., Clark, N. M., Simons-Morton, B. G., Forster, J., Connell, C. M., Altman, D., et al. (1995). Creating capacity: Establishing a health education research agenda for special population. *Health Education Quarterly, 22,* 390–405.

McTiernan, A. (1998a). Physical activity and cancer etiology: Associations and mechanisms. *Cancer Causes & Control, 9,* 487–509.

McTiernan, A. (1998b). Possible mechanisms mediating an association between physical activity and breast cancer. *Cancer, 83*(Suppl. 3), 621–628.

McTiernan, A. (2000). Associations between energy balance and body mass index and risk of breast carcinoma in women from diverse racial and ethnic backgrounds in the U.S. *Cancer, 88,* 1248–1255.

McTiernan, A., Stanford, J., Weiss, N., Daling, J., & Voigt, L. (1996). Occurrence of breast cancer in relation to recreational exercise in women age 50–64 Years. *Epidemiology, 7,* 598–604.

McTiernan, A., Ulrich, C., Slate, S., & Potter, J. (1998). Physical activity and cancer etiology: associations and mechanisms. *Cancer Causes and Control, 9,* 487–509.

Montano, D. E., Kasprzyk, D., & Taplin, S. H. (1997). The theory of reasoned action and the theory of planned behavior. In K. Glanz, F. M. Lewis, & B. Rimer (Eds.), *Health behavior and health education, theory research and practice* (pp. 85–112.) San Francisco: Jossey-Bass.

Nestle, M., Wing, R., Birch, L. L., DiSogra, L., Arbor, A., Middleton, S., et al. (1998). Behavioral and social influences on food choice. *Nutrition Reviews, 56*(Suppl. 5), 50–64.

Nordevang, E., Ikkala, E., Callmer, E., Hallstrom, L., & Holm, L. E. (1990). Dietary intervention in breast cancer patients: effects on dietary habits and nutrient intake. *European Journal of Clinical Nutrition, 44,* 681–687.

Paffenbarger, R. S., Jr., Hyde, R. T., Wing, A. L., Lee, I. M., Jung, D. L., & Kampert. J. B. (1993). The association of changes in physical-activity level and other lifestyle characteristics with mortality among men. *New England Journal of Medicine, 328,* 538–545.

Pierce, J. P., Faerber, S., Wright, F. A., Newman, V., Flatt, S. W., Kealey, S., et al. (1997). Feasibility of a randomized trial of a high-vegetable diet to prevent breast cancer recurrence. *Nutrition and Cancer, 28,* 282–288.

Potter, J. D. (1996). Nutrition and colorectal cancer. *Cancer Causes and Control, 7,* 127–146.

Powell, K. E., & Blair, S. N. (1994). The public health burden of sedentary habits: Theoretical but realistic estimates. *Medical Science and Sports Exercise, 26,* 851–856.

Prochaska, J. O. (1994). *Staging: A revolution in health promotion.* Paper presented at the Society for Behavioral Medicine, Boston, MA.

Resnicow, K., Davis-Hearn, M., Smith, M., Baranowski, T., Lin, L. S., Baranowski, J., et al. (1997). Social-cognitive predictors of fruit and vegetable intake in children. *Health Psychology, 16,* 272–276.

Reynolds, K. D., Gillum, J. L., Hyman, D. J., Byers, T., Moore, S. A., Paradis, G., et al. (1997). Comparing two strategies to modify dietary behavior and serum cholesterol. *Journal of Cardiovascular Risk, 4,* 1–5.

Rockett, H. R., Wolf, A. M., & Colditz, G. A. (1995). Development and reproducibility of a food frequency questionnaire to assess diets of older children and adolescents. *Journal of the American Dietetic Association, 95,* 336–340.

Rockhill, B., Willett, W. C., Hunter, D., Manson, J., Hankinson, S., Spiegelman, D., et al. (1998). Physical activity and breast cancer risk in a cohort of young women. *Journal of the National Cancer Institute, 90,* 1155–1159.

Rodgers, A. B., Kessler, L. G., Portnoy, B., Potosky, A. L., Patterson, B., Tenney, J., et al. (1994). "Eat for Health:" A supermarket intervention for nutrition and cancer risk reduction. *American Journal of Public Health, 84,* 72–76.

Rohan, T. E., Howe, G. R., Friedenreich, C. M., Jain, M., & Miller, A. B. (1993). Dietary fiber, vitamins A, C, and E, and risk of breast cancer: A cohort study. *Cancer Causes and Control, 4,* 29–37.

Sallis, J., Owen, N., & Fotheringham, M. J. (2000). Behavioral epidemiology: A systematic framework to classify phases of research on health promotion and disease prevention. *Annals of Behavioral Medicine, 22,* 294–298.

Sallis, J., & Saelens, B. E. (2000). Assessment of physical activity by self-report: Status, limitations, and future directions. *Research Quarterly for Exercise & Sport, S-71*(Suppl. 1), 1–13.

Sallis, J. F., & Owen, N. (1997). Ecological models. In K. Glanz and B. K. Rimer, & F. M. Lewis (Eds.), *Health behavior and health education: Theory, research, and practice* (2nd ed., pp. 403–424). San Francisco: Jossey-Bass.

Schultz, S. (1993). Educational and behavioral strategies related to knowledge of and participation in an exercise program after cardiac positron emission tomography. *Patient Education and Counseling, 22,* 47–57.

Shephard, R. (1996). Worksite fitness and exercise programs: A review of methodology and health impact. *American Journal of Health Promotion, 10,* 436–452.

Shephard, R. J., & Shek, P. N. (1998). Associations between physical activity and susceptibility to cancer. *Sports Medicine, 26,* 293–315.

Sherwood, N. E. (2000). The behavioral determinants of exercise: Implications for physical activity interventions. *Annual Review of Nutrition, 20,* 21–44.

Simon, M. S., Heilbrun, L. K., Boomer, A., Kresge, C., Depper, J., Kim, P. N., et al. (1997). A randomized trial of a low-fat dietary intervention in women at high risk for breast cancer. *Nutrition and Cancer, 27,* 136–142.

Simons-Morton, D. G. (1998). Effects of interventions in health care settings on physical activity or cardiorespiratory fitness. *American Journal of Preventive Medicine, 15*, 413–430.

Sorensen, G., Morris, D. M., Hunt, M. K., Hebert, J. R., Harris, D. R., Stoddard, A., et al. (1992). Work-site nutrition intervention and employees' dietary habits: The Treatwell program. *American Journal of Public Health, 82*, 877–880.

Sorensen, G., Thompson, B., Glanz, K., Feng, Z., Kinne, S., DiClemente, C., et al. (1996). Work site-based cancer prevention: primary results from the Working Well Trial. *American Journal of Public Health, 86*, 939–947.

Steinmetz, K. A., & Potter, J. D. (1996). Vegetables, fruit, and cancer prevention: A review. *Journal of the American Dietetic Association, 96*, 1027–1039.

Stolley, M. R., & Fitzgibbon, M. L. (1997). Effects of an obesity prevention program on the eating behavior of African American mothers and daughters. *Health Education and Behavior, 24*, 152–164.

Strychar, I. M., Champagne, F., Ghadirian, P., Bonin, A., Jenicek, M., & Lasater, T. M. (1998). Impact of receiving blood cholesterol test results on dietary change. *American Journal of Preventive Medicine, 14*, 103–110.

Swinburn, B., Walter, L., Arroll, B., Milyard, M., & Russell, D. (1998). The green prescription study: A randomized-controlled trial of written exercise advice in general practice. *American Journal of Public Health, 88*, 288–291.

Taylor, W. C. (1998). Physical activity interventions in low-income ethnic minority, and populations with disability. *American Journal of Preventive Medicine, 15*, 334–343.

Thompson, F., & Byers, T. (1994). Dietary assessment resource manual. *Journal of Nutrition, 124*(Suppl. 11), 2245–2317.

Thune, I. (1996). Physical activity and risk of colorectal cancer in men and women. *British Journal of Cancer, 73*, 1134–1140.

Thune, I., & Lund, E. (1994). Physical activity and the risk of prostate and testicular cancer: A cohort study of 53,000 Norwegian men. *Cancer Causes & Control, 5*, 549–556.

Tilley, B. C., Glanz, K., Kristal, A. R., Hirst, K., Li, S., Vernon, S. W., et al. (1999). Nutrition intervention for high-risk auto workers: Results of the Next Step Trial. *Preventive Medicine, 28*, 284–292.

U.S. Department of Health and Human Services. (2000). *US Department of Health and Human Services. Healthy people 2010: Conference edition.* Washington, D.C.

Verhoeven, D. T., Assen, N., Goldbohm, R. A., Dorant, E., van't Veer, P., Sturmans, F., et al. (1997). Vitamins C and E, retinol, beta-carotene and dietary fiber in relation to breast cancer risk: A prospective cohort study. *British Journal of Cancer, 75*, 149–155.

White, E., Shattuck, A. L., Kristal, A. R., Urban, N., Prentice, R. L., Henderson, M. M., et al. (1992). Maintenance of a low-fat diet: Follow-up of the Women's Health Trial. *Cancer Epidemiology, Biomarkers and Prevention, 1*, 315–323.

Whittemore, A. S., Kolonel, L. N., Wu, A. H., John, E. M., Gallagher, R. P., Howe, G. R., et al. (1995). Prostate cancer in relation to diet, physical activity, and body size in blacks, whites, and Asians in the United States and Canada. *Journal of the National Cancer Institute, 87*, 652–661.

Willett, W. (1998). *Nutritional epidemiology* (2nd ed.). New York: Oxford University Press.

Willett, W. (1995). Diet, nutrition, and avoidable cancer. *Environmental Health Perspectives, 103*, 165–170.

Willett, W. (1998). Is dietary fat a major determinant of body fat. *American Journal of Clinical Nutrition, 67*(Suppl.), 556–562.

Willett, W. (1999). Goals for nutrition in the year 2000. *CA Cancer Journal for Clinicians, 49*, 331–352.

Willett, W. C., & Trichopoulos, D. (1996). Nutrition and cancer: A summary of the evidence. *Cancer Causes and Control, 7*, 178–180.

Williamson, D. F., Pamuk, E., Thun, M., Flanders, D., Byers, T., & Heath, C. (1995). Prospective study of intentional weight loss and mortality in never-smoking overweight US white women aged 40–64 years. *American Journal of Epidemiology, 141*, 1128–1141.

Wood, T. (2000). Issues and future directions in assessing physical activity: An introduction to the conference proceedings. *Research Quarterly for Exercise and Sport, S-71*(Suppl. 2), ii–vii.

World Cancer Research Fund and American Institute for Cancer Research. (1997). *Food, nutrition and the prevention of cancer: A global perspective.* Washington, D.C.: American Institute for Cancer Research.

Young, K. J., & Lee, P. N. (1998). Intervention studies on cancer. *European Journal of Cancer Prevention, 8*, 91–103.

Ziegler, R. G., Mayne, S. T., & Swanson, C. A. (1996). Nutrition and lung cancer. *Cancer Causes and Control, 7*, 157–177.

# 3

# Cancer Screening

**Victoria L. Champion**
**Susan M. Rawl**
**Celette Sugg Skinner**

Cancer screening, as a secondary prevention measure, has significant potential for discovering certain cancers early and may reduce mortality and morbidity (Reintgen & Clark, 1996). Screening is testing an asymptomatic, primarily healthy person to identify the risk of developing cancer. Once an individual is identified as high risk by a positive screening test, further tests are necessary to diagnose cancer. Thus, cancer screening is an attempt to discover cancer early, so that medical treatment can be initiated and morbidity or mortality of the disease may be altered. Screening also makes intuitive sense; if we can discover cancer early and treat it by surgery, radiation, or chemotherapy, lives should be saved and suffering decreased.

Several epidemiological criteria must be met prior to recommending cancer screening for large numbers of people. First, the disease must be sufficiently common and result in sufficient morbidity and mortality. Secondly, if the cancer is discovered early, an effective treatment must take place. Without a treatment option, medical care providers have only extended the time during which the individual is aware of the diagnosis without altering the outcome. Third, a test must be done that can detect the cancer with few errors; the test must have three key measures of validity: sensitivity, specificity, and positive predictive value. Fourth, the test must be acceptable to the physician and client, and be feasible for large numbers of people.

Finally, the costs of the screening should be outweighed by the benefits. Not all cancer-screening tests meet these criteria; when this is the case, decision aids can help physicians and clients make the best possible personal decisions in the absence of well-accepted screening recommendations, and in light of uncertain and/or competing risks and benefits.

Cancer screening for cervical and breast cancer has been used for several decades with resulting decreases in mortality. Colorectal cancer screening, with the advent of fecal occult blood tests (FOBTs) and sigmoidoscopy or colonoscopy, has only begun to be widely accepted but also has the potential to dramatically reduce mortality. Currently, breast, cervical, and colorectal cancers are widely recommended for population screening and are supported by the American Cancer Society (ACS) and National Cancer Institute (NCI). Adherence to screening recommendations varies widely.

This chapter reviews interventions for increasing adherence to breast, cervical, and colorectal cancer-screening techniques to summarize the effectiveness of current interventions. First, the strategies used to identify and review references are described, followed by a section that describes theories commonly used in intervention research. Following the presentation of these introductory issues, the chapter is divided into three sections covering breast, cervical, and colorectal cancer screening. The chapter concludes with a summary of recommendations for further research.

## INTERVENTION STUDY SELECTION STRATEGIES AND COMMONLY USED THEORIES

### Selection Strategies

Intervention studies that had mammography, Pap, and colorectal screening as their outcome were identified from searches using multiple databases such as MEDLINE®, reviews of current literature in the area, and personal bibliographies. Mammography and Pap smear studies published since 1995 were selected. Because an extensive review of colorectal cancer-screening studies was published in 1997 (Vernon, 1997), only colorectal screening studies published after 1996 were included here. Only intervention studies that used quasi-experimental or experimental designs (randomized controlled trials) were included. For mammography, Pap smears, and colorectal screening, interventions targeted the individual, healthcare provider, community, or a combination of the three.

## Current Theory

Before addressing the individual screening tests, a review of behavioral theories commonly used in intervention research is provided. The importance of using empirically tested theoretical models to drive intervention research cannot be overstated. If researchers use prescriptive theories to frame interventions, we not only increase the probability of having a successful intervention, but also the probabilities of understanding why the intervention was successful and of having a model for repeating findings (Maibach & Parrott, 1995). The best intervention studies have been guided by well-supported theories. Current thoughts about using theoretical models to target and/or tailor interventions are also included.

### Health Belief Model (HBM)

The Health Belief Model (HBM) was one of the first theories to gain widespread use in developing interventions to increase cancer screening. Hochbaum (1958) conceptualized behavior as being dependent upon perceptions of susceptibility, severity, and the benefits of taking action, as well as the cues to taking action. Rosenstock (1974) further developed predictive concepts and added barriers to taking action. *Perceived susceptibility* was defined as a person's perceived risk of developing a disease. *Severity* was defined as the perceived consequences of the disease on the person's well being. *Perceived benefits and barriers* were defined as the positive and negative effects related to a specific health action. In 1988, Rosenstock added self-efficacy to the HBM. *Self-efficacy*, which had been frequently combined with HBM constructs in predicting screening behavior or developing interventions to increase screening, relates to an individual's confidence in his or her ability to take action. The constructs presented in the HBM represent cognitive variables that are additive in effect for explaining behavior.

One of the largest problems in assessing the effect of the HBM on behavior change has been the inconsistent measurement of variables. Studies have operationalized variables in very different ways, many using only one or two items. Another problem has been the failure of many researchers to use the entire complement of HBM variables when developing interventions. Nonetheless, the use of the HBM in screening interventions has demonstrated many significant findings (Ronis, 1992; Rosenstock, Strecher, & Becker, 1994).

TRANSTHEORETICAL MODEL (TTM)

The Transtheoretical Model (TTM) was developed and has been tested by Prochaska and DiClemente (1983) to understand how individuals progress toward adopting behaviors that result in more optimal health. A major innovation with this model has been the conceptualization of change as progressive and dynamic. Core constructs include stages of change, processes of change, and decisional balance. *Stages of change* refers to behavior and includes precontemplation, contemplation, preparation, action, maintenance, and termination. Precontemplation is defined as the stage in which a person does not intend to take action in the immediate future, usually defined as 6 months. Contemplation is defined as the stage in which a person decides to take action within the next 6 months. Preparation is the stage in which an individual prepares to take action in the immediate future; this may involve making an appointment or other preparation for action, such as obtaining nicotine replacement therapy. Action is defined as the point at which an individual has taken specific action to create behavioral change. Maintenance and termination follow action and are respectively defined as the period of time in which a person works to maintain behavior and the point at which behavior is so ingrained that there is no chance of relapse. Time frames for each stage vary depending on the behavior being addressed. For colorectal cancer screening, the correct interval for repeating a behavior may be as long as 10 years, whereas for physical activity, behavior maintenance involves frequent action (Prochaska et al., 1994).

*Processes of change* are defined as activities people use to progress through the stages of change. These include consciousness-raising, dramatic relief, self-reevaluation, environmental reevaluation, self-liberation, social liberation, counter-conditioning, stimulus control, contingency management, and helping relationships. Researchers have used the processes of change in intervention strategies to promote change. For example, consciousness-raising could include providing education and feedback regarding the benefits of screening or chances of developing the disease. Processes of change such as counter-conditioning and stimulus control involve altering the environment by learning healthier behaviors or removing cues that promote problematic behavior. *Decisional balance* refers to the pros and cons of taking action. These are conceptually similar to the benefits and barrier constructs in the HBM and refer to the positive and negative aspects of adopting a behavior.

The TTM has been used with studies involving mammography and colorectal screening. Most studies using this model have used the stages of change to define and measure outcome behaviors without using the entire model and incorporating processes of change. Interventions are reviewed under the appropriate screening sections later in the chapter (Prochaska, 1994b; Prochaska et al., 1994; Rakowski, Dube, & Goldstein, 1996).

SOCIAL LEARNING THEORY (SLT)

The Social Learning Theory (SLT) has been used alone and in combination with other theories to predict screening behavior. The theory includes the concepts of outcome expectations and efficacy expectations, which act in concert to predict behavior. *Outcome expectations* are defined as the belief that a given action will result in a desired outcome, while *efficacy expectations* are the belief that one has the ability to complete the action necessary to produce the outcome. Efficacy expectations vary depending on the task; efficacy expectations result from four areas—personal accomplishments, vicarious experiences, verbal persuasion, and physiological state—and a person can develop self-efficacy around a certain action in one of these four ways. Outcome expectations are the belief that the behavior will result in a certain state and is essentially indistinguishable from the benefit constructs of the HBM or the pros portion of the decisional-balance construct of the TTM.

## Use of Theory-Tailored or Targeted Interventions

The function of theory is to provide a structure that allows the prediction of behavior. Theoretical constructs are used to frame intervention strategies. To the extent that these strategies are based on individual psychological theories, one would assume that the more an intervention could be tailored to address factors influencing a particular individual's behavior, the more likely it would be to result in a behavior change in that person. For example, screening interventions often seek to reduce barriers that may discourage people from being screened and to convince them of screening benefits. An intervention focusing on benefits and barriers particularly important to an individual should be more effective than a message addressing potential barriers and benefits identified in a theoretical model but not important to that message recipient. Tailored interventions have generally been found to be more effective than messages designed for general audiences (Skinner, Campbell, Rimer, Curry, & Prochaska, 1999).

*Tailoring* has been defined as "Any combination of information or change strategies *intended to reach one specific person*, based on characteristics unique to that person, related to the outcome of interest, and *derived from an individual assessment*" (Kreuter, Farrell, Olevitch, & Brennan, 2000, p. 5). Tailored interventions are intended for one particular recipient and are based on individual-level features related to the behavior, which distinguish tailoring from targeted interventions. *Targeting* employs a single intervention approach or message "for a defined population subgroup" and "takes into account characteristics shared by the subgroup's members" (Kreuter & Skinner, 2000, p. 1). Tailored, targeted, and general interventions can address theoretical constructs that may affect behavior; the difference between these strategies lies in whether constructs are measured and then addressed at the individual, subgroup, or large-group level, respectively.

## RECOMMENDATIONS FOR POPULATION SCREENING

Currently, only three cancers—breast, cervical, and colorectal—are endorsed by virtually every agency for population screening. Breast cancer screening by mammography has accumulated the largest base of prospective randomized data supporting mortality benefit. Cervical cancer screening has never had large randomized trials, but retrospective evidence of mortality benefit is so great that it is universally endorsed. Colorectal cancer screening has had prospective randomized studies demonstrating mortality benefit to fecal occult blood screens and sigmoidoscopy; colonoscopy benefit is inferred.

### Breast Cancer Screening

Breast cancer is common in North America; in 2001, the American Cancer Society estimated that 192,000 women would be diagnosed with breast cancer and 40,600 would die from the disease (Greenlee, Hill-Harmon, Murray, & Thun, 2001). In 2002, an estimated 203,500 women will be diagnosed with breast cancer and 39,600 will die of the disease (American Cancer Society, 2002). The potential for mammography to decrease mortality through early detection has been demonstrated through prospective studies over the last 30 years. Eight major randomized controlled trials have been conducted for breast cancer screening, collectively including more than 500,000 women (Andersson et al., 1988; Collette, Rombach, Day, & DeWaard, 1984; Morrison, Brisson, & Khalid, 1988; Palli et al., 1986; Roberts et al., 1990; Shapiro, Venet, Strax, Venet, & Roeser, 1982; Tabar et al., 1985; Verbeek et al., 1984; Witte, 1994, 1995). Together these trials provide strong support for mortality decreases of up to 30% in women aged

50 or older who are screened at intervals of 1 to 2 years. Until recently, the benefits for women aged 40 to 50 were not as clear. However, in 1997 the ACS and NCI jointly recommended screening for asymptomatic women aged 40 to 75 (Eastman, 1997).

Although breast cancer screening by mammography is widely recommended, achieving compliance with yearly screening has been a challenge. Fortunately, however, behavioral research during the last decade has increased compliance to over 73% (Morbidity and Mortality Weekly Report, 2000). As a result, mortality for breast cancer is slowly decreasing (Mettlin, 1999). The remainder of this section will review the intervention work done to increase mammography screening. Twenty-four randomized intervention studies completed since 1994 are presented and summarized in Table 3.1.

PATIENT- AND PROVIDER-DIRECTED BREAST CANCER INTERVENTIONS

In 1994, Rimer reviewed interventions that ranged from personal counseling to media campaigns, finding substantial support for planned interventions to increase mammography compliance. Most of the studies combined messages regarding personal risk, perceived benefits and barriers to screening, and fear-increasing messages. The message delivery was addressed but not systematically studied. Rimer advocated the use of theories to inform the development of interventions and the investigation of message delivery strategies.

Many studies using patient or physician reminders used a combination of patient reminders, physician reminders, and personal counseling either alone or in combination. Burack et al. (1996) completed a large randomized control trial comparing patient letter reminders and physician letter reminders. A total of 2,368 women were eligible and randomly assigned to various combinations of reminders. Patient reminders had a limited impact on visitation; physician reminders were more effective, but their effectiveness differed by physician. Sharp, Peters, and Bartholomew (1996) contrasted a letter from a general practitioner with a nurse counseling session. Intervention groups were not significantly different than controls. Another study compared usual care, a mailed reminder, and a mailed reminder plus nurse counseling (Margolis & Menart, 1996). Although mailed reminders improved mammography appointment-keeping by 5%, this was not significant and the addition of nurse counseling had no effect.

Richardson, Mondrus, Danley, Deapen, and Mack (1996) tested a more complex mailed reminder system, where three different modules were tested. The first module was designed to increase perceived risk and provide

**TABLE 3.1  Breast-Cancer-Screening/Mammography Interventions**

| | Theoretical/ conceptual framework | Design | Sample | Measures | Results |
|---|---|---|---|---|---|
| Bastani, Maxwell, Bradford, Das, & Yan (1999) | None reported | Randomized control trial (RCT), 2-group design; mailed invitation with personalized risk | $N = 901$ with at least one first-degree relative from statewide cancer registry | Mammography risk assessment | 8% intervention group advantage for mailed intervention with personal risk assessment. |
| Bernstein, Mutschler, & Bernstein (2000) | None reported | Pre- and post-test; motivational interview at time of emergency department visit | $N = 151$ culturally and racially diverse older women | Whether or not mammography was obtained | 60% had postintervention mammogram. |
| Burack et al. (1996) | None reported | RCT; patient/physician reminders individually, together, or neither | $N = 2,368$ women | Whether or not mammography was obtained | Patient reminder had no effect; physician reminder effective at one site ($p = .001$). |
| Champion et al. (in press) | HBM and TTM | RCT; combination of physician reminder, telephone counseling, and in-person counseling | $N = 808$ women aged 50+ | Whether or not mammography was obtained | All intervention groups except physician reminder alone were significantly different than control group. |

| | Theoretical/ conceptual framework | Design | Sample | Measures | Results |
|---|---|---|---|---|---|
| Champion, Ray, Heilman, & Springston (2000) | HBM | RCT | $N = 301$ low-income women | Whether or not mammography was obtained | For women who had not had a mammogram, adherence was significantly higher in the experimental group (50%) than in control (18%). |
| Clover et al. (1996) | None reported | Quasi-experimental; physician promotion or community media intervention | Women from selected communities | Whether or not mammography was obtained | Community media intervention had 63% compliance versus 34%; physician involvement intervention had 68% versus 51%. |
| Costanza et al. (2000) | None reported | RCT; scripted call from counselor/MD; education and office staff training improving skills | $N = 1,655$ women from HMOs, aged 50–80, underusers of mammography | Whether or not mammography and repeat mammography were obtained | 44% in each intervention group became regular users, compared to 42% in control group. |
| Crane et al. (1998) | TTM | RCT, 3-group design; telephone outcall or advance card and outcall | Outcalls to CIS localities | Whether or not mammography was obtained | Successfully reached women but required intensive effort. |

(continued)

**TABLE 3.1  Breast-Cancer-Screening/Mammography Interventions (*continued*)**

| | Theoretical/ conceptual framework | Design | Sample | Measures | Results |
|---|---|---|---|---|---|
| Davis et al. (1998) | None reported | RCT; letter; letter and brochure; and letter, brochure, and 12-minute motivational videotape | $N = 445$ women in public hospital setting | Whether or not mammography was obtained | Group receiving letter, brochure, and motivational education had 29% compliance; letter alone 21%; letter and brochure 18%. |
| Duan, Fox, Derose, & Carson (2000) | None reported | RCT; peer telephone counseling | 30 churches, African-American, Latino, and white from Los Angeles county | Whether or not mammography was obtained | Mammography adherence from baseline adherent participants; nonadherence rates were from 23% to 60%. |
| Flynn et al. (1997) | None reported | Quasi-experimental; community intervention, educational program and mammography van | Individuals from communities in rural regions of Vermont | Whether or not mammography was obtained | Mammography was higher in program communities at 82% versus 72% in control. |

| | Theoretical/ conceptual framework | Design | Sample | Measures | Results |
|---|---|---|---|---|---|
| Goldberg et al. (2000) | None reported | Quasi-experimental, nonrandomized; computer-generated preventive reminders | $N = 42$ providers; 2,655 patients | Whether or not mammography was obtained | Increase over time for women receiving reminder versus time period in which no reminder received ($p = \leq .03$). |
| Janz et al. (1997) | None reported | RCT; physician letter followed by phone call | $N = 460$ women from private physician practices | Whether or not mammography was obtained | Intervention increased mammography 22% over standard care. |
| Kadison, Pelletier, Mounib, Oppedisano, & Poteat (1998) | None reported | Pre- and post-test; telephone counsel | $N = 189$ women who called for breast cancer risk assessment | Whether or not mammography was obtained | Increase in mammography from initial to follow-up call ($p = .057$). |
| King et al. (1998) | None reported | RCT; flyer; flyer and educational program; flyer, program, and transportation | $N = 40$ senior citizen housing centers | Whether or not mammography was obtained | Not significant. |

*(continued)*

**TABLE 3.1  Breast-Cancer-Screening/Mammography Interventions (*continued*)**

| | Theoretical/ conceptual framework | Design | Sample | Measures | Results |
|---|---|---|---|---|---|
| Margolis, Lurie, McGovern, Tyrell, & Slater (1998) | None reported | RCT; lay health advisor recommended screening | $N = 1,483$ women aged 40+ attending appointments in nonprimary care outpatient clinics | Whether or not mammography was obtained | Mammography 69% in intervention group versus 63% in usual care ($p = .009$). |
| Mayer et al. (2000) | None reported | RCT; reminder letter from physician or from mammography facility | $N = 1,562$ women aged 50–74 | Whether or not mammography was obtained and patient returned for follow-up visit | Women receiving reminder letters from either physician or facility had 48% and 47% compliance with a return versus 23% for control. |
| Paskett et al. (1999) | None reported | Quasi-experimental; clinic-based educational screening strategies for providers and patients; follow-up interventions for abnormal screening and implications of computer tracking system | $N =$ African-American women aged 40+ | Whether or not mammography and Pap smear were obtained; assessed follow-up rates | Compliance rates for follow-up with abnormal results increased from 50% to 97%. |

| | Theoretical/ conceptual framework | Design | Sample | Measures | Results |
|---|---|---|---|---|---|
| Rakowski et al. (1998) | TTM | RCT; stage-matched materials, mailed and follow-up telephone interviews | $N = 1{,}864$ women | Whether or not mammography was obtained | Stage-matched groups, 64% compliance; no-materials group, 55% compliance. |
| Richardson, Mondrus, Danley, Deapen, & Mack (1996) | None reported | RCT; written and audiotaped materials designed to increase breast cancer screening | $N = 369$ twin sisters of breast cancer cases | Whether or not mammography was obtained | Mammograms 10.3% higher in intervention group than control. |
| Sharp, Peters, Bartholomew, & Shaw (1996) | None reported | RCT, 3-group control trial; nurse visit with and without education for general practice letter | $N = 799$ women aged 50–64 | Whether or not mammography was obtained | Not significant. |
| Somkin et al. (1997) | None reported | RCT; letter reminder on chart | $N = 7{,}077$ women aged 50–74 | Whether or not mammography was obtained | Women who received letter (25%) versus no letter (16%). |

*(continued)*

75

**TABLE 3.1  Breast-Cancer-Screening/Mammography Interventions (*continued*)**

| | Theoretical/ conceptual framework | Design | Sample | Measures | Results |
|---|---|---|---|---|---|
| Stockdale, Keeler, Duan, Derose, & Fox (2000) | None reported | RCT; telephone counseling, mailed counseling, control | Individuals recruited from community church | Whether or not mammography was obtained | A 7.5% increase in mammography maintenance was found in previously adherent women receiving telephone counseling, a status update interview, and supplemental mailed materials. |
| Taplin et al. (2000) | SLT | RCT; group intervention: motivational telephone, reminder telephone, and poster | N = 5,062 women aged 50–79 in HMO | Whether or not mammography was obtained | Women receiving either of the reminder calls were more likely to get mammograms than women viewing poster. |
| Weber & Reilly (1997) | None reported | RCT; community health educator plus reminder letter versus reminder letter | N = 376 women aged 32–77 | Whether or not mammography was obtained | Women in intervention group were 3 times as likely to receive mammograms. |

screening information, the second to provide information about breast self-examinations, and the third to provide information about mammography decisions. Mammograms were over 10% higher in intervention groups. Women used in this study were twin sisters of breast cancer cases.

Bastani, Maxwell, Bradford, Das, and Yan (1999) used a two-group design to evaluate a mailed intervention focused on personalized risk information to increase mammography for women with at least one first-degree relative with breast cancer. An 8% intervention group advantage was realized. Later, Taplin et al. (2000) tested motivational telephone calls to increase mammography in a stratified random sample of 5,062 women. All women received an initial reminder. After 2 months, 47% of the women had not scheduled a mammogram and were randomly assigned to a reminder postcard, a reminder telephone call, or a motivational telephone call. The motivational and reminder telephone calls had equivalent effects. Women with prior mammography use were more likely to get a mammogram, and women who received reminder calls were more likely to get a mammogram. Calls were more effective for women who had prior mammograms.

In 1997, Janz et al. reported on a two-step intervention to increase mammography among older women; 460 women were identified from private physician practices and randomized to a control or two-step intervention. The first step was a physician letter recommending a clinical breast exam and mammography. For women who did not obtain a mammogram in the first step, a second step was implemented in which counselors called women to discuss their primary reason for not scheduling a mammogram. The intervention increased mammography 22% over standard care.

Davis et al. (1998) compared groups who variously received a personal recommendation; a personal recommendation plus an NCI brochure; or a recommendation, brochure, and 12-minute interactive motivational program. Women who received all three interventions were most likely to obtain a mammography (29%), followed by those who received a recommendation and brochure (21%), or who received only the brochure. Goldberg et al. (2000) tested a computer-generated printout attached to patients' charts with clinical reminders for screening. Implementing reminder systems in community-practice settings was found to increase mammography screening by 154%.

Mayer et al. (2000) tested a personalized physician letter against a facility letter or no letter using a sample of 1,562 randomly assigned women. Both groups that received the mammography letter were more likely to have returned for a mammogram than those who received standard care, with no difference between reminder groups.

Tailored and stage-specific interventions are increasingly being used to increase mammography compliance. For instance, if a woman is in precontemplation for mammography, an intervention to increase perceived risk might be appropriate. If a woman were in contemplation (had thought about having a mammogram), specific barriers could be addressed. Rakowski et al. (1998) studied 1,864 women aged 40 to 74. Women were randomized in three groups: The first group did not receive educational materials, the second group received standard materials, and the third group received stage-matched materials. The stage-matched group had higher mammography compliance (64%) than the no-materials group (55%). The stage-matched group differed from the standard group in multivariate analyses.

Champion et al. (in press) tested physician reminders against telephone and in-person counseling or a combination of both using stage-matched interventions. A combination of the HBM and TTM directed the intervention content. A total of 808 economically and socially diverse women, aged 50 and older, participated. Women who randomized to the telephone intervention had a compliance rate of 30%, while in-person compliance was 33% and control compliance was 17%. Both telephone and in-person results were significantly different than control findings.

COMMUNITY-SETTING BREAST CANCER INTERVENTIONS

Several intervention studies have also been carried out in community settings. Somkin et al. (1997) used Pap smear and mammogram reminders with an HMO population. Women were randomized to receive a patient reminder, patient and provider reminders, or usual care. Both intervention groups were more likely to receive mammograms and Pap smears than the usual-care group. Duan, Fox, Derose, and Carson (2000) randomized 30 churches to telephone counseling or control. Results indicated that nonadherence decreased from 23% to 16% in the experimental group. Costanza et al. (2000) tested a randomized trial to increase mammography use with 1,655 underserved women. Women were randomized to receive reminders (control), barrier-specific telephone counseling, or a physician-based educational program. Forty-four percent in each intervention group became regular users compared to 42% in the reminder group. Results were significant for women who had prior but not recent mammograms.

King et al. (1998) randomized mammography interventions in 40 senior citizen housing centers. Facilities were randomized to (a) usual care, which included a Medicare mammography benefit flyer; (b) an educational flyer and community educational program; (c) a flyer, mammography appointment, and provision of transportation; or (d) all of the above. The community intervention increased mammography use slightly for those who already had a mammogram, but results were not significant. King et al. concluded that women who have never had a mammogram may need more personalized interventions.

A church-based intervention program to promote mammography screening was reported by Stockdale, Keeler, Duan, Derose, and Fox (2000). Three intervention aims were used: telephone counseling, mailed counseling, or control. The cost for each screened participant was $188 when using volunteers but substantially increased when using paid workers.

Flynn et al. (1997) had two matched sets of communities identified in rural regions of Vermont. Education programs were implemented in one community in addition to a mammography van. Mammography use was higher in the community that received the intervention; an increase of 72% to 82% was realized. Weber and Reilly (1997) used a group of urban women aged 50 to 75 to conduct a randomized control trial using community health educators versus usual care in six practices. Women in the intervention group had a significantly higher odds ratio of receiving a mammogram. Women in towns receiving the community participation intervention compared with matched-media promotion towns were more likely to have a mammogram (Clover, Redman, Forbes, Sanson-Fisher, & Callaghan, 1996). Community participation and family practitioner involvement were promising strategies for increasing mammography.

Minorities have been the focus of several studies. Bernstein, Mutschler, and Bernstein (2000) tested the effects of a brief motivational interview and mammography referral at the time of an emergency department visit. Data indicated that 60% of the 151 culturally and racially diverse older women had a follow-up mammogram and, of these, 69% were first-time users. More than 90% planned a repeat mammogram the following year. Additionally, of those who did not receive a mammogram, many requested a second try appointment. Champion, Ray, Heilman, and Springston (2000) described the effect of in-person counseling on low-income African-American women. For women who had not had a mammogram, adherence was significantly higher in the experimental group (50%) than the control group (18%). Champion et al. targeted messages toward women based on their individual barriers and perceived risk.

Whether certain interventions are more effective in one cultural group versus another must be determined. This will require a large randomized study that includes sufficient numbers of African-American and Caucasian women randomized to the same interventions.

SUMMARY AND RECOMMENDATIONS
FOR BREAST CANCER SCREENING INTERVENTIONS

The last decade has provided a wealth of research on mammography-adherence interventions. Many of the reported studies have demonstrated statistically significant interventions with effect sizes varying from a 5% to greater than 25% difference in adherence by the intervention group. Because overall adherence for mammography is relatively high, research must concentrate on nonadherent women. Researchers also need to determine if—depending on a woman's predisposition to get a mammogram as measured by the stage of change—less complex or more complex interventions can be implemented. Recently, concentrated efforts at tailoring information specific to individuals have begun. With the advent of user-friendly technology, interventions need to be tested that can target specific needs and be cost effective. Finally, current interventions need to be tested in real-life settings with intent-to-treat designs.

## Cervical Cancer Screening

The American Cancer Society estimated that 12,900 American women would be diagnosed with cervical cancer in 2001, and 4,400 would die from the disease; the ACS predicted that in 2002, 13,000 women would be diagnosed with cervical cancer, and 4,100 would die from the disease (American Cancer Society, 2002). Although death from cervical cancer in the United States has decreased, it is still a leading cause of cancer death worldwide. It is estimated that the annual reduction of invasive cancer would be approximately 80% if women were screened every 5 years (Sherlau-Johnson, Gallivan, & Jenkins, 1997). Although cervical cancer is more of a problem outside of the United States, the incidence of invasive cervical cancer has been increasing by 3% a year in the United States since 1986 (Marcus & Crane, 1998). Most cervical cancers occur in young women. Sexually transmitted disease is thought to play a predominant role in the development of this cancer. Screening for cervical cancer was initiated in

1941, and in the early 1950s, cervical cancer screening was widely accepted in the United States (Ayre, 1947).

Although cervical cancer screening does not have the multitude of prospective randomized trials that accompany mammography screening, the evidence for cervical screening lies in the fact that mortality has been dramatically decreased with the advent of the Pap smear (Adami et al., 1994; Bocciolone, La Vecchia, Levi, Lucchini, & Franceschi, 1993; DiBonito et al., 1993; van der Graaf, Vooijs, Gaillard, & Go, 1987). The studies reviewed in the following section are summarized in Table 3.2.

PATIENT-DIRECTED CERVICAL CANCER INTERVENTIONS

Interventions to increase cervical cancer screening have varied from individualized interventions targeting specific women to community-based strategies. Yancey, Tanjasiri, Klein, and Tunder (1995) tested a video developed to increase cervical cancer screening in low-income African-American women. The video was a documentary designed to decrease barriers to breast and cervical cancer screening and emphasize relevant cultural dynamics. Utilization for Pap smears increased approximately 6% during the intervention.

Campbell, Peterkin, Abbott, and Rogers (1997) tested a computer intervention program; the intervention tested the impact of computer-generated feedback on cervical screening among underscreened women. Differences were not significant, but for women aged 50 to 70, the intervention significantly increased the chances of obtaining a Pap smear. Somkin et al. (1997) studied the effect of patient and provider reminders on both mammography and Pap smears. Women were randomized to receive either a letter inviting them to make an appointment for a mammogram or Pap smear, and a reminder was placed on the patient's medical chart. Women who received the letter were more likely to obtain Pap smears (20% versus 9%) in the 6 months following the study.

Further testing of invitations was done by Segnan, Senore, Giordano, Ponti, and Ronco in 1998. A series of four different invitation systems were tested with women randomized to four groups. The first group had a letter signed by a general practitioner with a prefixed appointment. A second group had an open-ended invitation signed by a general practitioner prompting the women to contact the screening center for an appointment. The third group had a letter with a prefixed appointment signed by the program coordinator. The fourth group had a letter highlighting the benefits of

**TABLE 3.2 Cervical-Cancer-Screening Interventions**

| | Theoretical/ conceptual framework | Design | Sample | Measures | Results |
|---|---|---|---|---|---|
| Campbell, Peterkin, Abbott, & Rogers, (1997) | None reported | RCT; computerized summary of cervical cancer screening | N = 679 women from general practice clinics | Whether or not Pap smear was obtained | Unable to determine effect because of the small number of responses. |
| Campbell, MacDonald, & McKiernan (1996) | None reported | Nonrandomized; visit from health visitor | N = 162 women | Whether or not Pap smear was obtained | 37% of those visited by a health visitor attended for a Pap smear. |
| Dignan et al. (1996) | None reported | RCT; lay health worker | N = 996 Cherokee Indian women | Whether or not Pap smear was obtained | Women who received intervention were more likely to have had a Pap smear. |
| Jenkins et al. (1999) | None reported | Quasi-experimental; media-led community educational intervention | N = 876 Vietnamese-American women | Whether or not Pap smear was obtained | Significant effect for client to have Pap smears. |

| | Theoretical/ conceptual framework | Design | Sample | Measures | Results |
|---|---|---|---|---|---|
| Lantz et al. (1995) | None reported | RCT; physician reminder letter and telephone contact | $N = 1,105$ women from low-income managed care program | Whether or not Pap smear was obtained | Women in control group were significantly more likely to have received a Pap smear. |
| Margolis, Lurie, McGovern, Tyrell, & Slater (1998) | None reported | Random assignment; invitation to participate by lay health advisors | $N = 1,693$ attending nonprimary care outpatient clinics | Whether or not Pap smear was obtained | Significant intervention effect for Pap smear for white women. |
| Paskett et al. (1999) | None reported | Quasi-experimental; educational session, media, and church programs | $N = 248$ women at baseline, 302 women at 3-year follow-up; predominantly African-American aged 40+ | Whether or not Pap smear was obtained | The proportion of women reporting regular use of Pap smear screening improved 14% and declined 7% in the comparison study. |
| Paskett et al. (1998) | None reported | Quasi-experimental; community health-center-based strategies; educational interventions for providers | African-American women aged 40+ residing in low-income housing | Whether or not Pap smear was obtained | Increase of almost 20% Pap smear utilization. |

early cancer detection signed by a general practitioner with a prefixed appointment. Differences appeared with women who received a personal invitation letter signed by their general practitioner and who had preallocated appointments.

Many studies have been directed toward low-income or multiethnic populations because these women have a lower rate of cervical cancer screening. Margolis, Lurie, McGovern, Tyrell, and Slater (1998) tested an intervention with women aged 40 or over who were attending appointments at nonprimary care outpatient clinics. Lay health advisors assessed participant breast and cervical cancer screening and offered women in the intervention group who were due for screening an appointment with a female nurse practitioner. Significant differences were found for both mammographies and Pap smears, although the difference between groups was small (7%). Another study tested adherence among 321 low-income, inner-city African-American women for breast and cervical cancer screening. Intervention group women were visited in their homes up to three times by a lay health worker who provided culturally sensitive educational programs. Although the intervention seemed to improve the rate of mammography, no change was found in women receiving Pap smears (Sung et al., 1997).

The NCI sought to increase screening for cervical cancer among Native American women in North Carolina. Cherokee Tribe Alliance households were mapped to ensure the maximum coverage of women 18 or older (Dignan et al., 1996). Female Cherokee lay health educators delivered an individualized health education program. Participants were randomly assigned to receive the intervention or standard care. Six months after receiving the educational program, women in all four groups received a post-test questionnaire; 73% of women in the program had a Pap smear, compared to 64% in usual care.

A randomized trial evaluated a physician reminder letter and telephone contact on the use of Pap smears in a low-income, managed-care program (Lantz et al., 1995). Women past due for screening were randomly assigned to the intervention or usual-care group. At follow-up, the odds of receiving cancer screening were four times higher for women in the intervention group (22% versus 4%).

COMMUNITY-DIRECTED CERVICAL CANCER INTERVENTIONS

Jenkins et al. (1999) launched a media-led education campaign to increase breast and cervical cancer screening among Vietnamese-American women.

Over a 24-month period, women in the intervention were significantly more likely to have had a Pap smear. Marcus and Crane (1998) reviewed many interventions related to cervical cancer screening, concluding that letters mailed to populations were effective, especially in promoting interval screening. Both physician and patient prompts were shown to be effective; mass-media campaigns worked best when multiple media sources were used.

Paskett et al. (1998) used a community health clinic as the setting for interventions to promote mammography and Pap smears to low-income African-American women. A quasi-experimental study tested interventions, including visual prompts in examination rooms and in-service education to primary care professionals. Interventions for providers included visual prompts, standardized protocols for receiving test results, educational games, and conferences. The number of women who subsequently obtained Pap smears was significantly higher in the intervention condition. Later, Paskett et al. (1999) reported a quasi-experimental study to increase breast and cervical cancer screening in low-income African-American women. The intervention included educational sessions and media programs in church and community settings. The proportion of women using regular Pap smears increased from 73% to 87% in participating counties, but the comparison counties noticed a decrease of 67% to 60%.

SUMMARY AND RECOMMENDATIONS FOR
CERVICAL CANCER SCREENING INTERVENTIONS

Cervical cancer screening is widely accepted as an effective method of preventing invasive cervical cancer. Cervical cancer screening enjoys wide acceptance with the majority of women being adherent. Strategies such as personal invitation, visual prompts, and preset appointments have been effective. Theory-based interventions are conspicuously absent. Future research needs to test tailored interventions that are framed by theory and tested through randomized designs.

Although screening in the United States has decreased morbidity, cervical cancer has increased in incidence in the States. Interval screening is especially problematic. Particular ethnic and age groups are less likely to have had adequate screening. These include women over 65 and low-income African-American, Latino, or Vietnamese women. Future work needs to be done to determine the most cost-effective approach for maintaining annual screening in the United States as well as implementing general screening.

## Colorectal Cancer Screening

In the United States, colorectal cancer is the second most common cause of cancer death in men and women, second only to lung cancer. Declines in incidence and mortality are more evident for Caucasians than for African-Americans, who are disproportionately burdened by this disease. Without preventive action, approximately 6%, or 1 in 17 Americans, will develop colorectal cancer during their lifetime. If colorectal cancer is diagnosed at an early stage, 5-year survival is over 90%. Unfortunately, only 37% of colorectal cancer cases are diagnosed while the cancer is still localized (Greenlee et al., 2001). Colorectal cancer exacts a substantial toll on our society in terms of healthcare costs and morbidity. Fortunately, the opportunity exists to substantially decrease this burden through screening. It has been estimated that, if current screening recommendations were employed, 50% of the deaths from colorectal cancer could be prevented annually (Progress Review Group, 2000).

Approximately 75% of all colorectal cancer occurs in people at average risk, that is, in those who have no known risk factors other than age; advancing age is the most common risk factor (Winawer et al., 1997). According to NCI Surveillance, Epidemilogy, and End Results (SEER) data, the highest age-specific incidence rates occur in men and women 70 years or older (Greenlee et al., 2001). Other risk factors include having a family history of colorectal cancer or adenomas (polyps) and a personal history of adenomas or inflammatory bowel disease. Some of the dietary factors implicated in the development of colorectal cancer include red meat consumption, a diet high in animal fat, a sedentary lifestyle, smoking, and chronic alcohol consumption. Protective dietary and lifestyle factors include vegetable consumption, nonsteroidal anti-inflammatory drugs (NSAIDs), hormone replacement therapy (HRT), and regular exercise (Cuzick, 1999; Potter, 1999). Inherited genetic syndromes such as familial adenomatous polyposis (FAP) and hereditary nonpolyposis colorectal cancer (HNPCC) increase the risk of developing colorectal cancer. Persons with FAP have an almost 100% chance of developing the disease. Gene–environment interactions are believed to play an important role in the development of colorectal cancer (Cuzick, 1999; Potter, 1999).

Randomized clinical trials have demonstrated a 15% to 33% mortality benefit from annual screening with FOBTs (Hardcastle et al., 1996; Kronborg, Fenger, Olsen, Jorgensen, & Sondergaard, 1996; Mandel et al., 1993). Evidence from a case-control study indicates that having a flexible sigmoidoscopy every 5 years is an effective screening test. Significant mortality reductions have been reported for cancers within the reach of the sigmoidoscope, as well as a lower incidence of colorectal cancer for those with a history of screening sigmoidoscopy (Kavanagh, Giovannucci, Fuchs, & Colditz, 1998; Newcomb, Norfleet, Storer, Surawicz, & Marcus, 1992; Selby, Friedman, Quesenberry, & Weiss, 1993). Two large randomized trials are currently under way to evaluate the efficacy of screening by a flexible sigmoidoscopy. Annual FOBT *combined with* sigmoidoscopy has been found to increase the benefits of screening above either test alone. Mortality was reduced for participants of all age groups screened with FOBT and sigmoidoscopy, from 0.63 per 1,000 per year for the control group to 0.36 for the study group (Winawer et al., 1993).

The ACS recently revised their screening recommendations for colorectal cancer (Smith et al., 2001). These guidelines provide five options for screening average-risk individuals: (a) annual FOBT, (b) flexible sigmoidoscopy every 5 years, (c) annual FOBT *plus* sigmoidoscopy every 5 years, (d) double contrast barium enema every 5 years, and (e) colonoscopy every 10 years. Although screening for colorectal cancer saves lives, participation in screening among the general population remains low. Data from the Behavioral Risk Factor Surveillance System (BRFSS) indicated that only 44% of screening-eligible persons received an FOBT and/or sigmoidoscopy/colonoscopy in the recommended time frame. For individual tests, 20.6% of the respondents had an FOBT in the preceding year, and only 33.6% reported having had a sigmoidoscopy within the preceding 5 years (MMWR, 2001). The Centers for Disease Control have recommended that "efforts to address barriers and promote screening should be intensified" (MMWR, p. 162).

Vernon (1997) published an extensive review of literature on the adherence to colorectal cancer screening with FOBT and sigmoidoscopy. The review included 18 intervention studies designed to increase participation in screening with FOBT and 4 intervention studies focusing on sigmoidoscopy. The intervention strategies tested ranged from letters of invitation from personal physicians that included FOBT kits to intensive follow-ups in person or through telephone counseling. Such interventions increased participation up to 50%, and mailed follow-up reminders increased participation in all studies that used them. The limitations of colorectal cancer screening intervention studies included (a) the lack of theoretically driven studies (only five investigators used theory-based interventions), (b) the use of volunteers as study participants, and (c) the lack of attention to repeat adherence to screening. Readers can refer to Vernon's work for a detailed discussion of studies published prior to 1997.

Peterson and Vernon (2000) subsequently reviewed literature focused on interventions directed at increasing physician adherence to colorectal cancer screening guidelines. Of the 18 studies reviewed, most interventions consisted of some type of screening reminder system. Computer-generated reminder systems generally outperformed manual reminder systems in increasing physician adherence to colorectal cancer screening guidelines, with postintervention adherence rates increasing 31% to 90% for FOBT and 40% to 64% for sigmoidoscopy.

Intervention studies published since 1996 that focus on increasing both patient and provider participation in colorectal cancer screening are reviewed here. Of the eight colorectal cancer intervention studies identified through searches of the MEDLINE and PsychINFO electronic databases, two were patient-directed interventions (Hart et al., 1997; Wolf & Schorling, 2000), two were conducted with community-based samples (Powe & Weinrich, 1999; Weinrich, Weinrich, Atwood, Boyd, & Greene, 1998), one was conducted in a worksite (Tilley et al., 1999), and three were directed at providers (Hillman et al., 1998; Schroy et al., 1999; Zubarik et al., 2000). These studies are summarized in Table 3.3.

PATIENT-DIRECTED COLORECTAL CANCER SCREENING INTERVENTIONS

Hart et al. (1997) conducted a randomized controlled trial of an educational brochure with 1,571 residents of a suburban/rural area in Britain. All were patients of a large practice staffed by 10 physicians. The educational brochure contained information on colorectal cancer incidence, screening with FOBT, and reasons for noncompliance (obtained from detailed interviews with 82 participants noncompliant with a previous screening program). All participants were sent a letter signed by the senior partner of the practice, inviting them to receive a free FOBT. Half were randomly assigned to receive the educational leaflet. Those who accepted screening were then sent an FOBT kit with instructions to return it to the hospital lab for processing. The intervention resulted in increased compliance, with the largest intervention effect observed among older men. However, no intervention effect was observed for women of either age group (38% versus 36% and 31% versus 31%, respectively). A significantly greater proportion of women in the control group complied with colorectal cancer screening than men (33% versus 25%, $p < .02$).

**TABLE 3.3  Colorectal-Cancer-Screening Interventions**

| | Theoretical/ conceptual framework | Design | Sample | Measures | Results |
|---|---|---|---|---|---|
| Hart et al. (1997) | None reported | RCT; physician letter offering free FOBT with (experimental) or without (control) health education brochure on colorectal cancer screening | $N = 1,571$ participants in a single practice group | Whether or not FOBT was obtained | Effects differed by age and gender; men who received brochure had significantly higher rates of compliance with FOBT—largest intervention effect for older men: aged 61–65 years, 36% versus 27%; and aged 66–70 years, 39 versus 23%; no intervention effect for women; both groups equally compliant. *(continued)* |

**TABLE 3.3  Colorectal-Cancer-Screening Interventions** (*continued*)

| | Theoretical/ conceptual framework | Design | Sample | Measures | Results |
|---|---|---|---|---|---|
| Hillman et al. (1998) | None reported | RCT; semiannual performance feedback to providers, financial bonuses for compliance with cancer-screening guidelines | 52 primary care sites in an HMO | Whether or not FOBT, colonoscopy, and sigmoidoscopy were obtained | Although intervention groups had higher compliance scores for colorectal cancer screening, intervention effects were not significant. |
| Powe & Weinrich (1999) | Powe Fatalism Model | Pre- and post-test; intervention group: 20-minute videotape designed to increase colorectal cancer screening; control group: 13-minute ACS videotape on colorectal cancer screening; both groups received free FOBT test kits analyzed free of charge | *N* = 70 predominantly African-American women attendees at rural senior citizen centers | Whether or not FOBT was obtained | No significant intervention effect on FOBT compliance; overall compliance high in both groups (60% intervention group, 68% control); significant reduction in cancer fatalism in intervention group (*p* = .003). |

| | Theoretical/ conceptual framework | Design | Sample | Measures | Results |
|---|---|---|---|---|---|
| Schroy et al. (1999) | None reported | Quasi-experimental; 4-phase procedural training program to enhance primary care providers' utilization of sigmoidoscopy, including the on-site provision of services and training | 9 neighborhood health centers (4 intervention sites, 5 comparison sites) | Whether or not sigmoidoscopy was obtained | Interventions sites had a 36% increase in sigmoidoscopy compliance versus a 7% increase at comparison sites ($p = .001$). |
| Tilley et al. (1999) | HBM; Social Cognitive Theory; Theory of Reasoned Action | RCT; colorectal-cancer-screening promotion and nutrition interventions; screening intervention consisted of (a) mailed screening invitation with tailored educational booklet, (b) follow-up telephone counseling based on booklet, (c) quarterly newsletters, and (d) booster intervention (1 and 2 repeated) 1 year later | 28 worksites (15 intervention, 13 control) with 5,042 employees | Whether or not FOBT and sigmoidoscopy was obtained | Intent-to-treat analyses showed modest but significant intervention effects for screening with FOBT (26% versus 23% in year 1 and 21% versus 19% in year 2) and with sigmoidoscopy (30% versus 25% in year 1 and 23% versus 18% in year 2). |

*(continued)*

**TABLE 3.3  Colorectal-Cancer-Screening Interventions (*continued*)**

| | Theoretical/ conceptual framework | Design | Sample | Measures | Results |
|---|---|---|---|---|---|
| Weinrich, Weinrich, Atwood, Boyd, & Greene (1998) | Orem's Self-Care Model | Quasi- experimental; 4 educational interventions tested: (a) nurse-delivered ACS slide-tape presentation on colorectal cancer; (b) elderly educators matched to age and race presented advantages of FOBT and demonstrated test procedure; (c) nurse-delivered ACS slide-tape presentation adapted for aging changes plus FOBT kit demonstration, return instructions with take-home written reminders; and (d) interventions a and b; free FOBT kits and return instructions provided to all | *N* = 211 from 14 congregate meal sites in South Carolina | Whether or not FOBT was obtained | Elderly educator intervention not significant; Adapted for Aging intervention was significant (*p* = .01); combined intervention was significant (*p* = .04). |

| | Theoretical/ conceptual framework | Design | Sample | Measures | Results |
|---|---|---|---|---|---|
| Wolf & Schorling (2000) | None reported | RCT; 3 in-person interventions to provide screening information; intervention groups received either (a) *relative* risk information or (b) *absolute* risk information; controls received no colorectal cancer risk information | *N* = 399 patients aged 65+ visiting 4 general internists for routine care | Intent to begin or continue FOBT, flexible sigmoidoscopy, or both. | No significant intervention effects. |
| Zubarik et al. (2000) | None reported | Cohort study; educational program directed at primary care physicians and nurses; telephone and written reminders to patients due for repeat sigmoidoscopy | 1 urban hospital and satellite clinics serving inner-city residents | Whether or not sigmoidoscopy was obtained | 42% increase in number of sigmoidoscopies performed in 5 months postintervention compared to 5 months prior. |

93

Wolf and Schorling (2000) randomized 399 patients to receive one of three colorectal cancer informational scripts delivered in person by a trained research assistant during routine care visits to their general internist. The control script briefly described FOBT and flexible sigmoidoscopy. The Relative Risk Reduction (RRR) script provided a 3-minute discussion of FOBT, flexible sigmoidoscopy, the test characteristics, evidence supporting mortality benefits described in terms of RRR (with graph), and the uncertain benefit of screening older people. The Absolute Risk Reduction (ARR) script contained information identical to the RRR except that colorectal cancer mortality benefit was described in terms of absolute risk. Scripts were reviewed by a panel of gastroenterologists for accuracy and content validity, and were pilot tested. No intervention effects were observed for either the RRR or ARR interventions.

### COMMUNITY-BASED AND WORKPLACE COLORECTAL CANCER INTERVENTIONS

Powe and Weinrich (1999), using a pre-/post-test design, randomized 70 attendees (42 intervention, 28 controls) at senior citizen centers to receive a videotaped intervention designed to decrease cancer fatalism and increase participation in colorectal cancer screening among African-Americans. The intervention video was 20 minutes long and designed to model the desired behavior of colorectal cancer screening. The majority of actors in the video were African-Americans who incorporated the study population's dress, food preferences, customs, traditions, and beliefs. The control group viewed a 13-minute ACS video. A significant intervention effect was observed for cancer fatalism scores as measured by the Powe Fatalism Inventory. Mean pretest scores were essentially equivalent (9.90 and 9.89). Post-test fatalism scores obtained 1 week later had decreased to 8.5 ($SD = 4.2$) for the intervention group and remained unchanged (9.79, $SD = 5.0$) in the control group. After controlling for differences in race and income with analyses of covariance, this difference was significant ($F = 9.23$, $p = .003$). Significant intervention effects were also observed for changes in colorectal cancer knowledge ($F = 3.95$, $p = .04$). No significant intervention effect was found in the rate of participation in FOBT; participation for both groups was high (60% and 68%, respectively).

Weinrich et al. (1998) conducted a replication study to test four educational interventions designed to increase participation in FOBT among 211 socioeconomically disadvantaged elderly. A quasi-experimental design was used; 14 congregate meal sites were randomly selected and assigned to 1 of 4 types of educational interventions. The traditional educational intervention consisted of a nurse presenting an ACS slide presentation on colorectal cancer screening. The second intervention involved elderly educators who gave testimony regarding the advantages of FOBT and demonstrated the test procedure. In the third intervention condition, titled Adaptation for Aging Changes, the traditional presentation was modified to accommodate normal aging changes and provided opportunities for participants to practice the FOBT test procedure with peanut butter. The fourth intervention combined the elderly educator and the Adaptation for Aging Changes intervention. Following all interventions, participants were given free FOBT kits with dietary restriction instructions and told to return completed tests. Results indicated a high level of compliance overall, with 65% of the participants completing FOBT. Logistic regression techniques were used to examine intervention effects. The investigators reported significant intervention effects for the Adaptation for Aging Changes intervention ($p = .01$) and the combined intervention group ($p = .04$).

The Next Step Trial was a randomized controlled trial designed to increase colorectal cancer screening and dietary change among workers at high risk (Tilley et al., 1999). Interventions were tested at 28 worksites with 5,042 employees of the automotive industry. Thirteen worksites ($N = 2,802$ high-risk employees) received usual care, which included a long-standing worksite colorectal cancer screening program offered by the employer. The program included digital rectal exams (DREs), FOBT, and flexible sigmoidoscopy. Eligible workers were notified each time a new round of screening was being offered through letters mailed to their homes and flyers posted at work. Because only 35% of those eligible were participating, this randomized trial was conducted to increase screening in this high-risk group.

Fifteen intervention worksites ($N = 2,240$ high-risk employees) received the standard screening program plus a tailored educational intervention consisting of a mailed invitation to screen accompanied by a personally tailored educational booklet that included information about the employees' screening history and individualized screening recommendations. This mailing was followed by a 5- to 7-minute telephone counseling session where an interviewer highlighted messages from the booklet, answered questions, and encouraged scheduling a screening appointment. Employees at intervention worksites also received a quarterly newsletter that included nutrition and screening information and interviews with coworkers who had been screened.

Results indicated that, after adjusting for baseline and worksite characteristics, modest but significant intervention effects were observed for both screening compliance ($OR = 1.46$, 95% $CI = 1.1$ to $2.0$) and coverage ($OR = 1.33$, 95% $CI = 1.1$ to $1.6$). Tilley et al. (1999) concluded that, given the relatively high rates of previous screenings and awareness of colorectal cancer risk, it was not surprising that the intervention effects were modest for this high-risk population. The investigators hypothesized that higher intervention effects might be observed if this intervention was tested in other work settings (without worksite screening programs) or with individuals not at increased risk for colorectal cancer.

PROVIDER-DIRECTED COLORECTAL CANCER INTERVENTIONS

Interventions to enhance physician adherence to colorectal cancer screening recommendations usually focus on education. Schroy et al. (1999) tested the effects of a practice-oriented educational program that included training in flexible sigmoidoscopy. Four neighborhood health centers served as intervention sites and five other centers served as comparison sites. The intervention had four phases: (a) a baseline provider survey and didactic seminar on colorectal cancer screening; (b) for over 12 months, a provision of on-site flexible sigmoidoscopy services provided by university gastroenterologists; (c) for 12 to 24 months, procedural training for sigmoidoscopy with 1 to 6 interested providers at each site; and (d) the establishment of free-standing flexible sigmoidoscopy programs staffed by primary care providers.

A follow-up was conducted at 12 months and self-reported adherence rates increased by an average of 36% at intervention sites (a range of 7% to 92%) compared to only 7% at comparison sites (a range of 8% to 50%). Examining utilization rates rather than self-reported adherence showed that adherence remained significantly higher for intervention sites (47% versus 4%, $p < .001$). The investigators concluded that provision of on-site sigmoidoscopies was a critical success factor, as was the regular presence of a gastroenterologist-fostered interaction, formal and informal consultations, and intellectual exchange.

In a randomized controlled study, Hillman et al. (1998) tested regular performance feedback and financial incentives as interventions to increase physician adherence to the guidelines, including colorectal cancer, in one managed-care organization; provider sites were paid by capitation. Fifty-two sites were randomly assigned to the intervention or usual care. Providers in the intervention group received semiannual feedback regarding adherence to screening guidelines and financial incentives for those who were adherent. Data were collected from audits conducted at baseline and every 6 months for 18 months.

Baseline compliance scores for all types of cancer screening were low and did not differ between groups. The mean compliance score for colorectal cancer screening was the lowest of all cancer screening types, with only 15% compliance at baseline in the intervention group and 11% in the control group. For comparison purposes, mammography compliance rates were also low, at only 41% and 34% in each group, respectively. Repeated measure analyses demonstrated significant changes over time, with colorectal cancer screening compliance rates increasing from 15% to 44% in the intervention group and from 11% to 37% in the control group. Unfortunately, a significant intervention (group × time) effect was not observed. Investigators credited the changes in practice to the increased emphasis on preventive care occurring on a national level. The investigators acknowledged that, although screening compliance improved dramatically during the study, compliance remained suboptimal, with approximately 60% of eligible women not receiving annual colorectal cancer screening.

Another study of provider education designed to enhance the use of sigmoidoscopy was conducted by Zubarik et al. (2000). In addition to educating healthcare providers, this intervention also incorporated a nurse-initiated telephone reminder and counseling contact to all patients due for repeat sigmoidoscopy. A pre-/post-test cohort design was used to examine screening utilization rates 5 months before and 5 months after a 1-month educational initiative. The intervention consisted of (a) didactic sessions on colorectal cancer screening conducted by gastroenterologists, presented formally in a monthly lecture format and informally at weekly morning reports to all medical house staff; (b) written materials and education about colorectal cancer screening provided by gastroenterology nurses to clinic nurses; and (c) phone contact and education by gastroenterology nurses for patients due for repeat sigmoidoscopies.

In the 5-month period following the intervention, a 42% increase in the number of screening sigmoidoscopies performed was observed, an increase from 50 to 71. Part of the intervention effect was likely due to the direct telephone counseling contacts with patients due for repeat screening sigmoidoscopies. However, when patients due for repeat sigmoidoscopies were excluded, there was still a 15% increase. Although the statistical significance of this change was not reported, the investigators concluded that the provider-directed educational interventions were effective.

## SUMMARY AND RECOMMENDATIONS FOR COLORECTAL CANCER SCREENING

Although examining colorectal cancer screening specific to each behavior separately is critical, it is also important to understand the interdependency of screening tests. Past research is now limited by a narrow focus on two screening tests: FOBT and flexible sigmoidoscopy. Colonoscopy is increasingly being used for screening rather than diagnostic purposes. Colorectal cancer intervention studies will focus on three screening modalities: FOBT, flexible sigmoidoscopy, and colonoscopy.

Efficacy studies currently under way or planned will guide the refinement of colorectal cancer screening recommendations and ultimately will influence intervention research. Participation in FOBT, flexible sigmoidoscopy, and colonoscopy screening behaviors will need to be examined in relation to one another. For example, individuals who have regular colonoscopies no longer need to have an annual FOBT. Vernon (1997) has begun to address this interdependency issue by suggesting the measurement of both colorectal cancer screening compliance (participation in all recommended screening tests) and coverage (participation in at least one screening test). More work is needed to clarify the measurement of colorectal cancer screening participation and examine the processes and constructs that may mediate intervention effectiveness.

Currently, colorectal cancer screening participation rates are unacceptably low, providing both challenges and opportunities for behavioral scientists. Investigators of colorectal cancer screening behaviors have begun to apply knowledge gained from intervention work on mammography screening. As the first part of this chapter indicates, theoretically based, tailored interventions increase screening (Champion et al., in press; Saywell et al., 1999; Tilley et al., 1999). In studies reviewed to date, colorectal cancer screening interventions have been directed at individuals, providers, and communities using in-person delivery, telephone delivery, and mailed print interventions. Multiple intervention modalities were often combined in a single study, making it difficult to determine which part(s) of the intervention was most effective. Few theoretically based intervention strategies have been tested.

No intervention studies addressed the issue of cost effectiveness; cost-effective methods for delivering interventions to appropriate populations must be identified. Technology holds great promise for tailoring interventions that can be delivered via interactive computer programs or through the Internet. Screening must be increased among populations at risk for colorectal cancer, such as patients with a history of polyps or a family history of colorectal cancer, and research efforts must then be focused appropriately. Intervention research to increase colorectal cancer screening is an important frontier for behavioral oncology that holds great potential for decreasing colorectal morbidity and mortality.

## DIRECTIONS FOR CANCER SCREENING RESEARCH

Investigators need to examine whether interventions designed to increase other types of cancer screening, such as mammography, can be translated to colorectal cancer screening. Research has already demonstrated that many of the theoretical variables important in mammography research are also associated with colorectal cancer screening (Peterson & Vernon, 2000; Rawl, Menon, Champion, Foster, & Skinner, 2000; Vernon, 1997). The next step is to adequately operationalize theoretical constructs, such as benefits, barriers, and self-efficacy specific to colorectal cancer screening. Progress in intervention research is dependent on reliable and valid measures of both mediators and outcomes. Psychometric testing of some of these measures has been conducted (Menon, 2000; Rawl, Champion, et al., 2001). Because colorectal cancer screening modalities differ greatly in the barriers to use, each modality must be addressed carefully and separately. For instance, barriers to FOBT may include the unpleasantness of obtaining a stool sample, while a significant barrier to colonoscopy is the preparation. Researchers must carefully identify issues specific to each screening behavior.

## REFERENCES

Adami, H. O., Ponten, J., Sparen, P., Bergstrom, R., Gustafsson, L., & Friberg, L. G. (1994). Survival trend after invasive cervical cancer diagnosis in Sweden before and after cytologic screening. 1960–1984. *Cancer, 73*, 140–147.

American Cancer Society (2002). *Cancer facts & figures: 2001–2002.* Available: http://www.cancer.org/downloads/STT/CancerFacts&Fugures2002TM.pdf [Accessed: November 11, 2002].

Andersson, I., Aspegren, K., Janzon, L., Landberg, T., Lindholm, K., Linell, F., et al. (1988). Mammographic screening and mortality from breast cancer: The Malmo Mammographic Screening Trial. *British Medical Journal, 297*, 943–948.

Ayre, J. E. (1947). Selective cytology smear for diagnosis of cancer. *American Journal of Obstetrics and Gynecology, 53*, 609.

Bastani, R., Maxwell, A. E., Bradford, C., Das, I. P., & Yan, K. X. (1999). Tailored risk notification for women with a family history of breast cancer. *Preventive Medicine, 29*, 355–364.

Bernstein, J., Mutschler, P., & Bernstein, E. (2000). Keeping mammography referral appointments: Motivation, health beliefs, and access barriers experienced by older minority women. *Journal of Midwifery and Women's Health, 45*, 308–313.

Bocciolone, L., La Vecchia, C., Levi, F., Lucchini, F., & Franceschi, S. (1993). Trends in uterine cancer mortality in the Americas, 1955–1988. *Gynecologic Oncology, 51*, 335–344.

Burack, R., Gimotty, P., George, J., Simon, M., Dews, P., & Moncrease, A. (1996). The effect of patient and physician reminders on use of screening mammography in a health maintenance organization. Results of a randomized controlled trial. *Cancer, 78*, 1708–1721.

Campbell, E., Peterkin, D., Abbott, R., & Rogers, J. (1997). Encouraging underscreened women to have cervical cancer screening: The effectiveness of a computer strategy. *Preventive Medicine, 26*, 801–807.

Campbell, H., MacDonald, S., & McKiernan, M. (1996). Promotion of cervical screening uptake by health visitor follow-up of women who repeatedly failed to attend. *Journal of Public Health Medicine, 18*, 94–97.

Champion, V. L., Menon, U., Seshadri, R., Anzalone, D., Rawl, S., Skinner, C. S., et al. (in press). Comparisons of tailored mammography interventions at two months post intervention. *Annals of Behavioral Medicine.*

Champion, V. L., Ray, D., Heilman, D., & Springston, J. (2000). A tailored intervention for mammography among low-income African-American women. *Journal of Psychosocial Oncology, 18*(4), 1–13.

Clover, K., Redman, S., Forbes, J., Sanson-Fisher, R., & Callaghan, T. (1996). Two sequential randomized trials of community participation to recruit women for mammographic screening. *Preventive Medicine, 25*, 126–134.

Collette, H. J. A., Day, N. E., Rombach, J. J., & deWaard, F. (1984). Evaluation of screening for breast cancer in a non-randomised study (The Dom Project) by means of a case-control study. *Lancet, 1*, 1224–1226.

Costanza, M. E., Stoddard, A. M., Luckmann, R., White, M. J., Spitz-Avrunin, J., & Clemow, L. (2000). Promoting mammography: Results of a randomized trial of telephone counseling and a medical practice intervention. *American Journal of Preventive Medicine, 19*, 39–46.

Crane, L. A., Leakey, T. A., Woodworth, M. A., Rimer, B. K., Warnecke, R. B., Heller, D., et al. (1998). Cancer information service-initiated outcalls to promote screening mammography among low-income and minority women: Design and feasibility testing. *Preventive Medicine, 27*(Suppl. 5), 29–38.

Cuzick, J. (1999). *Colorectal cancer.* New York: Marcel Dekker, Inc.

Davis, T. C., Berkel, H. J., Arnold, C. L., Nandy, I., Jackson, R. H., & Murphy, P. W. (1998). Intervention to increase mammography utilization in a public hospital. *Journal of General Internal Medicine, 13*, 230–233.

DiBonito, L., Falconieri, G., Tomasic, G., Colautti, I., Bonifacio, D., & Dudine, S. (1993). Cervical cytopathology. An evaluation of its accuracy based on cytohistologic comparison. *Cancer, 72*, 3002–3006.

Dignan, M., Michielutte, R., Blinson, K., Wells, H. B., Case, L. D., Sharp, P., et al. (1996). Effectiveness of health education to increase screening for cervical cancer among eastern-band Cherokee Indian women in North Carolina. *Journal of the National Cancer Institute, 88*, 1670–1671.

Duan, N., Fox, S. A., Derose, K. P., & Carson, S. (2000). Maintaining mammography adherence through telephone counseling in a church-based trial. *American Journal of Public Health, 90*, 1468–1471.

Eastman, P. (1997). NCI adopts new mammography screening guidelines for women. *Journal of the National Cancer Institute, 89*, 538–540.

Flynn, B. S., Gavin, P., Worden, J. K., Ashikaga, T., Gautam, S., & Carpenter, J. (1997). Community education programs to promote mammography participation in rural New York state. *Preventive Medicine, 26*, 102–108.

Goldberg, H. I., Neighbor, W. E., Cheadle, A. D., Ramsey, S. D., Diehr, P., & Gore, E. (2000). A controlled time-series trial of clinical reminders: Using computerized firm systems to make quality improvement research a routine part of mainstream practice. *Health Services Research, 34*, 1519–1534.

Greenlee, R. T., Hill-Harmon, M. B., Murray, T., & Thun, M. (2001). Cancer statistics, 2001. *CA-A Cancer Journal for Clinicians, 51*, 15–36.

Hardcastle, J. D., Chamberlain, J. O., Robinson, M. H. E., Moss, S. M., Amar, S. S., Balfour, T. W., et al. (1996). Randomised controlled trial of faecal-occult-blood screening for colorectal cancer. *Lancet, 348*, 1472–1477.

Hart, A. R., Barone, T. L., Gay, S. P., Inglis, A., Griffin, L., Tallon, C. A., et al. (1997). The effect on compliance of a health education leaflet in colorectal cancer screening in general practice in central England. *Journal of Epidemiology and Community Health, 51*, 187–191.

Hillman, A. L., Ripley, K., Goldfarb, N., Nuamah, I., Weiner, J., & Lusk, E. (1998). Physician financial incentives and feedback: Failure to increase cancer screening in Medicaid managed care. *American Journal of Public Health, 88*, 1699–1701.

Hochbaum, G. (1958). *Public participation in medical screening programs: A sociopsychological study.* Washington, D.C.: U.S. Government Printing Office.

Janz, N. K., Schottenfeld, D., Doerr, K. M., Selig, S. M., Dunn, R. L., Strawderman, M., et al. (1997). A two-step intervention of increase mammography among women aged 65 and older. *American Journal of Public Health, 87*, 1683–1686.

Jenkins, C. N., McPhee, S. J., Bird, J. A., Pham, G. Q., Nguyen, B. H., Nguyen, T., et al. (1999). Effect of a media-led education campaign on breast and cervical cancer screening among Vietnamese-American women. *Preventive Medicine, 28*, 395–406.

Kadison, P., Pelletier, E. M., Mounib, E. L., Oppedisano, P., & Poteat, H. T. (1998). Improved screening for breast cancer associated with a telephone-based risk assessment. *Preventive Medicine, 27*, 493–501.

Kavanagh, A. M., Giovannucci, E. L., Fuchs, C. S., & Colditz, G. A. (1998). Screening endoscopy and risk of colorectal cancer in United States men. *Cancer Causes & Control, 9*, 455–462.

King, E., Rimer, B. K., Benincasa, T., Harrop, C., Amfoh, K., Bonney, G., et al. (1998). Strategies to encourage mammography use among women in senior citizens' housing facilities. *Journal of Cancer Education, 13*, 108–115.

Kreuter, M., & Skinner, C. (2000). Tailoring: What's in a name. *Health Education Research, 15*, 1–4.

Kreuter, M. W., Farrell, D., Olevitch, L., & Brennan, L. (2000). *Tailoring health messages: Customizing communication with computer technology.* Mahwah, NJ: Lawrence Erlbaum Associates.

Kronborg, O., Fenger, C., Olsen, J., Jorgensen, O. D., & Sondergaard, O. (1996). Randomised study of screening for colorectal cancer with faecal-occult-blood test. *Lancet, 348*, 1467–1471.

Lantz, P. M., Stencil, D., Lippert, M. T., Beversdorf, S., Jaros, L., & Remington, P. L. (1995). Breast and cervical cancer screening in a low-income managed care sample: The efficacy of physician letters and phone calls. *American Journal of Public Health, 85*, 834–836.

Maibach, E., & Parrott, R. (1995). *Designing health messages.* Thousand Oaks, CA: Sage.

Mandel, J. S., Bond, J. H., Church, T. R., Snover, D. C., Bradley, G. M., Schuman, L. M., et al. (1993). Reducing mortality from colorectal cancer by screening for fecal occult blood. Minnesota Colon Cancer Control Study. *New England Journal of Medicine, 328*, 1365–1371.

Marcus, A. C., & Crane, L. A. (1998). A review of cervical cancer screening intervention research: Implications for public health programs and future research. *Preventive Medicine, 27*, 13–31.

Margolis, K. L., & Menart, T. C. (1996). A test of two interventions to improve compliance with scheduled mammography appointments. *Journal of General Internal Medicine, 11*, 539–541.

Margolis, K. L., Lurie, N., McGovern, P. G., Tyrell, M., & Slater, J. S. (1998). Increasing breast and cervical cancer screening in low-income women. *Journal of General Internal Medicine, 13*, 515–521.

Mayer, J. A., Lewis, E. C., Slymen, D. J., Dullum, J., Kurata, H., Holbrook, A., et al. (2000). Patient reminder letters to promote annual mammograms: A randomized controlled trial. *Preventive Medicine, 31*, 315–322.

Menon, U. (2000). *Factors associated with colorectal cancer screening in an average-risk population.* Unpublished dissertation, Indiana University School of Nursing, Indianapolis.

Mettlin, C. (1999). Global breast cancer mortality statistics. *CA: A Cancer Journal for Clinicians, 49*, 138–144.

Morbidity and Mortality Weekly Report. (2001). State-specific prevalence of selected health behaviors by race and ethnicity. *MMWR—Morbidity & Mortality Weekly Report 49.*

Morrison, A. S., Brisson, J., & Khalid, N. (1988). Breast cancer incidence and mortality in breast cancer detection demonstration project. *Journal of the National Cancer Institute, 80*, 1540–1547.

Newcomb, P. A., Norfleet, R. G., Storer, B. E., Surawicz, T. S., & Marcus, P. M. (1992). Screening sigmoidoscopy and colorectal cancer mortality. *Journal of the National Cancer Institute, 84*, 1572–1575.

Palli, D., Del-Turco, M. R., Buiatti, E., Carli, S., Ciatto, S., Toscani, L., et al. (1986). A case control study of the efficacy of a non-randomized breast cancer screening program in Florence (Italy). *International Journal of Cancer, 38*, 501–504.

Paskett, E. D., McMahon, K., Tatum, C., Velez, R., Shelton, B., Case, L. D., et al. (1998). Clinic-based interventions to promote breast and cervical cancer screening. *Preventive Medicine, 27*, 120–128.

Paskett, E. D., Tatum, C. M., D'Agostino, R., Rushing, J., Velez, R., Michielutte, R., et al. (1999). Community-based interventions to improve breast and cervical cancer screening: Results of the Forsyth County cancer screening (FoCaS) project. *Cancer Epidemiology, Biomarkers & Prevention, 8*, 453–459.

Peterson, S., & Vernon, S. (2000). A review of patient and physician adherence to colorectal cancer screening guidelines. *Seminars in Colon & Rectal Surgery, 11*, 1–17.

Potter, J. D. (1999). Colorectal cancer: Molecules and populations. *Journal of the National Cancer Institute, 91*, 916–932.

Powe, B. D., & Weinrich, S. (1999). An intervention to decrease cancer fatalism among rural elders. *Oncology Nursing Forum, 26*, 583–588.

Prochaska, J. O. (1994a). *Staging: A revolution in health promotion.* Paper presented at the Society for Behavioral Medicine, Boston, MA.

Prochaska, J. O. (1994b). Strong and weak principles for progressing from precontemplation to action on the basis of twelve problem behaviors. *Health Psychology, 13*, 47–51.

Prochaska, J. O., & DiClemente, C. C. (1983). Stages and processes of self-change of smoking: Toward an integrative model of change. *Journal of Consulting and Clinical Psychology, 51*, 390–395.

Prochaska, J. O., Velicer, W. F., Rossi, J. S., Goldstein, M. G., Marcus, B. H., Fiore, C., et al. (1994). Stages of change and decisional balance for twelve problem behaviors. *Health Psychology, 13*, 39–46.

Progress Review Group. (2000). *Conquering colorectal cancer: A blueprint for the future.* Bethesda, MD: National Cancer Institute.

Rakowski, W., Ehrich, B., Goldstein, M. G., Rimer, B. K., Pearlman, D. N., Velicer, W. F., et al. (1998). Increasing mammography among women aged 40–74 by use of a stage-matched, tailored intervention. *Preventive Medicine, 27*, 748–756.

Rakowski, W., Dube, C. E., & Goldstein, M. G. (1996). Considerations for extending the transtheoretical model of behavior change to screening mammography. *Health Education Research, 11*, 77–96.

Rawl, S. M., Menon, U., Champion, V. L., Foster, J. L., & Skinner, C. S. (2000). Colorectal cancer screening beliefs. Focus Groups with first-degree relatives. *Cancer Practice, 8*, 32–35.

Rawl, S., Champion, V., Menon, U., Loehrer, P., Vance, G., Skinner, C. S., et al. (2001). Validation of scales to measure benefits and barriers to colorectal cancer screening. *Journal of Psychosocial Oncology, 19*(3/4), 47–63.

Reintgen, E., & Clark, R. (1996). *Cancer Screening.* St. Louis, MO: Mosby.

Richardson, J. L., Mondrus, G. T., Danley, K., Deapen, D., & Mack, T. (1996). Impact of a mailed intervention on annual mammography and physician breast examinations among women at high risk of breast cancer. *Cancer Epidemiology, Biomarkers & Prevention, 5,* 71–76.

Rimer, B. K. (1994). Mammography use in the U.S.: Trends and the impact of interventions. *Annals of Behavioral Medicine, 16,* 317–326.

Roberts, M. M., Alexander, F. E., Anderson, T. J., Chetty, U., Donnan, P. T., Forrest, P., et al. (1990). Edinburgh trial of screening for breast cancer: Mortality at seven years. *Lancet, 335,* 241–246.

Ronis, D. L. (1992). Conditional health threats: Health beliefs, decisions, and behaviors among adults. *Health Psychology, 11,* 127–134.

Rosenstock, I. M. (1974). Historical origins of the Health Belief Model. *Health Education Monograph, 2,* 328–335.

Rosenstock, I. M. (1988). Adoption and maintenance of lifestyle modifications. *American Journal of Preventive Medicine, 4,* 349–352.

Rosenstock, I. M., Strecher, V. J., & Becker, M. H. (1994). *The Health Belief Model and HIV risk behavior change.* New York: Plenum.

Saywell, R. M., Jr., Champion, V. L., Skinner, C. S., McQuillen, D., Martin, D., & Maraj, M. (1999). Cost-effectiveness comparison of five interventions to increase mammography screening. *Preventive Medicine, 29,* 374–382.

Schroy, P. C., Heeren, T., Bliss, C. M., Pincus, J., Wilson, S., & Prout, M. (1999). Implementation of on-site screening sigmoidoscopy positively influences utilization by primary care providers. *Gastroenterology, 117,* 304–311.

Segnan, N., Senore, C., Giordano, L., Ponti, A., & Ronco, G. (1998). Promoting participation in a population screening program for breast and cervical cancer: A randomized trial of different invitation strategies. *Tumori, 84,* 348–353.

Selby, J. V., Friedman, G. D., Quesenberry, C. P., & Weiss, N. S. (1993). Effect of fecal occult blood testing on mortality from colorectal cancer. A case-control study. *Ann Intern Med, 118,* 1–6.

Shapiro, S., Venet, W., Strax, P., Venet, L., & Roeser, R. (1982). Ten- to fourteen-year effect of screening on breast cancer mortality. *Journal of the National Cancer Institute, 69,* 349–355.

Sharp, D. J., Peters, T. J., Bartholomew, J., & Shaw, A. (1996). Breast screening: A randomised controlled trial in UK general practice of three interventions designed to increase uptake. *Journal of Epidemiology and Community Health, 50,* 72–76.

Sherlau-Johnson, C., Gallivan, S., & Jenkins, D. (1997). Evaluating cervical cancer screening programmes for developing countries. *International Journal of Cancer, 72,* 210–216.

Skinner, C. S., Campbell, M. K., Rimer, B. K., Curry, S., & Prochaska, J. O. (1999). How effective is tailored print communication? *Annals of Behavioral Medicine, 21,* 290–298.

Smith, R. A., von Eschenbach, A. C., Wender, R., Levin, B., Byers, T., Rothenberger, D., et al. (2001). American Cancer Society guidelines for the early detection of cancer: Update of early detection guidelines for prostate, colorectal, and endometrial cancers. *CA-A Cancer Journal of Clinicians, 51*, 38–70.

Somkin, C. P., Hiatt, R., Hurley, L. B., Gruskin, E., Ackerson, L., & Larson, P. (1997). The effect of patient and provider reminders on mammography and Papanicolau smear screening in a large health maintenance organization. *Archives of Internal Medicine, 157*, 1658–1664.

Stockdale, S. E., Keeler, E., Duan, N., Derose, K. P., & Fox, S. A. (2000). Costs and cost-effectiveness of a church-based intervention to promote mammography screening. *HSR: Health Services Research, 35*, 1037–1057.

Sung, J. F. C., Blumenthal, D. S., Coates, R. J., Williams, J. E., Alema-Mensah, E., & Liff, J. M. (1997). Effect of a cancer screening intervention conducted by lay health workers among inner-city women. *American Journal of Preventive Medicine, 13*, 51–57.

Tabar, L., C. Fagerberg, J., Gad, A., Baldetorp, L., Holmberg, L. H., Grontoft, O., et al. (1985). Reduction in mortality from breast cancer after mass screening with mammography. Randomised trial from the Breast Cancer Screening Working Group of the Swedish National Board of Health and Welfare. *Lancet, 1*, 829–832.

Taplin, S. H., Barlow, W. E., Ludman, E., MacLehos, R., Meyer, D. M., Seger, D., et al. (2000). Testing reminder and motivational telephone calls to increase screening mammography: A randomized study. *Journal of the National Cancer Institute, 92*, 233–242.

Tilley, B. C., Vernon, S. W., Myers, R., Glanz, K., Lu, M., Hirst, K., et al. (1999). The Next Step Trial: Impact of a worksite colorectal cancer screening promotion program. *Preventive Medicine, 28*, 276–283.

van der Graaf, Y., Vooijs, G. P., Gaillard, H. L., & Go, D. M. (1987). Screening errors in cervical cytologic screening. *Acta Cytologica, 31*, 434–438.

Verbeek, A. L. M., Hendriks, J. H. C. L., Holland, R., Mravunac, M., Sturmans, F., & Day, N. E. (1984). Reduction of breast cancer mortality through mass screening with modern mammography. First results of the Nijmegan Project, 1975–1981. *Lancet, 1*, 1222–1224.

Vernon, S. W. (1997). Participation in colorectal cancer screening: A review. *Journal of the National Cancer Institute, 89*, 1406–1422.

Weber, B. E., & Reilly, B. M. (1997). Enhancing mammography use in the inner city. A randomized trial of intensive case management. *Archives of Internal Medicine, 157*, 2345–2349.

Weinrich, S. P., Weinrich, M. C., Atwood, J., Boyd, M., & Greene, F. (1998). Predictors of fecal occult blood screening among older socioeconomically disadvantaged Americans: A replication study. *Patient Education and Counseling, 34*, 103–114.

Winawer, S. J., Flehinger, B. J., Schottenfeld, D., & Miller, D. G. (1993). Screening with colorectal cancer with fecal occult blood testing and sigmoidoscopy. *Journal of the National Cancer Institute, 85*, 1311–1318.

Winawer, S. J., Fletcher, R. H., Miller, L., Godlee, F., Stolar, M. H., Mulrow, C. D., et al. (1997). Colorectal cancer screening: Clinical guidelines and rationale. *Gastroenterology, 112*, 594–642.

Witte, K. (1994). Fear control and danger control: A test of the extended parallel process model (EPPM). *Communication Monographs, 61*, 113–134.

Witte, K. (1995). Fishing for success: Using the persuasive health message framework to generate effective campaign messages. In E. Maibach & R. L. Parrott (Eds.), *Designing health messages: Approaches from communication theory and public health practice* (pp. 145–166). Thousand Oaks, CA: Sage Publications.

Wolf, A. M. D., & Schorling, J. B. (2000). Does informed consent alter elderly patients' preferences for colorectal cancer screening? *Journal of General Intern Medicine, 15*, 24–30.

Yancey, A. K., Tanjasiri, S. P., Klein, M., & Tunder, J. (1995). Increased cancer screening behavior in women of color by culturally sensitive video exposure. *Preventive Medicine, 24*, 142–148.

Zubarik, R., Eisen, G., Zubarik, J., Teal, C., Benjamin, S., Glaser, M., et al. (2000). Education improves colorectal cancer screening by flexible sigmoidoscopy in an inner city population. *The American Journal of Gastroenterology, 95*, 509–512.

# 4

# Smoking Cessation in Cancer Patients: Never Too Late to Quit

**Ellen R. Gritz**
**Damon J. Vidrine**
**Amy B. Lazev**

In 2002, cancer incidence is estimated at 1,248,900 cases and a total of 555,500 deaths will occur. Of these deaths, 170,000 will be related to tobacco use (Jemal, Thomas, Murray, & Thun, 2002). Respiratory system cancers alone (larynx, lung and bronchus, and other respiratory organs) will claim 67,300 lives, oral cavity and pharynx malignancies another 2,500, and cancers of the urinary bladder 4,000 deaths. The 5-year survival rate for all cancers is currently 62%, and 8.9 million Americans with a history of cancer were alive in 1997 (Jemal et al., 2002).

Given the staggering figures on cancer incidence and mortality (more than 1,500 deaths per day in the U.S. alone) and the increasing overall survival rate, it is important to examine the impact of smoking behavior on cancer patients beyond etiological relationships. This is an understudied population; many oncology clinicians still do not believe it is a priority to intervene regarding tobacco use or do not feel they have the skills to do so effectively. The prevalence of smoking among adult Americans 18 years of age and older is 23.5%; in the age groups most likely to experience cancer (45 to 64, and 65 and older), smoking prevalence rates are 23.3% and 10.6%, respectively. Smoking prevalence is much higher among those diagnosed with smoking-related tumors (e.g., 39.0% to 59.8%; Gritz, Carr et al., 1991; Lippman et al., 2001) than tumors not related to smoking, in which prevalence would be expected to be at population levels. Thus, smoking cessation interventions have the potential to benefit a substantial portion of persons diagnosed with and treated for cancer.

In this chapter, the adverse impact of smoking on cancer treatment and survival are reviewed, as well as smoking's effects on quality of life. The quality of life section will provide an in-depth discussion of smoking, smoking cessation, and quality of life in cancer patient and other medical populations. In the final section, an overview of research on smoking cessation in cancer patient populations is presented, as well as a summary of theoretical perspectives, models, and state-of-the-art guidelines for intervention. This latter discussion will consider the tailoring and modifications of cessation treatments for cancer patients and survivors. Finally, limitations of the research to date and recommendations for future directions are presented.

## ADVERSE EFFECTS OF SMOKING ON THE OUTCOMES OF CANCER TREATMENT

Although most smoking cessation efforts have been aimed at the primary prevention of cancer, a growing stream of evidence indicates substantial medical benefits for individuals who quit smoking after they are diagnosed with cancer. These studies indicate that continued smoking: (a) reduces the effectiveness of treatment while causing complications with healing as well as exacerbating treatment side effects, (b) increases the risk of developing a second primary malignancy, and (c) decreases overall survival rates.

### Decreased Effectiveness of Medical Treatment due to Smoking

Smoking may result in complications for the major cancer treatment modalities: surgery, radiation, and chemotherapy. It may also compromise the efficacy of chemoprevention interventions. Quitting smoking prior to treatment is therefore recommended for all smokers. Patients may believe that quitting smoking after a cancer diagnosis is futile. However, an understanding of the potential benefits outlined here may increase patient motivation to quit smoking and help those interested in quitting maintain their abstinence.

SURGERY

Smoking cessation is advised for patients undergoing surgery and provides both peri- and postoperative benefits. For patients undergoing general anesthesia for surgery, cessation is advised to decrease sputum production (Thawley & Panje, 1987) and increase the oxygen-carrying capacity of the blood by decreasing carboxyhemoglobin levels (USHHS, 1983). Smokers also have a higher rate of general complications postsurgery. Nicotine and carbon monoxide cause vasoconstriction, which can compromise capillary blood flow. Smoking a single cigarette can produce skin vasoconstriction for up to 90 minutes (Smith & Fenske, 1996); persons who smoke at least 1 pack per day experience significant tissue hypoxia for up to 15 to 20 hours per day (Jensen, Goodsen, Hopf, & Hunt, 1991). Consequently, smoking increases the risk of wound infection (Hussey, Hynan, & Leeper, 2001) and is detrimental to wound healing (for a full review, see Smith & Fenske, 1996).

Other evidence related to poor wound healing and surgical complications is reported in studies involving reconstructive procedures for breast cancer. The impact of smoking on treatment for breast cancer is significant. Procedures such as the pedicled transverse rectus abdominis myocutaneous (TRAM) flap for breast reconstruction have been found to involve a higher risk of complications for smokers. Therefore, the free TRAM flap for breast construction, which maximizes blood flow, is recommended for smokers (Chang et al., 2000). However, even with this procedure, smokers have a higher rate of complications, including TRAM flap necrosis, abdominal flap necrosis, and hernia (Chang et al., 2000). Further, the overall complication rate following TRAM flap surgery is significantly higher among smokers (39.4%) when compared with ex-smokers (25.0%) and nonsmokers (25.9%; Padubidri et al., 2001).

Stopping smoking, even shortly before surgery, reduces complication rates. When comparing smokers and former smokers, donor site complications were significantly reduced in the latter group (25.6% among smokers versus 10.0% among former smokers; Chang et al. 2000). Another way to reduce wound complications among smokers is to delay reconstruction. Delay allows for skin flap vascularity to increase and also provides patients with an opportunity to quit smoking. In the TRAM flap reconstruction study, smokers who underwent immediate reconstruction had a significantly higher incidence of mastectomy skin flap necrosis (21.7%) than smokers who underwent delayed reconstruction (0%; Chang et al., 2000). Patients with a smoking history of greater than 10 pack-years (1 pack-year is equivalent to smoking one pack of cigarettes per day for a year) were especially at high risk for perioperative complications. Evidence was so striking that researchers urged other clinicians to consider this as a relative contraindication for free TRAM flap breast reconstruction (Chang et al., 2000).

This in-depth discussion of breast reconstruction is included because surveys suggest that women are significantly more concerned about breast cancer than lung cancer (American Legacy Foundation, 2001) despite the fact that since 1987 lung cancer mortality has substantially surpassed breast cancer mortality in American women (Parker, Tong, Bolden, & Wingo, 1996). Smokers may be unaware that quitting smoking has a positive impact on breast cancer treatment, thus providing a "teachable moment" for cessation. Smokers can benefit greatly from cessation for multiple reasons, including the potential adverse impact on the primary treatments for breast cancer and breast reconstruction as well as the later risk for second primary tumors and poorer overall health status.

RADIATION THERAPY

Smoking also impacts treatment with radiation: Studies conducted with head and neck cancer patients show decreased treatment response for smokers. For example, patients who continued to smoke during radiation treatment had a significantly lower rate of a complete response to radiation therapy (45% versus 74%; Browman et al., 1993).

In addition to decreased treatment effectiveness, cancer patients who continue to smoke during treatment also experience more severe treatment side effects. Oral mucositis, loss of taste, and xerostomia are all exacerbated by smoking. Among patients with advanced head and neck cancer receiving radiation therapy, those who continue to smoke suffer mucositis for an extended time (Rugg, Saunders, & Dische, 1990). This is in comparison to patients who quit at the time of radiation therapy and remain abstinent or those who remain abstinent for at least a month after treatment. Studies indicate that extended mucositis may be associated with a permanent alteration in appearance (Rugg et al., 1990) in addition to the pain and discomfort associated with mucositis.

Lung cancer patients who smoke have an increased risk for clinical radiation pneumonitis (Monson et al., 1998). Long-term complications exacerbated by smoking have also been found, including soft tissue and bone necrosis (Million & Cassisi, 1984) and the inability to regain satisfactory voice quality following radiation for laryngeal carcinoma (Karim, Snow, Siek, & Njo, 1983).

Radiation treatment for Hodgkins disease has been linked to the development of second primary tumors, with an increased risk for smokers (Travis et al., 2002; van Leeuwen et al., 1995). A dose–response relationship has been reported, with patients who smoked more than 10 pack-years after diagnosis having a six-fold increase for lung cancer compared to patients who smoked less than 1 pack-year. Although smoking after diagnosis (around the time of radiation treatment) has a significant impact, smoking prior to diagnosis and treatment is not significantly related to the development of lung cancer (van Leeuwen et al., 1995).

CHEMOTHERAPY

Chemotherapy produces numerous side effects, including immune suppression, weight loss, fatigue, pulmonary toxicity, and cardiac toxicity. Smoking may be especially detrimental in these cases. Immune suppression may be the result of an underlying malignancy or of antineoplastic therapy, especially when this includes corticosteroids, cytotoxic chemotherapy, or irradiation (De Vita, Hellman, & Rosenberg, 1989). In healthy individuals, smoking has been associated with a decrease in the number of circulating natural killer cells and an increase in the number of chromosomal abnormalities in circulating lymphocytes (Tollerud et al., 1989).

Smoking may increase weight loss by speeding up the metabolism, decreasing appetite, serving as a substitute for eating, and increasing satiety by delaying gastric emptying (Gritz, Klesges, & Meyers, 1989; Klesges, Meyers, Winders, & French, 1989). Individuals who quit smoking often experience increased appetite and weight gain (Gritz et al., 1989). These outcomes are frequently cited as barriers to smoking cessation; however, in cancer patients, these outcomes may actually be beneficial (Flegal, Troiano, Pamuk, Kuczmarski, & Campbell, 1995; Gritz, 1991). In a study designed to identify variables associated with cancer-related cachexia among a sample of lung cancer patients, multivariate analysis indicated that current smoking, older age, and female gender were significant predictors of weight loss after controlling for the stage of disease (Brown, 1993). Given that death may be accelerated by malnutrition and cachexia (De Vita et al., 1989), the impact of smoking on weight is important.

Fatigue, induced by both the physiological mechanisms of cancer and its therapy, is among the most common complaints of cancer patients

(Simon & Zittoun, 1999). Cigarette smoking is also associated with increased fatigue. The mechanism underlying smoking-induced fatigue is believed to be increased carbon monoxide levels, displacing oxygen-binding sites on hemoglobin, resulting in a decrease in the blood's ability to deliver oxygen to tissue throughout the body (Glantz & Parmley, 1995). Disease and treatment induced anemia might combine with decreased oxygen availability due to smoking to contribute to fatigue.

Pulmonary and cardiac toxicity are known side effects of numerous, commonly used antineoplastic agents, including bleomycin, busulfan, carmustine, cyclophosphamide, and doxorubicin (U.S. FDA, 2001). Cancer patients receiving such agents who also smoke experience more cardiopulmonary toxicities than nonsmokers (Brockstein, Smiley, Al-Sadir, & Williams, 2000; Nysom, Holm, Hertz, & Hesse, 1998). Smokers also experience more postoperative pulmonary complications (McCulloch, Jensen, Girod, Tsue, & Weymuller, 1997).

In addition to chemotherapy, smoking can also reduce the effectiveness of many other medications used with cancer patients such as beta-blockers, bronchodilators, analgesics, benzodiazepines, and phenothiazines (Lippman, 1985). Smoking increases the hepatic metabolism, which may decrease the effectiveness of many drugs by reducing the therapeutic level of the drug (Dresler & Gritz, 2001).

In summary, smoking decreases treatment effectiveness and increases treatment complications and side effects. Quitting smoking after a cancer diagnosis is beneficial to the treatment process and offers a window of opportunity to improve both short- and long-term health. As detection and treatment for cancer occur earlier in the disease process, the opportunity to offer cessation interventions will increase as well.

## Increased Risk of Second Malignancy due to Smoking

The risk for the development of a second malignancy, at both the same and other sites, is increased in smokers (Johnson, 1998). In studies involving survivors of small cell lung cancer (primarily stage I and II), the risk of a second cancer is 3.5- to 4.4-fold above the general population (Richardson et al., 1993; Tucker et al., 1997). For those who stopped smoking at the time of diagnosis, the relative risk (RR) of a second lung cancer was 11.0 (CI, 4.4 to 23.0); for those who continued to smoke, the RR was 32 (CI, 12.0 to 69.0). One study did not find a significant increase in second primary tumors in patients with nonsmall cell lung cancer who were current or former smokers, compared to those who have never smoked (Lippman et al., 2001). Tucker et al. (1997) found an interaction between chest irradiation and smoking ($RR = 21.0$) and alkylating agents and smoking ($RR = 19.0$). Patients with oral and pharyngeal cancers who smoke also have an exceptionally high rate of second primary cancers because of field carcinogenesis (Lippman & Spitz, 2001). Among long-term heavy smokers (2 packs or more per day for 20+ years), the risk of a second cancer increased with continued smoking almost 5 times (odds ratio $= 4.7$, $CI = 1.4–16.0$) for all aerodigestive cancers (Day et al., 1994). In another smoking-related site, bladder cancer, patients who smoke are also at risk for the development of second primary cancers (Fleshner et al., 1999).

Stopping smoking, even at the time of diagnosis, can have a significant impact on decreasing secondary cancers (Tucker et al., 1997). Kawahara et al. (1998) reported that patients with small cell lung cancer who survive at least 2 years greatly reduce their likelihood of a second cancer if they quit smoking.

## Decreased Survival Rates

Smoking has an adverse effect upon survival. This finding has been documented in terms of the prognostic impact of smoking history on survival, the timing of smoking cessation relative to diagnosis and treatment, and the impact of continuing to smoke.

Cigarette smoking pack-years is an independent prognostic factor for overall survival in patients with a stage I nonsmall cell lung cancer (Fujisawa et al., 1999). The number of nonmalignant and malignant causes of death is significantly greater in patients with primary resected stage I nonsmall cell lung cancer with 30 or more pack-years of cigarette smoking (compared with less than 30 pack-years). An 83.0% overall survival at 10 years is reported for patients with less than 30 pack-years, compared to 36.7% for those with more than 30 pack-years. It should be noted, however, that resuming cigarette smoking following surgery is not related to cause of death, but smoking before surgery greatly influences long-term survival (Fujisawa et al., 1999). Lippman et al. (2001) also report a higher mortality rate among stage I and II nonsmall cell lung cancer patients who were current or former smokers, compared to those who had never smoked.

Among former smokers, mortality from head and neck cancer has been shown to be influenced by the length of time between quitting and treatment, with a risk reduction of 40% for patients who quit less than 12 weeks before diagnosis and 70% for patients who quit more than 1 year before diagnosis (Browman et al., 1993).

A study of small cell lung cancer patients reports that those who stopped smoking prior to diagnosis (on average 2.5 years) had prolonged survival compared to those who continued to smoke (Johnston-Early et al., 1980). Poorer survival rates have also been found for patients with prostate cancer (Bako, Dewar, Hanson, & Hill, 1982) and cervical cancer (Kucera, Enzelberger, Eppel, & Weghaupt, 1987) who continue to smoke. A greater 5-year, tumor-specific mortality rate among continuing smokers with prostate stage D2 disease (88% versus 63%) or nonstage A disease (39% versus 17%) has also been cited (Daniell, 1995).

Continued smoking after diagnosis also has a pronounced effect on survival rates for patients with head and neck cancer (Stevens, Gardner, Parkin, & Johnson, 1983). Those who stop smoking have double the chance of survival, irrespective of the extent of disease at diagnosis. After 2 years, the survival of quitters approaches that of those who have never smoked.

## SMOKING AND QUALITY OF LIFE

### Background

Although numerous definitions of quality of life can be found in the literature, most include the concept of an individual's subjective perception of health status (Leplege & Hunt, 1997). Quality of life is a multidimensional concept that typically incorporates the influence of physical, psychological, and social health on individuals' subjective perception of health or well-being (Cella et al., 1993). These constructs are influenced not only by cancer and cancer treatment, but also by numerous personal characteristics (e.g., past experiences) and environmental characteristics (e.g., socioeconomic status; Testa & Simonson, 1996).

Quality of life can be conceptualized as existing on a proximal–distal continuum, with disease onset and symptom status representing the proximal variables and overall quality of life representing a distal variable. Personal and environmental characteristics exert influence throughout this continuum, further altering quality of life (Brenner, Curbow, & Legro, 1995; Wilson & Cleary, 1995). This model, modified to illustrate the influence of smoking on quality of life in cancer patients (see Figure 4.1), suggests that interventions directed at the level of personal characteristics (e.g.,

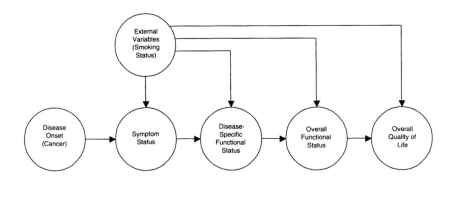

**FIGURE 4.1**   **Theoretical framework for the relationship between quality of life and smoking in cancer patients**

smoking cessation) may not only alter the disease process, but may also improve a patient's quality of life.

## Relationship Between Smoking and Quality of Life in the General Population

Perhaps because the causal relationship between smoking and numerous diseases (e.g., cancer, heart disease, and chronic obstructive pulmonary disease) has been overwhelmingly established and the decrease in quality of life brought about from disease is equally well-established, relatively few studies have sought to directly link smoking with quality of life. Less common are efforts to demonstrate improvements in quality of life due to smoking cessation and to demonstrate how these improvements may change with increasing the time since cessation. The first step in exploring the relationship between smoking and quality of life in cancer patients is to consider the relationship between these two variables among representative population samples. Investigators indirectly examined the relationship between smoking and quality of life by examining the relationship between smoking and disability (Nusselder, Looman, Marang-van de Mheen, van de Mheen, & Mackenbach, 2000). Nusselder et al. (2000) examined the relationship between smoking and disability among large cohorts in the Netherlands and the U.S. The findings, based on an analysis of longitudinal data, indicated that smoking was not only associated with a shorter life, but was also associated with more disability and a greater number of years lived with disability. In addition, episodes of disability among nonsmokers were compressed into shorter periods of time. A lower incidence of disability and shorter periods of disability among nonsmokers were associated with a higher quality of life.

Several other researchers have more directly assessed the relationship between smoking and quality of life in general populations. The measure most often utilized in these investigations is the Medical Outcomes Survey 36-Item Short Form (SF-36; Ware & Sherbourne, 1992). This well-validated and extensively used instrument measures quality of life on eight subscales: physical functioning, role limitations due to physical problems, role limitations due to emotional problems, vitality, mental health, social functioning, bodily pain, and general health, as well as two summary measures—the physical component summary and the mental component summary (Ware & Sherbourne, 1992). The associations identified in these studies are, for the most part, quite consistent: Nonsmokers report higher levels of quality of life than do smokers.

In a recent study of smoking status and quality of life in a large, representative sample, significant differences were observed between current smokers, ex-smokers, and those who had never smoked. The latter group reported the highest, ex-smokers reported lower, and current smokers reported the lowest quality of life. Perhaps most compelling, the authors also observed a significant dose–response relationship among current smokers between the number of cigarettes smoked per day and quality of life, with quality of life being inversely related to the level of cigarette consumption (Wilson, Parsons, & Wakefield, 1999).

Similar findings were observed among a representative population sample from the Netherlands. Current smokers reported significantly poorer quality of life as compared to ex-smokers; however, the quality of life of ex-smokers and those who had never smoked did not differ significantly. A dose–response relationship was also observed, with heavy smokers reporting the lowest quality of life. The authors did not observe a significant association between the time since smoking cessation and the quality of life (Mulder, Tijhuis, Smit, & Kromhaut, 2001).

Data collected in the Nurses' Health Study also provided evidence of a dose–response relationship between smoking and quality of life (Michael, Colditz, Coakley, & Kawachi, 1999). Women in the highest smoking intensity category (25 or more cigarettes per day) consistently reported the lowest levels of physical functioning, the most bodily pain, and the lowest vitality. This association was even more prominent among women aged 65 years or older.

A pair of similarly designed yet somewhat more limited cross-sectional surveys yielded similar results. Researchers compared the quality of life of current smokers and ex-smokers (individuals who had been abstinent for at least 5 years) among subjects randomly selected from several general practice clinics. The results indicated that ex-smokers had a higher quality of life than did the current smokers (Tillmann & Silcock, 1997). In the second survey, smoking and quality of life status between ever-smokers (individuals who had ever smoked for a period of at least 6 months) and never smokers were compared. The study sample was systematically selected from persons in the Family Health Service Authority. Never smokers had a significantly higher quality of life on four of the eight SF-36 subscales (general health, physical functioning, bodily pain, and vitality), but no significant differences were found between the groups on the remaining four subscales (role limitations due to physical problems, role limitations due to emotional problems, social functioning, and mental health; Lyons, Lo, & Littlepage, 1994).

Canadian researchers examining quality of life in a representative sample of older adults found similar results (Hirdes & Maxwell, 1994). Although quality of life was not assessed by a commonly used and previously validated scale, common domains (i.e., physical functioning, psychological functioning, and social functioning) were measured. The findings indicated that current smokers (defined as daily smokers) reported a significantly poorer quality of life than did participants who had never smoked. Also of note, while the quality of life of ex-smokers who had been abstinent *for 10 years or less* did not differ significantly from that of current smokers, the quality of life of ex-smokers who had been abstinent *for more than 10 years* was equivalent to the quality of life of those who had never smoked (Hirdes & Maxwell, 1994). These findings demonstrate that the potential increases in quality of life obtainable through smoking cessation might not be appreciable in the first several years after cessation.

Further analyses indicated that the effects of smoking cessation on quality of life were not necessarily the same for men and women. Among men, current smokers reported significantly poorer mobility and higher levels of stress than ex-smokers. Among women, current smokers reported lower levels of happiness and more dissatisfaction with social relationships (Maxwell & Hirdes, 1993).

Because these studies of the relationship between smoking and quality of life in the general population utilized a cross-sectional design, certain limitations are inherent. As the temporal relationship is unknown, it is not possible to directly attribute changes in quality of life to smoking status. For example, these findings do not address the question of whether stopping smoking leads to a higher quality of life or whether individuals with a higher quality of life are less likely to smoke. Moreover, among participants categorized as ex-smokers, the reasons for quitting are unknown. Some ex-smokers may have quit smoking in response to the onset of a smoking-related disease. Such occurrences could reduce the strength of the indicated association between smoking status and quality of life or could even result in findings indicating that recent smoking cessation may temporarily worsen certain life-quality outcomes (Halpern & Warner, 1994). Several comorbid behaviors are associated with smoking, including increased alcohol consumption, lack of physical exercise, and poor diet. These factors may also contribute to lower quality of life. Finally, the lack of uniform measurement of quality of life and the variation in smoking-status definitions make direct comparisons across these studies somewhat difficult. Despite these limitations, the implications suggested by these studies are quite clear:

- Nonsmokers have a higher quality of life than do current smokers.
- Ex-smokers have a higher quality of life than do current smokers.
- As smoking intensity (the number of cigarettes smoked per day) increases, quality of life decreases.

## Relationship Between Smoking and Quality of Life in Patients With Chronic Disease

Additional evidence for the association between smoking and one's quality of life comes from studies involving patients with chronic disease. Few studies in patients with chronic disease have examined the relationship between smoking status and quality of life, but the findings of these studies are generally in agreement with those of the general population cross-sectional surveys, indicating that smoking is adversely associated with quality of life.

In a study examining quality of life and the need for hospital-based care in a cohort of asthma patients, researchers found that smoking cigarettes and exposure to environmental tobacco smoke were associated with lower quality of life (Sippel, Pedula, Vollmer, Buist, & Osborne, 1999). Exposure to tobacco smoke (both direct and environmental exposure) remained a significant and independent predictor of quality of life after a statistical adjustment for possible confounders (e.g., age, gender, asthma severity, and income). In addition, baseline exposure to tobacco smoke was an independent predictor of subsequent hospital-care utilization.

In prospective studies considering quality of life as a result, the same relationship between smoking and quality of life status has been observed. Among a group of patients with coronary heart disease, the baseline smoking status was an independent predictor of quality of life 5 years later (Denollet, Vaes, & Brutsaert, 2000). In another study of patients with coronary heart disease, current smokers undergoing percutaneous coronary revascularization (PTCA) reported a lower quality of life at 6 months and 1 year after the procedure, while ex-smokers (defined as individuals who had abstained from smoking for at least 1 year prior to PTCA) reported life-quality levels similar to those who had never smoked (Taira et al., 2000). An association between smoking and life-quality status was also observed among patients undergoing limb salvage surgery for osteomyelitis (Siegel, Patzakis, Holtom, Sherman, & Sheperd, 2000). In this study, at a mean follow-up time of 5 years, smoking status was a significant predictor of quality of life, with current smokers reporting poorer functional status and more pain than did ex-smokers and those who had never smoked.

## Relationship Between Smoking and Quality of Life in Cancer Patients

Few published studies of the relationship between smoking status and quality of life in cancer patients exist. However, indirect evidence on this relationship can be gleaned by studying potential links between smoking and conditions that commonly affect quality of life in cancer patients.

Clearly, cancer and cancer treatment (e.g., surgery, chemotherapy, and/or radiation therapy) can adversely affect quality of life and not only the more generic dimensions of life quality (physical, psychological, and social functioning), but also cancer-related quality of life constructs. Although many of these cancer-related constructs are specific to the site of the disease (e.g., swallowing and speaking difficulties among patients with head and neck cancer, sexual dysfunction among patients with prostate cancer, or hot flashes among patients with breast cancer), others are experienced more universally. Among the quality of life constructs most commonly affected by cancer are pain, anorexia/cachexia, and fatigue (Aaronson et al., 1993). Presently, no studies have directly investigated whether an association exists between smoking and these cancer-specific constructs, but evidence shows such an association may exist.

Pain, frequently reported among cancer patients, is associated with decreased physical, psychological, and social functioning, as well as diminished global quality of life (Owen, Klapow, & Casebeer, 2000). Nicotine is known to exert analgesic effects; thus, cigarettes may theoretically represent a form of self-medication helping to ameliorate pain symptoms experienced by cancer patients (Decker & Meyer, 1999; Picciotto, Caldarone, King, & Zachariou, 2000). As discussed earlier, researchers have observed a significant association between smoking and mucositis, a common and painful side effect of cancer treatment. An intervention that helps to minimize mucositis (e.g., smoking cessation) may also improve one's quality of life (McCarthy, Awde, Ghandi, Vincent, & Kocha, 1998). Future research is needed to fully explore the association between smoking and pain among cancer patients.

In addition to the evidence that smoking may be associated with pain, cachexia, and fatigue in cancer patients, evidence shows that smoking may be associated with increased cardiopulmonary toxicity in cancer patients. The measurement of quality of life has not yet been incorporated into the design of studies assessing the association between smoking and cardiopulmonary toxicity, but it appears probable that these toxicities would adversely affect both functional status and the physical dimension of overall life quality. Future research efforts should thoroughly explore this possible association.

Despite the evidence suggesting an association between smoking and quality of life among cancer patients, only one published study to date has examined this subject. In that study, Gritz, Carmack, et al. (1999) prospectively investigated the results in patients with head and neck cancer, all of whom at baseline were current smokers or had stopped smoking within the prior 12 months. The results of this analysis indicated that study participants who were ex-smokers by the 1-year follow-up reported a higher quality of life than patients who had not stopped smoking. Although only a single study, the findings are in agreement with those of the other patient populations. Future studies of cancer treatment that include quality of life measurements should routinely assess smoking status and determine its effect on both treatment outcome and quality of life.

## SMOKING INTERVENTION STUDIES AMONG CANCER PATIENTS: TRANSLATING RESEARCH INTO PRACTICE

### Quitting Following Diagnosis

The interest and motivation for quitting smoking are greatly increased following cancer diagnosis. Disease site, disease stage, treatment, education, age, readiness to change, and past smoking history have all been identified as predictors of cessation postdiagnosis (Gritz, 1991; Gritz et al., 1993; Ostroff et al., 1995). The disease site has been identified as the strongest predictor of quitting (Ostroff et al., 1995), with higher quit rates reported for cancers strongly related to smoking such as head and neck (Gritz et al., 1993) and lung cancer (Gritz, Nisembaum, et al., 1991). In a population of stage I nonsmall cell lung cancer patients, 83.2% of smokers made a quit attempt in the first year following surgery, with 53% achieving continuous abstinence at the end of the first year (Gritz, Nisembaum, et al., 1991).

In contrast, studies of patients with cancers less strongly associated with smoking typically find moderate to high quit rates, but lower continuous abstinence rates (e.g., 31% among bladder cancer patients; Ostroff et al., 2000). Reasons for the lower sustained cessation may include a lack of awareness of the link between certain types of cancer (e.g., bladder) and smoking, minimization of the risk of continued smoking due to higher cure rates, shorter and fewer hospitalizations (where smoking is not permitted), and less interference with smoking due to the disease or treatment (Ostroff et al., 2000).

Despite the high quit rates among patients with smoking-related cancers, some head and neck cancer patients continue to smoke or relapse following initial quit attempts. However, among these smokers, many are interested in quitting and make multiple attempts to do so. One study found that among smokers who continued to smoke postsurgery, 92% reported an interest in quitting, 84% made at least one quit attempt, and 69% had made multiple quit attempts (Ostroff et al., 1995).

This increased interest in quitting can be used as a window of opportunity to intervene and provide assistance in the quitting process. However, despite the established benefits derived from smoking cessation and the increased interest in quitting among cancer patients, very few cessation interventions among cancer patients have been completed.

## Current Interventions

An extensive literature search yielded only five studies specifically examining cessation interventions for cancer patients. The most scientifically rigorous of these studies involved a randomized trial of a surgeon-/dentist-delivered intervention for 186 patients newly diagnosed with the first primary squamous cell carcinoma of the upper aerodigestive tract (Gritz, Carmack, et al., 1991; Gritz et al., 1993; Gritz et al., 1994). In this study, all patients received personalized risk factor information and strong personalized advice from their surgeon or maxillofacial prosthodontist to quit smoking. Although the intervention group's quit rates were not significantly increased by the addition of booster sessions, specially tailored booklets, reminder postcards, and contracts, the high quit rates for all participants (64.6% continuous abstinence at the 12-month follow-up) suggests that brief advice given in the context of medical care is a powerful tool. The authors suggested that a "stepped care" approach may be most useful with medical practitioners incorporating advice to quit smoking into usual care and, for those patients who have difficulty quitting, more intensive treatment, including adjunctive pharmacological treatment.

Four smaller studies examined nurse-delivered interventions for cancer patients. A small pilot study with 26 surgical oncology patients examined the effect of a nurse-delivered structured intervention (Stanislaw & Wewers, 1994). The intervention consisted of three in-hospital visits, an ACS stop smoking booklet, and an American Lung Association audiotape, followed by five phone calls postdischarge. At follow-up, 75% of those who received the intervention were abstinent, compared to 43% of the usual-care control participants. Although this difference only approached statistical significance due to the small sample size, the results suggests that hospital-based cessation interventions may play an important role. A similar study by Wewers, Bowen, Stanislaw, and Desimone (1994) used the same intervention for 80 smokers and found slightly lower abstinence rates: 64.3% for the intervention group compared to 50.0% for the usual-care group at the 5- to 6-week follow-up.

Another nurse-delivered intervention pilot study examined cessation in lung cancer patients (Wewers, Jenkins, & Mignery, 1997). Using the same intervention as Stanislaw and Wewers (1994), the cessation rate at the 6-

week follow-up was 40%. In this study, however, no control group was used, so the effectiveness of the intervention could not be tested.

A nurse-delivered minimal cessation intervention consisting of only one in-hospital visit, an ACS stop smoking guide, and five post-discharge calls for hospitalized cancer patients reported lower rates of abstinence (Griebel, Wewers, & Baker, 1998). In this study, only 21% of the intervention group and 14% of the usual-care group were abstinent at the 6-week follow-up. The authors concluded that a more intensive intervention might be needed.

The four nurse-delivered interventions illustrate the need for larger, more rigorous studies. The small sample sizes decreased the power to find significant differences and evaluate the effectiveness of the intervention. Although the intervention used in these studies was very similar, the cessation rates varied greatly. This difference may have been due to variations in the samples used. For example, the highest abstinence rates (75%) were found by Stanislaw and Wewers (1994), with a sample that consisted of 80% head and neck cancer patients. Griebel et al. (1998) found much lower abstinence rates (21%); however, only 7% of their sample were head and neck cancer patients. Cancer site has been established as a significant predictor of cessation (e.g., Ostroff et al., 1995) and may account for the differences in the abstinence rates in these studies.

In a review of health behavior change following cancer diagnosis, Pinto, Eakin, and Maruyama (2000) noted the need for more rigorous studies, which include larger, more racially diverse samples that better represent the larger population of smokers with cancer. They further suggested the need for data on the timing of interventions as well as longer follow-up periods. The nurse-delivered intervention studies used a 5- to 6-week follow-up period compared to the 1-year follow-up in the Gritz et al. (1993) study, which is the standard follow-up period for smoking cessation interventions. Twelve-month or longer follow-up periods are needed to examine the true impact of cessation interventions.

Relapse rates for those who quit following treatment and for those who quit prior to treatment are in need of further exploration. No participant who was an ex-smoker at baseline relapsed in the Gritz et al. (1993) head and neck trial during the 12-month follow-up, perhaps due to the standardized intervention in both conditions. The natural course of relapse has been reported in a study examining relapse rates and patterns in resected stage I nonsmall cell lung cancer patients (Gritz, Schacherer, et al., 1991): 43.4% of current smokers at baseline exhibited multiple periods of smoking and abstinence, suggesting that smoking status fluctuates greatly. However, rates appeared to stabilize at 47.0% continuous abstinence and 59.6% point-prevalence abstinence by the 2-year follow-up point. Patterns of relapse also varied based on the time of cessation, with more recent quitters exhibiting more instability in their smoking status. Gritz (1991; Gritz et al., 1993) recommended the inclusion of recent ex-smokers in observational and intervention trials due to the high risk of relapse. Careful attention is clearly needed in the definition and inclusion of patients based on their smoking status (e.g., ex-smoker or nonsmoker).

Because the total number of studies on smoking cessation in cancer patients is still small, recommendations for this group must be based on the evidence from smoking cessation studies conducted in the general population and other patient groups. Recognizing the complexity of tobacco use is a necessary first step in developing effective cessation interventions and successful prevention trials. The biobehavioral model of nicotine addiction and tobacco-related cancers (NCI, 1998) presents the complex interplay of social, psychological, and biological factors that influence tobacco use and addiction (see Figure 4.2). These very factors in turn mediate dependence, cessation, and relapse in every individual. Treatment, therefore, has been developed to address many of the factors noted in this model.

The Agency for Healthcare Research and Quality (AHRQ) has produced a clinical practice guideline containing a series of recommendations to assist all healthcare providers in delivering treatment to combat tobacco

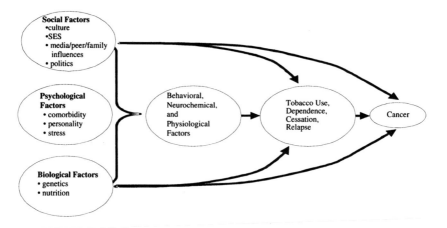

**FIGURE 4.2    Biobehavioral model of nicotine addiction and tobacco-related cancers**

use and dependence based on the systematic review and analysis of scientific literature. The guidelines (cited in Fiore et al., 2000) note:

- Tobacco dependence is a chronic condition that often requires repeated interventions. However, effective treatments exist that can produce long-term or even permanent abstinence.
- Because effective tobacco treatments are available, every patient who uses tobacco should be offered treatment.
- Brief tobacco dependence treatment is effective, and every patient who uses tobacco should be offered at least brief treatment.
- There is a strong dose–response relation between the intensity of tobacco dependence counseling and its effectiveness. (pp. 3–4)

The diagnosis of cancer provides a teachable moment during which healthcare providers can offer patients as well as their family members cessation treatment. During this period, patients are highly motivated for recovery and the prevention of further disease. Therefore, a brief cessation message can effectively change smoking behavior (Gritz et al., 1993). Brief physician advice to quit smoking has been shown to be an effective intervention, even when the advice is as minimal as 3 minutes (Fiore et al., 2000).

The AHRQ guideline outlines a five-step approach in promoting cessation. Healthcare providers should: (a) systematically identify all tobacco users, (b) strongly urge all tobacco users to quit, (c) determine willingness to make a quit attempt, (d) aid patients in quitting, and (e) schedule follow-up contact. These steps have been termed the five A's: Ask, Advise, Assess, Assist, and Arrange (see Table 4.1). Due to the chronic relapsing nature of tobacco dependence, healthcare providers should provide patients with brief relapse prevention treatment. Relapse prevention reinforces the patient's decision to quit, reviews the benefits of quitting, and assists the patient in resolving any problems arising from quitting (Fiore et al., 2000). The outlined strategy has been termed the five R's (refer to Table 4.1): Relevance, Risks, Rewards, Roadblocks, and Repetition.

Providers should be familiar with other behavioral aspects of smoking cessation treatment, particularly because all individuals are not equally motivated to quit. A feasible and highly effective model for behaviorally based counseling is the Transtheoretical Model (TTM) of change. This model classifies smoking behavior as a function of five stages of change: (a) precontemplation, (b) contemplation, (c) preparation, (d) action, and

**TABLE 4.1    The Five A's and Five R's for Brief Smoking Intervention**

| | | |
|---|---|---|
| Five A's | Ask about tobacco use | Identify and document tobacco use status for every patient at every visit. |
| | Advise to quit | Urge every tobacco user to quit in a clear, strong, and personalized manner. |
| | Assess willingness to make a quit attempt | Assess whether or not the tobacco user is willing to make a quit attempt at this time. |
| | Assist in quit attempt | Use counseling and/or pharmacotherapy with the patient willing to make a quit attempt to help him or her quit. |
| | Arrange follow-up | Schedule follow-up contact, preferably within the first week after the quit date. |
| Five R's | Relevance | Encourage the patient to indicate why quitting is personally relevant, being as specific as possible. |
| | Risk | Ask the patient to identify the potential negative consequences of tobacco use, including acute risks (e.g., short breath), long-term risks (e.g., cancer), and environmental risks (e.g., cancer among family). |
| | Rewards | Request that the patient identify potential benefits of stopping tobacco use (e.g., improved health, improved sense of smell, money saved, reduced effects on skin). |
| | Roadblocks | Ask the patient to identify barriers or impediments to quitting and note the elements of treatment that could address such barriers (e.g., withdrawal symptoms, fear of failure, lack of support). |
| | Repetition | Repeat the motivational intervention every time an unmotivated patient visits the clinic setting. |

(Adapted from Fiore et al. 2000)

(e) maintenance. These stages reflect the individual's current smoking behavior and readiness to stop smoking. This type of strategy has practical applications for healthcare providers to offer appropriate intervention strategies, tailored to each individual (see Table 4.2).

## TABLE 4.2    Stages of Change

| Stage | Defining characteristics | Applicable strategies |
|---|---|---|
| Precontemplation | Not considering quitting in the next 6 months | • Promote recognition of problem.<br>• Inform and discuss effects on disease state.<br>• Emphasize benefits of stopping smoking. Use empathic listening and understanding techniques. |
| Contemplation | Considering quitting in the next 6 months | • Discuss pros and cons of smoking and why it is important to quit smoking<br>• Use persuasive messages.<br>• Emphasize that patient must make the choice to quit.<br>• Provide support and acknowledge difficulty of the decision.<br>• Commend the patient who considers quitting.<br>• Help identify or enlist significant others to provide encouragement and support.<br>• Increase awareness of pharmacological methods to assist quitting. |
| Preparation | Ready to quit in the next month; has made at least one 24-hour quit attempt in the past year | • Commend patient's readiness to quit.<br>• Help set goals.<br>• Discuss a plan of action and methods of cessation.<br>• Reinforce availability of pharmacological methods to assist quitting.<br>• Inquire about support.<br>• Set a quit date. |

*(continued)*

**TABLE 4.2    Stages of Change** *(continued)*

| Stage | Defining characteristics | Applicable strategies |
|---|---|---|
| Action | Taking steps toward cessation; quit date and cessation plan implemented | • Solicit a commitment to quit for good.<br>• Discuss and provide specific skills for quitting.<br>• Continue support by praising efforts.<br>• Help the patient recognize and avoid situations that might trigger a relapse.<br>• Enlist the help of family and friends.<br>• Reinforce small successes. |
| Maintenance | Has not smoked for at least 6 months | • Continue supportive role.<br>• Provide reinforcement.<br>• Remind patient to be wary of cues to relapse.<br>• Explain that maintenance is a continuous process of learning new ways to cope.<br>• Reinforce importance of continued support from family and friends. |

By assessing the stage of change status over time, providers are able to match strategies to patients' needs, assisting in movement through the stages. Using the TTM, the outcome is reconceptualized as movement through the stages as opposed to a dichotomous goal of nonsmoker versus smoker. With this more realistic goal, more successful experiences occur as the patient moves from precontemplation to contemplation and eventually to action (Prokhorov, Hudmon, & Gritz, 1997). The physician can monitor patient progress, reinforcing change, which decreases the self-perceived pressure to criticize patients who have not yet achieved successful abstinence.

When assisting patients to quit smoking, physicians should be aware of the many types of effective treatment currently available. Research has shown that three types of counseling are especially effective and should be used with all patients attempting to quit smoking: practical counseling (problem solving/skills training), social support as part of treatment, and social support outside of treatment. In addition, numerous effective phar-macotherapies (see Table 4.3) for smoking cessation are available (Fiore et al., 2000), including both nicotine replacement therapy (nicotine patch,

**TABLE 4.3   Recommended FDA Approved First-line Pharmacotherapies**

| Pharmacotherapy | Daily dosage | Side effects | Contraindications/recommendations |
|---|---|---|---|
| Bupropion Hydrochloride Wellbutrin® Zyban | 150 mg/day for 3 days and then increase to 300 mg/day for 7 to 12 weeks | Insomnia, dry mouth | Contraindicated in individuals with a history of seizure disorder. Not to be taken with Wellbutrin® and Wellbutrin® SR. Higher incidence of seizures in patients treated for bulimia and anorexia. |
| Nicotine Polacrilex (Gum) Nicorette® Gum | 18 to 24 mg/day | Mouth soreness, jaw ache | Maximum of 24 pieces/day. Tailor dosage and duration to patient need. |
| Nicotine Inhaler Nicotrol Inhaler® | 6 to 16 cartridges/day (each cartridge delivers 4 mg of nicotine over 80 inhalations) | Local irritation of mouth and throat | Duration of therapy up to 6 months (taper dosage during final 3 months). |
| Nicotine Nasal Spray Nicotrol NS® | Minimum 8 doses/day, maximum 40 doses/day (Dose = 0.5 mg each nostril) | Nasal irritation | Duration of therapy 3 to 6 months. |
| Nicotine Patch Nicoderm CQ®; Nicotrol; generic varieties | 7 to 21 mg/day | Local skin irritation | Treatment of 8 weeks or less has been efficacious. |

Note: Adapted from AHRQ 2000.

gum, inhaler, and spray) and bupropion SR (Zyban®), which have been shown to significantly increase cessation rates by reducing nicotine withdrawal symptoms.

## Special Tailoring of Cessation Advice for Cancer Patients

Many factors influence the choice and delivery of smoking cessation interventions, such as whether or not interventions should be targeted or modified to the population under study. Although insufficient research adequately addresses this question, available research findings can be used to select from the array of available cessation treatments.

Although the limited research on cancer patients suggests that many of the factors that influence cessation are similar to those seen in the general population (e.g., the importance of the readiness to quit, education, and age), unique cancer-related concerns should be taken into account when delivering cessation advice to cancer patients. Cancer patients are highly motivated to quit smoking and—based on the finding that cancer site is related to cessation (Gritz, 1991; Ostroff et al., 1995)—the more aware patients become of the connection between their diagnosis and their smoking status, the greater the likelihood of quitting smoking. Healthcare professionals can educate patients regarding the connection between cancer and smoking, emphasizing that quitting has benefits with all cancer types.

Tailoring behavioral and pharmacological treatment for a cancer patient population involves careful assessment. The techniques and activities recommended to promote cessation or prevent a relapse among disease-free populations may need to be modified and adapted for use with cancer patients. For example, particular attention must be placed on the physical limitations brought about by disease and treatment. In this instance, suggestions regarding exercise regimens and dietary change would need to be modified among cancer patients (see Gritz et al., 1993; Gritz et al., 1994).

The primary cancer site can be an important determinant in selecting the appropriate pharmacological treatment. The wide range of nicotine replacement therapies currently available (patch, gum, spray, or inhaler) as well as the nicotine-free alternative (Zyban®) provides an array of treatment options. Patients may have medical contraindications to a specific type of nicotine replacement. For example, the nicotine patch may be the most appropriate alternative for patients with oral cancers who are unable to use oral forms of nicotine replacement such as the gum, spray, or inhaler. Cancer patients have reported similar withdrawal symptoms to the general population with relapsers reporting greater levels of anxiety and craving during withdrawal than nonrelapsers (Gritz, Schacherer, et al., 1999). Given the proven efficacy of pharmacological treatment for smoking cessation and the extensive alternatives available, efforts should be made to offer all patients pharmacological treatment for smoking cessation.

Psychological issues such as guilt, depression, anxiety, and stress must also be considered (Gritz, 1991). Care should be taken to avoid blaming patients for their illness, which has the potential to increase depression and decrease motivation for behavioral change, as well as to decrease social support. Instead, patients should be empowered with the knowledge that they can exert personal control and play a role in their recovery. Providers can also enlist the support of families and friends of the patient, thus increasing extra treatment support. It is recommended that providers work with the patient's family and friends to help them understand the psychological issues involved in cancer treatment and recovery (Gritz, 2000). This includes teaching positive support (e.g., reinforcement and coping skill assistance) and discouraging negative types of support (e.g., nagging or criticism).

Relapse after quitting is also an important concern. Smoking status fluctuates greatly following diagnosis and treatment (Gritz, Nisenbaum, et al., 1991). Although a relapse in healthy populations occurs mostly within the first week following cessation, the majority of head and neck cancer patients in the Gritz, Schacherer, et al. (1999) intervention study relapsed 1 to 6 months postsurgery. Although more research is needed to understand this delay, it is likely that patient motivation to remain abstinent may decrease over time following diagnosis and treatment. As patients return to their prediagnosis lifestyle, the importance of, and support for, cessation may decrease. However, physicians can use the delay in relapse as an opportunity for relapse prevention. Physicians should assess smoking status and motivation to remain abstinent at *all* follow-up visits, and provide appropriate support and interventions.

Combining the latest advances in the treatment of nicotine dependence and behavioral therapy, a randomized clinical trial is investigating a state-of-the-art smoking cessation intervention among completely resected stage I and II nonsmall cell lung cancer survivors who are current smokers (Gritz et al., 2002). This multicenter study separately compares in men and women the effect of adding an antidepressant (bupropion-Zyban) versus a placebo to a behavioral intervention that includes a nicotine replacement. The specially targeted written materials (AHRQ-based tip sheets, etc.) and behavioral advice are delivered by healthcare providers, including physicians and nurses. This trial will provide much needed data describing the relationships among treatment groups, smoking cessation, gender-related information, and emotional functioning. It also will explore standard clinical outcome measures (e.g., second malignancies and survival). Symptom improvement and quality of life will be measured using a symptom distress scale and a psychosocial questionnaire, which includes measures of anxiety, depression, and perceived stress. Additionally, researchers have developed a genetic substudy that explores the relationship of genetic indicators of susceptibility to nicotine dependence with smoking, treatment outcome, gender, and pharmacologic agents. Genetic indicators of nicotine susceptibility may provide a window of opportunity for smoking prevention and cessation interventions in the future.

## DIRECTIONS FOR THE FUTURE

As research in cancer prevention, early detection, and treatment advances, further opportunities to study and intervene upon smoking behavior will arise. Examples are provided by research in chemoprevention, computed tomographic (CT) scanning for early stage lung cancer, and genetic biomarker testing for lung cancer risk (Ostroff, Buckshee, Mancuso, Yankelevitz, & Henschke, 2001). Research in chemoprevention to prevent second primary tumors and prolong survival holds great promise but is not without complexity (Hong et al., 1990; Lippman, Lee, & Sabichi, 1998). For example, in a study examining the efficacy of isotretinoin to prevent second primary tumors in stage I nonsmall cell lung cancer, Lippman et al. (2001) reported that isotretinoin was harmful for current smokers and beneficial for those who had never smoked. Another trial by Khuri et al. (2001) examined the efficacy of low-dose 13-cis-retinoic acid in the prevention of second primary tumors in patients with stage I or II squamous cell carcinoma of the larynx, oral cavity, or pharynx. Preliminary data show significantly higher rates of second primary tumors in current smokers compared to those who have never smoked. Future analyses at study completion will examine the impact of smoking status on the efficacy of chemoprevention.

Recent advances in genetic testing and low-dose helical computed tomographic (low-dose CT) scans have increased the interest in the screening and early detection of lung cancer for those at an elevated cancer risk. These advances also provide an opportunity for cessation interventions. However, concerns exist that if individuals are not found to be at an elevated risk or to have premalignant tissue changes, they may be less likely to quit smoking. Ostroff et al. (2001) examined this possibility in a sample of smokers following CT scans. Results suggest that the majority of smokers (74%) were motivated to quit smoking following the CT scan, with 23% quitting smoking and 27% decreasing the amount they smoked.

Genetic biomarker testing for cancer risk also offers an opportunity to reach smokers concerned about cancer risk. Interest in receiving this information has been reported (Ostroff et al., 1999) and initial research suggests that smokers report heightened risk and fear, as well as increased perceived benefits from quitting (Lerman, Gold, Audrain, & Lin, 1997). However, for the intended cessation to occur, smoking cessation counseling may be necessary (Audrain et al., 1997).

## CONCLUSIONS

Additional research is sorely needed on smoking cessation in cancer patient populations, both for smoking-related and nonsmoking-related tumors. The diagnosis of cancer is an underutilized teachable moment for cessation among patients, family, and significant others. Program dissemination of existing interventions, which is effective in healthy populations, is rarely undertaken in cancer-treatment centers that are focused on diagnosis, treatment, and rapid discharge.

Research must explore targeting interventions to specific cancer sites and tailoring them to the patient's readiness to quit, physical limitations, and psychological status. Potential differences exist among cancer sites and between smoking-related and nonsmoking-related tumors. New opportunities for targeting are developing all the time, such as among persons with elevated risk and susceptibility to a given type of cancer, to nicotine dependence, and to other comorbid conditions (e.g., substance use and depression). An assessment of quality of life should be included in cancer patient smoking cessation trials to evaluate potential changes in life quality following intervention, and to counter concerns that intervention is taking away one of the few remaining pleasures left to the patient. Future studies must introduce standardized assessment tools and sound methodology well established in the smoking cessation literature on healthy populations. The inclusion of follow-up periods of an adequate length (e.g., at least 1 year) is important to assess the duration of the effect.

A great need exists to educate providers regarding the appropriateness of intervention and the importance of prioritizing cessation along with other treatment adjuvants. Interventions delivered to patients with nonsmoking-related cancers, for whom the need for intervention appears less obvious, must be increased. Facilitating the rationale for smoking cessation intervention—the knowledge base of medical, psychosocial, and general health benefits—along with providing theoretically grounded and effective interventions and assisting clinicians in their tasks, will greatly enhance this field of research and practice.

## REFERENCES

Aaronson, N. K., Ahmedzai, S., Bergman, B., Bullinger, M., Cull, A., Duez, N. J., et al. (1993). The European Organization for Research and Treatment of Cancer QLQ-C30: A quality-of-life instrument for use in international clinical trials in oncology. *Journal of the National Cancer Institute, 85*, 365–376.

American Legacy Foundation. (2001). *Women and lung cancer survey.* Washington, D.C.: American Legacy Foundation.

Audrain, J., Boyd, N. R., Roth, J., Main, D., Caporaso, N. E., & Lerman, C. (1997). Genetic susceptibility testing in smoking-cessation treatment: One year outcomes of a randomized trial. *Addictive Behaviors, 22*, 741–751.

Bako, G., Dewar, R., Hanson, J., & Hill, G. (1982). Factors influencing the survival of patients with cancer of the prostate. *Journal of the Canadian Medical Association, 127*, 727–729.

Brenner, M. H., Curbow, B., & Legro, M. W. (1995). The proximal-distal continuum of multiple health outcome measures: The case of cataract surgery. *Medical Care, 33*(Suppl. 4), 236–244.

Brockstein, B. E., Smiley, C., Al-Sadir, J., & Williams, S. F. (2000). Cardiac and pulmonary toxicity in patients undergoing high-dose chemotherapy for lymphoma and breast cancer: Prognostic factors. *Bone Marrow Transplant, 25*, 885–894.

Browman, G. P., Wong, G., Hodson, I., Sathya, J., Russell, R., McAlpine, L., et al. (1993). Influence of cigarette smoking on the efficacy of radiation therapy in head and neck cancer. *New England Journal of Medicine, 328*, 159–163.

Brown, J. K. (1993). Gender, age, usual weight, and tobacco use as predictors of weight loss in patients with lung cancer. *Oncology Nursing Forum, 20*, 466–472.

Cella, D. F., Tulsky, D. S., Gray, G., Sarafian, B., Linn, E., Bonomi, A., et al. (1993). The Functional Assessment of Cancer Therapy scale: Development and validation of the general measure. *Journal of Clinical Oncology, 11*, 570–579.

Chang, D. W., Reece, G. P., Wang, B., Robb, G. I., Miller, M. J., Evans, G., et al. (2000). Effect of smoking on complications in patients undergoing free TRAM flap breast reconstruction. *Plastic & Reconstructive Surgery, 105*, 2374–2380.

Daniell, H. (1995). A worse prognosis for smokers with prostate cancer. *Journal of Urology, 154*, 153–157.

Day, G. L., Blot, W. J., Shore, R. E., McLaughlin, J. K., Austin, D. F., Greenberg, R. S., et al. (1994). Second cancers following oral and pharyngeal cancers: Role of tobacco and alcohol. *Journal of the National Cancer Institute, 86*, 131–137.

De Vita, V. T., Jr., Hellman, S., & Rosenberg, S. A. (Eds.). (1989). *Cancer principles and practice of oncology* (3rd ed.). Philadelphia: J. B. Lippincott.

Decker, M. W., & Meyer, M. D. (1999). Therapeutic potential of neuronal nicotinic acetylcholine receptor agonists as novel analgesics. *Biochemical Pharmacology, 58*, 917–923.

Denollet, J., Vaes, J., & Brutsaert, D. L. (2000). Inadequate response to treatment in coronary heart disease: Adverse effects of type D personality and younger age on 5-year prognosis and quality of life. *Circulation, 102*, 630–635.

Dresler, C. M., & Gritz, E. R. (2001). Smoking, smoking cessation and the oncologist. *Lung Cancer, 34*, 315–323.

Fiore, M. C., Bailey, W. C., Cohen, S. J., Dorfman, S. F., Goldstein, M. G., Gritz, E. R., et al. (2000). *Treating tobacco use and dependence. Clinical practice guideline.* Rockville, MD: U.S. Department of Health and Human Services. Public Health Services. Public Health Service.

Flegal, K. M., Troiano, R. P., Pamuk, E. R., Kuczmarski, R. J., & Campbell, S. M. (1995). The influence of smoking cessation on the prevalence of overweight in the United States. *New England Journal of Medicine, 333*, 1165–1170.

Fleshner, N., Garland, J., Moadel, A., Herr, H., Ostroff, J., Trambert, R., et al. (1999). Influence of smoking status on the disease-related outcomes of patients with tobacco-associated superficial transitional cell carcinoma of the bladder. *Cancer, 86*, 2337–2345.

Fujisawa, T., Lizasa, T., Saitoh, Y., Sekine, Y., Motohashi, S., Yasukawa, T., et al. (1999). Smoking before surgery predicts poor long-term survival in patients with stage I non-small-cell lung carcinomas. *Journal of Clinical Oncology, 17*, 2086–2091.

Glantz, S. A., & Parmley, W. W. (1995). Passive smoking and heart disease. mechanisms and risk. *Journal of the American Medical Association, 273*, 1047–1053.

Griebel, B., Wewers, M. E., & Baker, C. A. (1998). The effectiveness of a nurse-managed minimal smoking-cessation intervention among hospitalized patients with cancer. *Oncology Nursing Forum, 25*, 897–902.

Gritz, E. R. (1991). Smoking and smoking cessation in cancer patients. *British Journal of Addiction, 86*, 549–554.

Gritz, E. R. (2000). Facilitating smoking cessation in cancer patients. *Tobacco Control, 9*(Suppl. 1), 50.

Gritz, E. R., Albain, K. S., Sarna, L., Pauler, D., Giarritta, S., Moinpour, C., et al. (2002). *Smoking cessation intervention (including bupropion-zyban versus placebo) for completely resected stage I and stage II non-small cell lung cancer survivors who are currently smokers, phase III* (current clinical trial). Southwest Oncology Group: A National Clinical Research Group.

Gritz, E. R., Carmack, C. L., de Moor, C., Coscarelli, A., Schacherer, C. W., Meyers, E. G., et al. (1999). First year after head and neck cancer: Quality of life. *Journal of Clinical Oncology, 17*, 352–360.

Gritz, E. R., Carr, C. R., Rapkin, D., Abemayor, E., Chang, L. J., Wong, W. K., et al. (1993). Predictors of long-term smoking cessation in head and neck cancer patients. *Cancer Epidemiology, Biomarkers, & Prevention, 2*, 261–270.

Gritz, E. R., Carr, C. R., Rapkin, D. A., Chang, C., Beumer, J., & Ward, P. H. (1994). A physician- and dentist-delivered smoking cessation intervention for head and neck cancer patients. In *Tobacco and the clinician: Interventions for medical and dental practice. Smoking and Tobacco Control Monograph, No. 5*. Rockville, MD: U.S. Department of Health and Human Services, Public Health Services, National Institutes of Health. NIH Publication No. 94-3693.

Gritz, E. R., Carr, C. R., Rapkin, D. A., Chang, C., Beumer, J., & Ward, P. H. (1991). A smoking cessation intervention for head and neck cancer patients: Trial design, patient accrual, and characteristics. *Cancer Epidemiology, Biomarkers, & Prevention, 1*, 67–73.

Gritz, E. R., Klesges, R. C., & Meyers, A. W. (1989). The smoking and body weight relationship: Implications for intervention and post cessation weight control. *Annals of Behavioral Medicine, 11*, 144–153.

Gritz, E. R., Nisenbaum, R., Elashoff, R. E., & Holmes, E. C. (1991). Smoking behavior following diagnosis in patients with stage I non-small cell lung cancer. *Cancer Causes Control, 2*, 105–112.

Gritz, E. R., Schacherer, C., Koehly, L., Nielsen, I.R., & Abemayor, E. (1999, August). Smoking withdrawal and relapse in head and neck cancer patients. *Head & Neck*, pp. 420–427.

Halpern, M. T., & Warner, K. E. (1994). Differences in former smokers' beliefs and health status following smoking cessation. *American Journal of Preventive Medicine, 10*, 31–37.

Hirdes, J. P., & Maxwell, C. J. (1994). Smoking cessation and quality of life outcomes among older adults in the Campbell's Survey on Well-Being. *Canadian Journal of Public Health, 85*, 99–102.

Hong, W. K., Lippman, S. M., Itri, L. M., Karp, D. D., Lee, J. S., Byers, R. M., et al. (1990). Prevention of second primary tumors with isotretinoin in squamous-cell carcinoma of the head and neck. *New England Journal of Medicine, 323*, 795–801.

Hussey, L.C., Hynan, L., & Leeper, B. (2001). Risk factors for sternal wound infection in men versus women. *American Journal of Critical Care, 10*, 112–116.

Jemal, A., Thomas, A., Murray, T., & Thun, M. 2002. Cancer statistics (2002). *CA: A Cancer Journal for Clinicians, 52*, 23–47.

Jensen, J. A., Goodsen, W. H., Hopf, H. W., & Hunt, T. K. (1991). Cigarette smoking decreases tissue oxygen. *Archives of Surgery, 126*, 1131–1134.

Johnson, B. E. (1998). Second lung cancers in patients after treatment for an initial lung cancer. *Journal of the National Cancer Institute, 90*, 1335–1345.

Johnston-Early, A., Cohen, M. H., Minna, J. D., Paxton, L. M., Fossieck, B. E., et al. (1980). Smoking abstinence and small cell lung cancer survival. *Journal of the American Medical Association, 244*, 2175–2179.

Karim, A. B., Snow, G. B., Siek, H. T., & Njo, K. H. (1983). The quality of voice in patients irradiated for laryngeal carcinoma. *Cancer, 51*, 47–49.

Kawahara, M., Ushijima, S., Kamimori, T., Kodama, N., Ogawara, M., Matsui, K., et al. (1998). Second primary tumors in more than 2-year disease-free survivors of small-cell lung cancer in Japan: The role of smoking cessation. *British Journal of Cancer, 78*, 409–412.

Khuri, F. R., Kim, E. S., Lee, J. J., Winn, R. J., Benner, S. E., Lippman, S. M., et al. (2001). The impact of smoking status, disease stage, and index tumor site on second primary tumor incidence and tumor recurrence in the head and neck retinoid chemoprevention trial. *Cancer Epidemiology, Biomarkers, & Prevention, 10*, 823–829.

Klesges, R. C., Meyers, A. W., Winders, S. E., & French, S. N. (1989). Determining the reasons for weight gain following smoking cessation: Current findings, methodological issues, and future directions for research. *Annals of Behavioral Medicine, 11*, 134–143.

Kucera, H., Enzelsberger, H., Eppel, W., & Weghaupt, K. (1987). The influence of nicotine abuse and diabetes mellitus on the results of primary irradiation in the treatment of carcinoma of the cervix. *Cancer, 60*, 1–4.

Leplege, A., & Hunt, S. (1997). The problem of quality of life in medicine. *Journal of the American Medical Association, 278*, 47–50.

Lerman, C., Gold, K., Audrain, J., & Lin T. H. (1997). Incorporating biomarkers of exposure and genetic susceptibility into smoking cessation treatment: Effects on smoking-related cognitions, emotions, and behavior change. *Health Psychology, 16*, 87–99.

Lippman, A. G. (1985). How smoking interferes with drug therapy. *Modern Medicine, 8*, 141–142.

Lippman, S. M., Lee, J. J., Karp, D. D., Vokes, E.E., Benner, S.E., Goodman, G. E., et al. (2001). Randomized phase III intergroup trial of Isotretinoin to prevent second primary tumors in stage I non-small-cell lung cancer. *Journal of the National Cancer Institute, 93*, 605–618.

Lippman, S. M., Lee, J. J., & Sabichi, A. L. (1998). Cancer chemoprevention: Progress and promise. *Journal of the National Cancer Institute, 90*, 1514–1528.

Lippman, S. M., & Spitz, M. R. (2001). Lung cancer chemoprevention: An integrated approach. *Journal of Clinical Oncology, 19*(Suppl. 90001), 74–82.

Lyons, R. A., Lo, S. V., & Littlepage, B. N. C. (1994). Perception of health amongst ever-smokers and never-smokers: A comparison using the SF-36 health survey questionnaire. *Tobacco Control, 3*, 213–215.

Maxwell, C. J., & Hirdes, J. P. (1993). The prevalence of smoking and implications for quality of life among the community-based elderly. *American Journal of Preventive Medicine, 9*, 338–345.

McCarthy, G. M., Awde, J. D., Ghandi, H., Vincent, M., & Kocha, W. I. (1998). Risk factors associated with mucositis in cancer patients receiving 5-fluorouracil. *Oral Oncology, 34*, 484–490.

McCulloch, T. M., Jensen, N. F., Girod, D. A., Tsue, T. T., & Weymuller, E. A., Jr. (1997). Risk factors for pulmonary complications in the postoperative head and neck surgery patient. *Head and Neck, 19*, 372–377.

Michael, Y. L., Colditz, G. A., Coakley, E., & Kawachi, I. (1999). Health behaviors, social networks, and healthy aging: Cross-sectional evidence from the Nurses' Health Study. *Quality of Life Research, 8*, 711–722.

Million, R. R., & Cassis, N. J. (Eds.). (1984). *Management of head and neck cancer: A multidisciplinary approach*. Philadelphia: J. B. Lippincott.

Monson, J. M., Stark, P., Reilly, J. J., Sugerbaker, D. J., Strauss, G. M., Swanson, S. J., et al. (1998). Clinical radiation pneumonitis and radiographic changes after thoracic radiation therapy for lung carcinoma. *Cancer, 82*, 842–850.

Mulder, I., Tijhuis, M., Smit, H. A., & Kromhout, D. (2001). Smoking cessation and quality of life: The effect of amount of smoking and time since quitting. *Preventive Medicine, 33*, 653–660.

National Cancer Institute. (1998). *Tobacco research implementation plan: Priorities for tobacco research beyond the year 2000.* Bethesda, MD: National Institutes of Health.

Nusselder, W. J., Looman, C. W., Marang-van de Mheen, P. J., van de Mheen, H., & Mackenbach, J. P. (2000). Smoking and the compression of morbidity. *Journal of Epidemiology and Community Health, 54*, 566–574.

Nysom, K., Holm, K., Hertz, H., & Hesse, B. (1998). Risk factors for reduced pulmonary function after malignant lymphoma in childhood. *Medical and Pediatric Oncology, 30*, 240–248.

Ostroff, J., Garland, J., Moadel, A., Fleshner, N., Hay, J., Cramer, L., et al. (2000). Cigarette smoking patterns in patients after treatment of bladder cancer. *Journal of Cancer Education, 15*, 86–90.

Ostroff, J. S., Buckshee, N., Mancuso, C. A., Yankelevitz, D. F., & Henschke, C. I. (2001). Smoking cessation following CT screening for early detection of lung cancer. *Preventive Medicine, 33*, 613–621.

Ostroff, J. S., Hay, J. L., Primavera, L. H., Bivona, P., Cruz, G. D., & LeGeros, R. (1999). Motivating smoking cessation among dental patients: Smokers' interest in biomarker testing for susceptibility to tobacco-related cancers. *Nicotine & Tobacco Research, 1*, 347–355.

Ostroff, J. S., Jacobsen, P. B., Moadel, A. B., Spiro, R. H., Shah, J. P., Strong, E. W., et al. (1995). Prevalence and predictors of continued tobacco use after treatment of patients with head and neck cancer. *Cancer, 75*, 569–576.

Owen, J. E., Klapow, J. C., & Casebeer, L. (2000). Evaluating the relationship between pain presentation and health-related quality of life in outpatients with metastatic or recurrent neoplastic disease. *Quality of Life Research, 9*, 855–863.

Padubidri, A. N., Yetman, R., Browne, E., Lucas, A., Papay, F., Larive, B., et al. (2001). Complications of postmastectomy breast reconstructions in smokers, ex-smokers, and nonsmokers. *Plastic & Reconstructive Surgery, 107*, 342–349.

Parker, S. L., Tong, T., Bolden, S., & Wingo, P. A. (1996). Cancer statistics, 1996. *Cancer Journal for Clinicians, 46*, 5–27.

Picciotto, M. R., Caldarone, B. J., King, S. L., & Zachariou, V. (2000). Nicotinic receptors in the brain: Links between molecular biology and behavior. *Neuropsychopharmacology, 22*, 451–465.

Pinto, B. M., Eakin, E., & Maruyama, N. C. (2000). Health behavior changes after a cancer diagnosis: What do we know and where do we go from here? *Annals of Behavioral Medicine, 22*, 38–52.

Prokhorov, A. V., Hudmon, K. S., & Gritz, E. R. (1997). Promoting smoking cessation among cancer patients: A behavioral model. *Oncology, 11*, 1807–1813.

Richardson, G. E., Tucker, M. A., Venzon, D. J., Linnoila, I., Phelps, R., Phares, J. C., et al. (1993). Smoking cessation after successful treatment of small-cell lung cancer is associated with fewer smoking-related second primary cancers. *Annals of Internal Medicine, 119*, 383–390.

Rugg, T., Saunders, M.I., & Dische, S. (1990). Smoking and mucosal reactions to radiotherapy. *British Journal of Radiology, 63*, 554–556.

Siegel, H. J., Patzakis, M. J., Holtom, P. D., Sherman, R., & Shepherd, L. (2000). Limb salvage for chronic tibial osteomyelitis: An outcomes study. *Journal of Trauma, 48*, 484–489.

Simon, A. M., & Zittoun, R. (1999). Fatigue in cancer patients. *Current Opinions in Oncology, 11*, 244–249.

Sippel, J. M., Pedula, K. L., Vollmer, W. M., Buist, A. S., & Osborne, M. L. (1999). Associations of smoking with hospital-based care and quality of life in patients with obstructive airway disease. *Chest, 115*, 691–696.

Smith, J. B., & Fenske, N. A. (1996). Cutaneous manifestations and consequences of smoking. *Journal of the American Academy of Dermatology, 34*, 717–732.

Stanislaw, A. E., & Wewers, M. E. (1994). A smoking cessation intervention with hospitalized surgical cancer patients: A pilot study. *Cancer Nursing, 17*, 81–86.

Stevens, M. H., Gardner, J. W., Parkin, J. L., & Johnson, L. P. (1983). Head and neck cancer survival and life-style change. *Archives of Otolaryngology, Head and Neck Surgery, 109*, 746–749.

Taira, D. A., Seto, T. B., Ho, K. K., Krumholz, H. M., Cutlip, D. E., Berezin, R., et al. (2000). Impact of smoking on health-related quality of life after percutaneous coronary revascularization. *Circulation, 102*, 1369–1374.

Testa, M. A., & Simonson, D. C. (1996). Assessment of quality-of-life outcomes. *New England Journal of Medicine, 334*, 835–840.

Thawley, S. E., & Panje, W. R. (Eds.). (1987). *Comprehensive management and head and neck tumors.* Philadelphia: W. B. Saunders.

Tillmann, M., & Silcock, J. (1997). A comparison of smokers' and ex-smokers' health-related quality of life. *Journal of Public Health Medicine, 19*, 268–273.

Tollerud, D. J., Clark, J. W., Bronn, L. M., Neuland, C. Y., Mann, D. L., Pankiw-Trost, L. K,. et al. (1989). Association of cigarette smoking with decreased numbers of circulating natural killer cells. *American Review of Respiratory Disease, 139*, 194–198.

Travis, L. B., Gospodarowicz, M., Curtis, R. E., Clarke, E. A., Andersson, M., Glimelius, B., et al. (2002). Lung cancer following chemotherapy and radiotherapy for Hodgkin's disease. *Journal of the National Cancer Institute, 94*, 182–192.

Tucker, M. A., Murray, N., Shaw, E. G., Ettinger, D. S., Mabry, M., Huber, M. H., et al. (1997). Second primary cancers related to smoking and treatment of small-cell lung cancer. *Journal of the National Cancer Institute, 89*, 1782–1788.

U.S. Department of Health and Human Services. (1983). *The health consequences of smoking: Cardiovascular disease: A report of the surgeon general.* Rockville, MD: Public Health Service, Office on Smoking and Health, DHHS Publication No. (PHS) 84-50204.

U.S. Food and Drug Administration. (2001). Drug information. Retrieved June 12, 2001 from www.fda.gov/cder/.

van Leeuwen, F. E., Klokman, W. J., Stovall, M., Hagenbeek, A., van Belt-Dusebout, A., Noyon, W. R., et al. (1995). Roles of radiotherapy and smoking in lung cancer following Hodgkin's disease. *Journal of the National Cancer Institute, 87,* 1530–1537.

Ware, J. E., Jr., & Sherbourne, C. D. (1992). The MOS 36-item short-form health survey (SF-36). I. Conceptual framework and item selection. *Medical Care, 30,* 473–483.

Wewers, M. E., Bowen, J. M., Stanislaw, A. E., & Desimone, V. B. (1994). A nurse-delivered smoking cessation intervention among hospitalized postoperative patients—influence of a smoking-related diagnosis: A pilot study. *Heart & Lung, 32,* 151–156.

Wewers, M. E., Jenkins, L., & Mignery, T. (1997). A nurse-managed smoking cessation intervention during diagnostic testing for lung cancer. *Oncology Nursing Forum, 24,* 1419–1422.

Wilson, D., Parsons, J., & Wakefield, M. (1999). The health-related quality-of-life of never smokers, ex-smokers, and light, moderate, and heavy smokers. *Preventive Medicine, 29,* 139–144.

Wilson, I. B., & Cleary, P. D. (1995). Linking clinical variables with health-related quality of life. A conceptual model of patient outcomes. *Journal of the American Medical Association, 273,* 59–65.

# 5

# Decision Aids for Cancer-Related Behavioral Choices

## Celette Sugg Skinner
## R. Brian Giesler

"Which choice is best?" is a complicated question with an easy answer, if the question is "Should I try or not try to stop smoking?" It is hard to imagine any context in which to not recommend cessation. "Should I have a mammogram?" also has an easy answer if a 55-year-old woman is considering mammography. We would encourage her to be screened. But what if the woman is in her mid-30s and has some family history of breast cancer? Before giving a recommendation, we would need to know more about her family history and other personal risk factors. Even then, the scientific evidence might not be strong enough to recommend a definite course of action. Rather than advocating a particular behavior, we should inform her about current scientific information and help her weigh the competing benefits and risks to make a personal decision. Health interventions with this goal are called *decision aids*.

This chapter discusses the emerging area of cancer-related decision aids. Decision aids are designed to facilitate decisions regarding health behaviors for which no definitive data exist indicating a benefit of one choice versus another. A decision aid is typically intended as an adjunct to usual care and can take multiple forms; it may consist of a printed brochure, videotape, interactive media, a special form of counseling, or some combination of methods. Although decision aids vary greatly in terms of their form and content, the one feature they all share is the provision of information specific to a decision problem (e.g., a decision aid for a Prostate-Specific Antigen [PSA] screening might provide information about the impact of prostate cancer therapies on life expectancy and quality of life). Decision aids may also suggest strategies that enable decision makers to more effectively use information (e.g., ways to organize information or improve communication with healthcare providers about preferred outcomes).

Decision aids can be used to facilitate behavioral decisions that span the cancer continuum, from prevention and early detection to treatment choices and end-of-life issues. Decision aids have been developed and evaluated for helping people choose drug therapies that may affect cancer risks (e.g., hormone replacement therapy [HRT]), genetic testing for cancer susceptibility (e.g., BRCA1/2 testing), cancer-screening modalities with uncertain benefits (e.g., PSA testing, some modalities of colorectal cancer screening, or mammography for young women), and cancer treatment options (e.g., treatment for localized breast cancer).

This chapter will (a) contrast decision aids with traditional behavior-change interventions, both in approach and intended results; (b) discuss the historical background and context of decision aids; (c) describe the theoretical underpinnings of decision aids; (d) summarize the literature and the state of the field of cancer-related decision aids; and (e) briefly outline important areas for future research. Because several excellent reviews and bibliographies have been recently published (Bekker, Thorton, et al., 1999; O'Connor, Drake, et al., 1997; O'Connor, Fiset, et al. 1999; O'Connor, Rostom, et al., 1999), it is neither our intent to review and evaluate all published studies to date nor to comprehensively review the literature regarding patient preferences or decision-making theory. This is, rather, a survey of cancer-related decision aids tested using a controlled trial or an equivalent methodology.

To determine which articles in the literature met these criteria, we used the following search strategy: First, keywords—*decision(s), decision-making, decision aid(s), treatment alternative(s), choice(s), decision support, patient preference(s),* and *decision theory*—were used to retrieve abstracts from MEDLINE®, CANCERLIT®, and PsychINFO. The keywords *cancer, treatment,* and *screening* were also used for the PsychINFO search. This resulted in a large collection of abstracts, which we reviewed for relevance to cancer-related decision-making by patients or potential consumers of health services. References from review articles focusing on the topic areas covered in this chapter (e.g., a PSA screening) were also examined. After retrieving the literature that met the initial criteria, empirical articles evaluating the effectiveness of a cancer-related decision aid using randomized or another type of controlled methodology were retained and incorporated into this chapter. Originally, articles that used healthy surrogate samples were excluded, but due to the relative paucity of articles meeting the previous criteria, these were reintroduced into the review.

## DECISION AIDS VERSUS BEHAVIOR-CHANGE INTERVENTIONS

As shown in Table 5.1, decision aids differ from traditional behavior-change interventions in several ways. Decision aids apply to scenarios in which the situation and scientific evidence are such that no one recommendation can be suggested with certainty. Deliberation is needed, either because outcomes associated with various choices are uncertain or because weighing the risks and benefits involves value judgments (Kassirer, 1994). Rather than indicating and steering people toward one particular decision, decision aids are aimed toward providing accurate information to an individual in order to facilitate selecting from among a set of alternatives. Contrast, for example, a postmenopausal woman's HRT and mammography decisions. Whereas the HRT benefits and risks are complex, competing, and

**TABLE 5.1   Comparison of Behavior-Change Interventions and Decision Aids**

| Behavior-change interventions | Decision aids |
| --- | --- |
| Definite behavioral recommendation based on epidemiologic evidence for | No best recommendation among alternatives due to |
| • Mortality reduction<br>• Morbidity reduction<br>• Quality of life | • Differential effects on quantity versus quality of life<br>• Differential effects for various disease<br>• Unknown effects |
| Intervention recommends specific behavior change | Intervention provides specific information to facilitate individualized decision |
| Behavior change is major outcome variable | Multiple outcome variables used to assess impact of decision aid |

uncertain, the evidence for the mammography's benefit is quite strong (30% mortality reduction with regular repeated use, and minimal risks and quality-of-life issues). Thus, a decision aid intervention would be more appropriate for the former decision scenario than the latter. Behavior-change and decision aid interventions also differ as to how they are evaluated. The success of most behavior-change interventions can be gauged by the degree to which the recommended behavior is enacted. Currently, no consensus exists as to how to evaluate the performance of a decision aid, with most studies using a variety of outcome variables. For example, some investigations focus on the ability of a decision aid to reduce decisional conflict, whereas others emphasize whether behavioral choices or quality-of-life results differ between decision aids and comparison groups. Because of its importance, this issue will be revisited several times over the course of this chapter.

## Historical Background and Context

Much of the impetus behind the development of modern decision aids was provided by the initial research on practice variation (Gramlich & Waitzfelder, 1998). Wennberg et al. (1988) were among the first to document that patients with similar diagnoses often received very different treatment depending on their geographical location. Such variations are especially likely to occur when no clear superior choice exists; this is the scenario for many types of cancer treatment. Without definitive guidelines or standards, physicians' idiosyncratic preferences can become the primary force driving decisions, resulting in treatment choices that may not maximize outcomes.

To remedy this situation, several authors have proposed that patients be informed of the benefits and risks of each treatment under consideration and then actively collaborate with their providers to generate treatment decisions. This strategy should enable patient preferences to inform health-care choices, thereby increasing the likelihood that patients experience the outcomes most important to them. Practically, this model requires altering the patient–physician encounter in a way that facilitates the communication of information and preferences in an efficient manner. Decision aids offer a potential means of achieving this goal.

A related factor driving the development of decision aids, particularly in oncology, is the recent explosion in the number of treatment alternatives offered to patients (Giesler, 2000), depending on the stage, grade, and patient age. Surgery and/or chemo, radiation, hormonal therapy, and other treatments may be used alone or in combination as prophylactic, first-line, adjuvant, neo-adjuvant, or salvage therapies. Because different therapeutic regimens differentially affect quantity and quality of life, it is often impossible to identify a single regimen that will maximize the benefits for all patients. These sorts of trade-offs between quantity and quality of life have implications for decision-making at every point along the cancer care continuum, from screening through palliative care.

The economic realities of modern healthcare also contribute to the need for decision aids (Cramer & Spilker, 1998). To achieve this goal, patient-centered outcomes have been increasingly used to justify policy planning, including which screening procedures and therapies will and will not be covered by third-party payers (Cramer & Spilker, 1998; Hunt, 1998). This process has been facilitated by the growth of patient/consumer movements, which recognize that disease and treatment often have highly individual effects on quality of life and therefore stress incorporating patient preferences for results into treatment decisions (Read, 1993). A concomitant increase has taken place in efforts to develop decision aids that enable the incorporation of patients' preferences and values into clinical practice.

## THEORETICAL UNDERPINNINGS OF DECISION AID CONSTRUCTION

What constitutes a good decision? Researchers and philosophers have yet to achieve consensus on this issue. Although it is beyond this chapter's scope to review the vast literature devoted to defining good versus poor decisions, it is worth noting that most randomized trials involving cancer-related decision aids use one or more of the following outcomes to assess effectiveness: knowledge, decisional conflict, decisional satisfaction, consistency of a decision with patient values and preferences, changes in decision alternatives chosen, and quality of life. Presumably, decision aids that produce positive changes in these outcomes are considered to facilitate good decisions. Two different but complementary theoretical perspectives on decision-making appear to have driven the use of these types of outcome variables (Chapman, Elstein, & Hughes, 1995). Although not always explicitly recognized, these two perspectives have provided the basis for much of the work in this area.

### Subjective Expected Utility (SEU) Perspective

The first perspective emerges from the classical decision-making literature and subjective expected utility (SEU) theory. This approach assumes that a good decision is one that maximizes an individual's expected utility (Feeny & Torrance, 1989; Torrance, 1986). In this context, *utility* refers to the value or desirability an individual perceives a set of outcomes to possess (e.g., the outcomes a person judges as possessing great utility would be said to be highly valued or preferred). For example, a form of chemotherapy accompanied by severe toxicity would be considered to have lower utility compared to a less toxic but equally effective regimen.

When formally using this approach, results likely to occur for each decision option and the probabilities of these results are identified from the literature or clinical practice. Results are presented, usually through written or mixed-media descriptions, and a person's utility for each is then elicited using, for example, standard gambles or rating scales (Kaplan, Feeny, Revicki, 1993). Utility elicitation techniques produce scores ranging from 0 (death) to 1 (perfect health; Feeny & Torrance, 1989; Kaplan et al., 1993). Utility scores thus indicate how patients value outcomes relative to death and perfect health. Consider the following imaginary scenario in which a patient must choose between chemotherapy and radiation:

| Result | Person's utility for results | Probability via chemotherapy | Probability via radiation |
|---|---|---|---|
| Cure with minimal side effects | .95 | 20% | 50% |
| Cure with severe side effects | .80 | 70% | 20% |
| No cure, recurrence in 1 year | .20 | 10% | 30% |

In this scenario, the patient will experience a cure with minimal side effects, a cure with severe side effects, or no cure and recurrence. Chemotherapy is most likely to cause a cure with severe side effects. To determine the subjective expected utility of chemotherapy versus radiation for each treatment type, the probability of each result is weighed by the patient's utility for that result and summated:

SEU (chemotherapy): $(.95) (.20) + (.80) (.70) + (.20) (.10) = .77$
SEU (radiation):     $(.95) (.50) + (.80) (.20) + (.20) (.30) = .70$

Given this person's preferences or utilities, the strict SEU perspective would recommend chemotherapy over radiation.

In actuality, few cancer-related decision aids adhere this closely to the classic SEU paradigm. Many assumptions underlying this approach have not been supported empirically, and measurement issues related to the validity of the utility scores have been raised (Cella, 1996; Cowen et al., 1998; Giesler et al., 1999; Hornberger, Redelmeier, & Petersen, 1992; Mulley, 1989). However, two basic assumptions underlying the SEU approach are pervasive in the decision aid literature: that a best decision alternative exists and that choosing the best alternative will lead to the best possible outcome. In other words, although researchers may disagree about how to identify the best alternative, producers of decision aids usually assume that one exists for a given patient and intend for their decision aid to guide that patient toward his or her optimal choice.

The second assumption underlying this approach, and one echoed in the health services literature, is that people require two types of information to make good decisions: knowledge about the possible outcomes linked to each decision option and their preferences or values for each possible outcome. Most decision aids are explicitly designed to provide the first type of information. Fewer provide methods to obtain the second type of information, usually leaving decision aid users to determine through self-reflection how they value different results. Fewer still provide any explicit mechanism to integrate these two types of information into decision-making, either leaving it to the patient or the patient–physician interaction.

## Social-Cognitive Perspective

The second perspective informing much of the work on decision aids emerges from the cognitive and social psychological literature and emphasizes the processes by which decisions are made, as opposed to identifying the optimal choice. From this perspective, decision aids are intended to accomplish two goals. The first goal is to place decision makers in a frame of mind that will help them make a reasoned decision (i.e., some aids are designed to provide information with the specific purpose of relieving uncertainty and anxiety, which in turn should result in more deeply considered decisions). The second goal is to encourage decision-making that will facilitate the operation of psychosocial processes that promote positive adaptation and coping.

Fostering positive adaptation can be achieved through many routes. For example, reducing decisional conflict and other negative effects should increase confidence in the decision and bolster a sense of control. An increased sense of control, in turn, should foster well-being and facilitate adaptation (e.g., Marks, Richardson, Graham, & Levine, 1986; Taylor, Lichtman, & Wood, 1984). Similarly, a decision aid that improves communication between the patient and physician should increase the likelihood that the patient will contact the physician after treatment for assistance with complications. These are just some of the many ways decision aids can affect outcomes through psychosocial routes. The key point is that, from this perspective, decision aids function not only to identify the best alternative, but they also facilitate the type of decision-making that will promote adaptive responses, regardless of which decision alternative is actually chosen.

## REVIEW OF EVIDENCE REGARDING DECISION AIDS

The studies described in the following sections are those that have evaluated decision aids for cancer-related behavioral decisions. *Cancer-related behavioral decisions* refers to behavioral choices that could affect the risk of either getting cancer or having a recurrence, that could influence the likelihood of detecting cancer, or that involve selecting a treatment from among alternatives. The reviewed studies are grouped by topic area (such as PSA screening), as indicated by the headings in the following sections. Note that many of the studies do not actually assess behavioral choice. Instead, related variables such as a preference for, or intention to perform, a behavior are often used as proxies for an actual choice.

### PSA Testing for Men

PSA screening for men has been the subject of considerable debate during the past decade (Coley, Barry, Fleming, & Mulley, 1997; Potosky, Miller, Albertsen, & Kramer, 1995). Although PSA screening, especially when coupled with digital rectal exams (DRE), can reliably detect prostate cancer, uncertainties regarding the natural history of this disease and the efficacy of treatment have resulted in conflicting standards and guidelines from health agencies (Flood et al., 1996). Studies suggest that more aggressive tumors will have already produced subclinical metastases by the time they are detected, which would also tend to reduce the beneficial effects of local control (Yang et al., 1998). Thus, men who undergo aggressive treatment after a positive screening may be exposing themselves to unnecessary risks, including side effects such as impotence, urinary incontinence, and bowel dysfunction.

Further complicating PSA screening decisions is the lack of evidence demonstrating any form of aggressive therapy as more effective in prolonging life than expectant management (i.e., watchful waiting; Albertsen, Fryback, Storer, Kolon, & Fine, 1995; Gerber et al., 1996). However, it is also probably true that certain subgroups of patients (e.g., those with aggressive tumors who could otherwise expect to live a relatively long life) would benefit from active treatment. Researchers are attempting to identify markers of aggressive versus indolent tumors to enable better decisions regarding screening and treatment. Even if such markers are reliably identified, however, it is unlikely that universally applicable guidelines will result. The decision to undergo screening appears to depend on patients' preferences for different potential results. For some men, the possible benefits of screening (e.g., increased life expectancy) will not outweigh the risks (e.g., decrements to quality of life). For others, the opposite will be true. Uncertainties surrounding the clinical aspects of prostate cancer coupled with variations in patient preferences led to the development of decision aids for PSA screening (reviewed in Table 5.2).

Flood et al. (1996) reported findings from two controlled trials comparing a specifically designed educational videotape against a generic videotape about PSA screening prepared by a pharmaceutical company in one study and against usual care (i.e., no videotape) in the other. The Prostate Program of Research and Treatment (PORT) video, introduced by C. Everett Koop, stresses shared decision-making and the pros and cons of screening, followed by presentations from two physician patients who reached conflicting conclusions about screening. A nonphysician patient who received a positive result but chose to not undergo active treatment explains his regret over having been screened. Men exposed to the intervention videos exhibited more accurate knowledge about prostate cancer, were less inclined to choose active treatment if prostate cancer was detected after screening, and were less likely to want PSA tests in the future. Most tellingly, men exposed to the intervention video were less likely to have a PSA test at the next available opportunity.

In a separate study, Volk, Cass, and Spann (1999) used the PORT video in a randomized controlled trial comparing the video plus a pamphlet to usual care. Patients completed self-report questionnaires prior to and after watching the videotape and then again 2 weeks later, after having taken home a pamphlet that summarized the video. At 2 weeks, the intervention group exhibited more accurate knowledge about prostate cancer and was less willing to undergo a PSA test. The video may have helped

**TABLE 5.2  Decision Aid Studies for PSA Testing**

| | Theoretical/ conceptual framework | Design | Sample | Measures | Results |
|---|---|---|---|---|---|
| Davison, Kirk, Degner, & Hassard (1999) | None reported | Randomized control trial (RCT), pre- and post-test; verbal and written information PSA versus no intervention | $N = 100$ patients presenting at primary care clinic | Preferred role in decision-making, anxiety, decisional conflict, actual use of PSA assessed after intervention | The information group exhibited a greater preference for more active role in decision-making and less decisional conflict; no difference in anxiety or actual use of PSA. |
| Flood et al. (1996) *study 1* | None reported | Quasi-experimental post; prostate PORT video versus Schering video | $N = 372$ patients attending free PSA screening clinic | Knowledge, treatment preference if diagnosed, intention to be tested in 2 years, actual use of PSA test | The PORT video group exhibited greater knowledge, preferred watchful waiting to active treatment, reported less intention to take future test, and were marginally less likely to undergo PSA test. |

| | Theoretical/ conceptual framework | Design | Sample | Measures | Results |
|---|---|---|---|---|---|
| Flood et al. (1996) *study 2* | None reported | Cross-over post; PORT video versus standard care | N = 196 patients with scheduled visit at primary care clinic | Knowledge, treatment preference if diagnosed, intention to be tested in 2 years, actual use of PSA test at next opportunity | The PORT video group exhibited greater knowledge, preferred watchful waiting to active treatment, reported less intention to take future test, and were less likely to undergo PSA test. |
| Schapira, McAuliffe, & Nattinger (2000) | None reported | RCT, prepost; illustrated pamphlet plus RA versus no intervention | N = 257 veterans with at least one outpatient visit during a 5-year period | Knowledge, how well-informed the patient felt, actual use of PSA assessed at 2 weeks | The pamphlet group exhibited greater knowledge and felt more informed; no difference in actual use of PSA. |
| Volk, Cass, & Spann (1999) | None reported | RCT, prepost; videotape and brochure versus standard care | N = 160 patients presenting at family health clinic | Knowledge, preference for PSA testing, assessed at 2 weeks | The videotape group exhibited greater knowledge, less willing to undergo PSA test. |
| Wolf, Nasser, Wolf, & Schorling (1996) | None reported | RCT post; RA-delivered scripted information about PSA versus single sentence | N = 205 patients presenting at primary care practice | Interest in PSA testing | The scripted information group expressed less interest in undergoing PSA test. |

*Note: No theoretical models reported to guide studies are summarized here; models are discussed in chapter text.

participants formulate decisions about screening that were consistent with their preferences.

In another trial, men were randomized to receive either a scripted overview about PSA screening read aloud by a research assistant or a brief statement regarding the availability of a test that can sometimes detect prostate cancer (Wolf, Nasser, Wolf, & Schorling, 1996). The scripted overview (i.e, the decision aid intervention) contained information about the lifetime probability of dying of prostate cancer, the known risk factors, the ability of a PSA test to detect prostate cancer, the probability of a positive result, the positive predictive value of the test, the uncertain effectiveness of active therapies, and the potential complications from active treatment. Participants in the intervention arm reported significantly less interest in having a PSA test, as assessed on a five-point, Likert-type scale.

Davison, Kirk, Degner, and Hassard (1999) reported the findings of a study in which men waiting in a clinic for a scheduled checkup either (a) received written and verbal information about the controversies surrounding screening that encouraged discussing screening issues with their doctor or (b) were asked about general health issues. Dependent measures were completed prior to randomization and then again after the primary care appointment. The intervention group reported a more active role in PSA decision-making and less decisional conflict. No significant differences were found on state anxiety levels or actual screening decisions.

In contrast to previous studies, Schapira, McAuliffe, and Nattinger (2000) used a more basic approach to improving decision-making for PSA screening. During a visit to a large, urban Veterans Affairs medical center, male patients completed the study's dependent measures and were then randomized to receive either (a) an illustrated decision aid pamphlet containing information about prostate cancer epidemiology and symptoms, screening methods and potential benefits, screening test operating characteristics, follow-up tests, and the uncertain efficacy of treatment, or (b) a pamphlet that was similar but did not contain information about the risks and benefits of screening. In both arms, a research assistant was available to answer questions or provide clarification. After 2 weeks, participants returned and again completed the study's dependent measures after which they were asked if they wanted to receive PSA and DRE tests. Men in the decision aid group reported more accurate knowledge about PSA screening, but the two groups did not differ in the percent requesting PSA and DRE screening.

In summary, controlled trials evaluating the effectiveness of decision aids for PSA screening have produced mixed results. Most decision aids appear capable of increasing knowledge about PSA screening, and the study by Davison et al. (1999) suggested that reducing decisional conflict and increasing patient involvement in decision-making could be accomplished relatively easily. However, relative to a comparison group, changes in actual screening behavior have occurred only after exposure to the PORT videotape. Across three studies, men exposed to this videotape were less likely to decide to undergo screening. Perhaps because the video conveys information in a more vivid manner (e.g., it uses a famous spokesperson and shows two physician patients talking about their personal experiences) compared to either pamphlets or scripted information read aloud, it was more likely to change actual screening choices. However, the video also closes with the personal account of a nonphysician patient who regrets having been screened. The lack of a countering viewpoint may be primarily responsible for the video's stronger effects on screening decisions relative to other types of decision aids.

## Other Cancer Screening

Rimer et al. (2000) began a mammography decision aid study in 1995, when there were no clear recommendations for women in their 40s. Women aged 40 to 49 were to discuss mammography with their physicians and decide whether screening was right for them (NCI, 1997). Tailored print materials supplemented by phone counseling resulted in greater knowledge about mammography and breast cancer risk, and more accuracy in perceived breast cancer risk. Although the communications were designed to facilitate decisions rather than to encourage mammography per se, women in the decision aid groups had more mammograms than those assigned to usual care.

Among elderly primary care patients, Wolf and Schorling (2000) compared groups receiving standard information about colorectal cancer screening test procedures with those receiving an informed consent type decision aid about potential risks and benefits. No differences were found in screening-related results, but postintervention those receiving the decision aid were more knowledgeable about the tests' predictive values.

## Cancer Treatment Decisions

Because recent technological advances have increased the number of treatment alternatives available for many types of cancer, patients and their physicians are increasingly faced with having to select among modalities with competing benefits and drawbacks (Giesler, 2000). One of the most common of these treatment decisions is faced by thousands of women each year—those diagnosed with stage I or II breast cancer who must choose between lumpectomy with radiation (often referred to as breast-conserving treatment) or mastectomy. Both approaches are potentially curative and neither confers a clear survival or quality-of-life advantage (Kiebert, de Haes, & van de Velde, 1991), but they differ in some critical respects. Mastectomy requires the removal of far more tissue and changes one's physical appearance. Lumpectomy, although less invasive, is associated with a somewhat higher rate of recurrence and must be paired with radiation therapy (which requires more clinic visits and is associated with side effects [Chapman et al., 1995; Nixon, Troyan, & Harris, 1996]).

In the absence of unequivocal data indicating the superiority of one treatment over another, many authors have recommended that patients' individual preferences drive decision-making (Chapman et al., 1995; Molenaar et al., 2001; Street, Voigt, Geyer, Manning, & Swanson, 1995). However, this approach requires that physicians communicate the full range of possible results and that patients evaluate and communicate which results they most value, with the resulting information integrated into a treatment plan. Decision aids are ideally suited for use in these types of scenarios, in which a complex exchange of information is performed and then used in an appropriate manner to guide treatment decisions. Cancer-related decision aid studies are summarized in Table 5.3.

LOCALIZED BREAST CANCER TREATMENT

Chapman et al. (1995) reported results from a randomized trial among college students and nurses who were asked to imagine that a friend had been diagnosed with localized breast cancer and needed help choosing between breast-sparing surgery with radiation, a mastectomy followed by reconstructive surgery, or a mastectomy followed by use of a breast prosthesis. Participants were randomized to receive a decision aid via eith r a videotape or booklet. A female physician who presented breast cancer information, an overview of treatment alternatives, and an in-depth discussion of the various treatment procedures narrated the 40-minute video. Positive and negative personal accounts from five breast cancer survivors were interspersed through the video. The booklet contained the text version of the video minus the women's personal accounts. Participants in both groups showed significant but equal gains in knowledge about breast cancer and its treatment and were equivalent in terms of how much they would

**TABLE 5.3  Decision Aid Studies for Cancer-Related Behavioral Decisions**

| | Theoretical/ conceptual framework | Design | Sample | Measures | Results |
|---|---|---|---|---|---|
| Chapman, Elstein, & Hughes (1995) | None reported | Choosing treatment for localized breast cancer; RCT pre- and post-test: video versus booklet | $N = 82$ healthy students and nurses | Knowledge; treatment preference assessed after the administration of intervention | No difference in knowledge; difference in treatment preference with video group expressing greater preference for lumpectomy |
| Lerman et al. (1997) | None reported | Choosing whether to receive BRCA1 testing; RCT; (a) education session including presentation, visual aids, and handouts; (b) education in group plus nondirective counseling; or (c) control group | $N = 400$ first-degree relatives of breast or ovarian cancer patients referred by affected relatives | Knowledge and testing; perceived risk of cancer; benefits and risks of testing; genetic testing intention and behavior | Increase in knowledge and testing in both education groups compared to control; decrease in perceived risk in first education group compared to control; no differences in benefits and risks of testing by group; no differences in genetic testing by group |

*(continued)*

155

**TABLE 5.3  Decision Aid Studies for Cancer-Related Behavioral Decisions** (*continued*)

| | Theoretical/ conceptual framework | Design | Sample | Measures | Results |
|---|---|---|---|---|---|
| Llweellyn-Thomas, McGreal, & Thiel (1995) | None reported | Choosing whether to participate in a hypothetical clinical trial; RCT post-test; written and aural information versus interactive, computerized presentation of information | N = 100 mixed-diagnosis cancer patients | Knowledge; satisfaction; decision to participate in trial | No differences in knowledge or satisfaction; computer group more likely to choose to participate |
| Molenaar et al. (2001) | None reported | Choosing treatment for localized breast cancer; quasi-experimental, prepost design; interactive media versus brochure | N = 180 breast cancer patients | Treatment choice; satisfaction; quality of life assessed at 3 and 9 months | No difference in treatment choice; media group reported greater satisfaction and quality of life |

| | Theoretical/ conceptual framework | Design | Sample | Measures | Results |
|---|---|---|---|---|---|
| Rimer et al. (2000) | None reported | Choosing whether to undergo mammography; RCT; (a) usual care, (b) tailored booklets, or (c) tailored booklets plus tailored phone counseling | $N = 1,127$ women in their early 40s and 50s, all members of Blue Cross Blue Shield | Knowledge regarding mammogram; risk perception accuracy; attitudes toward mammogram; decision satisfaction; mammogram use since decision aid | Knowledge greater, risk perception accuracy greater, attitudes toward mammogram, and mammogram use greater among print and phone decision aid group; no difference in decision satisfaction by group |
| Sebban et al. (1995) | None reported | Choosing treatment for chronic myeloid leukemia; RCT post-test; full decision board versus short-form of decision board | $N = 42$ healthy surrogates | Treatment preference; satisfaction assessed after administration of decision board | Marginal difference in treatment preference with full decision board group expressing greater preference for BMT; full board group more satisfied |

*(continued)*

**TABLE 5.3  Decision Aid Studies for Cancer-Related Behavioral Decisions** *(continued)*

|  | Theoretical/ conceptual framework | Design | Sample | Measures | Results |
|---|---|---|---|---|---|
| Sepucha, Belkora, Tripathy, & Esserman (2000) | None reported | Choosing treatment for breast cancer; sequential, controlled, pre- and post-test; consultation recording versus observation | N = 24 breast cancer patients | Decision quality; patient-doctor agreement of decision quality; satisfaction with consultation; consultation time; assessed after consultation | Consultation recording group achieved higher quality, more agreement, and marginally greater satisfaction; no difference in consultation time or number of consults |
| Skinner, Campbell, Rimer, Curry, & Prochaska (1999) | None reported | Choosing whether to receive BRCA1/2 testing; RCT; tailored decision aid or nontailored decision aid | N = 461 test candidates referred by physicians or identified through tumor registry | Knowledge regarding genetics and testing; perceived risk accuracy (of being mutation carrier); anxiety | Greater increase in knowledge regarding genetics and testing in tailored group; greater increase in tailored group of perceived risk accuracy (of being mutation carrier); no difference in anxiety by group |

| | Theoretical/conceptual framework | Design | Sample | Measures | Results |
|---|---|---|---|---|---|
| Street, Voigt, Geyer, Manning, & Swanson (1995) | None reported | Choosing treatment for localized breast cancer; RCT pre- and post-test; interactive media versus brochure | N = 60 breast cancer patients | Knowledge; optimism; patient involvement; treatment choice assessed after third consultation | Marginal difference in knowledge favoring media group; no difference in optimism or patient involvement; nonsignificant trend toward choosing lumpectomy in media group |
| Wolf & Schorling (2000) | None reported | Choosing whether to undergo colorectal cancer screening; RCT; (a) material describing screening, (b) informed-consent-type information giving relative risk, or (c) informed-consent-type information giving absolute risks | N = 399 elderly (65 years and older) primary care patients recruited during office visits | Interest in screening; intent to screen; knowledge regarding predictive value of screening | No differences in interest in screening by group; no differences in intent to screen; both informed consent groups greater than standard information group |

*Note: No theoretical models reported to guide studies are summarized here; models are discussed in chapter text.

recommend the mastectomy treatment options; those in the video group were more likely to recommend breast-sparing surgery.

Street et al. (1995) randomly assigned patients diagnosed with early-stage breast cancer to receive a decision aid in the form of an interactive multimedia program or brochure prior to discussing treatment options with their physicians. The 30- to 45-minute interactive program provided information about breast cancer and treatment options (i.e., lumpectomy with radiation or mastectomy) as well as eight audiovisual clips of women—half of whom had chosen lumpectomy—describing their experiences with breast cancer. During the presentation, women were urged to take an active role in the treatment decision process. The brochure contained the same information about breast cancer and treatment options, as well as provided encouragement to take an active role in treatment decision-making, but the personal accounts from the eight women were replaced by comments from four women describing how they reacted to their breast cancer diagnosis. Dependent measures were completed after intervention and again after physician consultation. Both groups exhibited increased knowledge, although the interactive program group's increase was marginally greater. Neither optimism nor patient involvement in decision-making differed by group. More women using the interactive decision aid chose breast-sparing surgery (76% versus 58%), but the difference was not statistically significant.

A trial conducted by Sepucha, Belkora, Tripathy, and Esserman (2000) took a more direct approach to increasing patient involvement in treatment decision-making. Women were randomized to (a) a decision aid group, in which a facilitator first met with a patient to identify concerns, and then led her and her physician through a structured discussion during the treatment consultation, or (b) a control group in which a researcher observed the consultation but did not otherwise participate. Consultation time did not differ between groups. In the decision aid group, the facilitator led the patient and physician through a five-stage process: deciding how to share decision-making responsibilities, setting an agenda, discussing the agenda, deciding what to do next to enact the agenda, and reviewing a printed summary of the consultation. Dependent measures were completed by patients prior to the first meeting with the facilitator, and before and after the treatment consultation. Although both groups reported improved scores on a measure of decision quality, a construct similar to decisional conflict, the decision aid group's improvement was significantly greater. The decision aid group also reported higher satisfaction with the consultation (although this was marginally significant), and there was greater concordance between patient and physician perceptions of the patient's decisional conflict.

Molenaar et al. (2001) conducted a prospective trial involving patients diagnosed with early-stage breast cancer who were choosing between having a lumpectomy with radiation or mastectomy. Women received either standard care (i.e., oral information and brochures) or an interactive CD-ROM decision aid during an outpatient visit after their initial physician consultation. The decision aid provided multimedia information concerning the pros and cons of each procedure presented by physicians and survivors. Using submenus, patients could choose whichever topics were of interest. Dependent measures were administered after the initial consultation and again at 3 and 9 months after hospital discharge. Equivalent numbers of patients in the decision aid and usual-care groups chose lumpectomy (75% versus 68%, respectively). At 3 and 9 months, decision aid patients reported greater satisfaction with the treatment choice and information received. At 9 months, the CD-ROM group also reported higher satisfaction with the decision-making process and communication with physicians. The decision aid group also reported better general health at 3 months and higher generic and disease-specific quality of life at 9 months.

The four studies summarized previously suggest that multimedia decision aids are more effective than written text methods in helping women make treatment decisions for breast cancer. All four studies demonstrated generally positive effects for multimedia decision aids across a diverse set of outcomes, including increased knowledge, greater satisfaction, lower decisional conflict, understanding differences in the chosen treatment, and higher quality of life. However, the inconsistent nature of these effects across studies (e.g., one aid increased knowledge whereas another did not) combined with the use of different types of samples and outcome variables precludes the drawing of specific conclusions about which aspects of multimedia aids might be most important. Of note, the trial conducted by Molenaar et al. (2001) is one of the few studies to demonstrate that a decision aid can improve quality of life despite there being no differences in the type of treatment chosen.

TREATMENT FOR LEUKEMIA

Sebban et al. (1995) reported the results of a trial to validate a decision aid for patients with early-stage chronic myeloid leukemia who must choose between bone marrow transplantation and chemotherapy. Healthy volunteers were asked to imagine they were patients who had to choose one of the treatments and received information via a full-length or shortened decision aid. In the former group, an interviewer described the decision problem, each type of treatment, and then four scenarios that could occur at different points in time following each treatment. After delivering morbidity and mortality information and their associated probabilities for each scenario, the interviewer placed a card summarizing the information on a decision board. In the decision aid group, two general scenarios were presented that contained primarily mortality probabilities at several points in time for each treatment. Dependent measures were administered after completing the decision aid. Participants in the full decision aid condition reported a marginally greater preference for chemotherapy and significantly greater satisfaction with their treatment choice. In both scenarios, when the interviewer altered the morbidity and mortality probabilities, participants tended to switch treatment choices in a manner logically consistent with the changing probabilities.

HORMONE REPLACEMENT THERAPY (HRT)

The use of HRT, postmenopause, can have competing benefits and risks, some of which are cancer related. In recent years, the HRT decision has become even more complicated (for a review, see Kenemans, van Unnik, Mijatovic, & van der Mooren, 2001). Strong scientific evidence shows that HRT reduces the climacteric symptoms associated with menopause and lowers the risk of osteoporosis, but it reduces mammographic sensitivity (Mandelson, Oestreicher, Porter, Taplin, & White, 2000; Rutter, Mandelson, Laya, & Taplin, 2001). Although a plethora of studies have been conducted, definitive information about the magnitude of disease risks and preventive effects associated with HRT is lacking. Some studies have suggested—but the evidence is weak or inconclusive—that long-term HRT use may lower the risk for heart disease and colon cancer, and delay the onset of Alzheimer's disease. However, HRT use may increase the risk for breast cancer (especially among lean women) and endometrial cancer (Kenemans et al., 2001; Writing Group, 2002). See Table 5.4 for a summary of HRT-related decision studies.

As if HRT decisions were not difficult enough, a great variation exists in information dissemination in light of the current state of scientific knowledge. For example, studies have shown that women are much more aware of HRT's potential to increase breast cancer risk than of its potential preventive effects for other diseases, including colon cancer. In light of these facts, guidelines suggesting that *all* postmenopausal women be counseled

**Table 5.4  Studies on HRT Decisions**

| | Theoretical/ conceptual framework | Design | Sample | Measures | Results |
|---|---|---|---|---|---|
| Holmes-Rovner et al. (1999) | None reported | RCT; (a) brochure, (b) lecture/ discussion, or (c) active decision support | $N = 248$ perimenopausal community volunteers aged 40 to 65 | Consistency between decision and expected utility of HRT; change in likelihood to take HRT pre- to post-intervention | Less decision consistency in brochure group than other two groups; no difference in decision to take HRT. |
| McBride et al. (2002) | None reported | RCT; tailored print decision aid material or no decision aid | $N = 581$ women aged 45 to 54 recruited from community sample by phone | Accuracy of perceived breast cancer risk; confidence to understand HRT risks and benefits; decision satisfaction | Decision aid group had greater accuracy, were more satisfied with decision, and had more confidence. |

*(continued)*

**Table 5.4  Studies on HRT Decisions (continued)**

| | Theoretical/ conceptual framework | Design | Sample | Measures | Results |
|---|---|---|---|---|---|
| Murray et al. (2001) | None reported | RCT; interactive multimedia program with booklet and printed summary or usual care | $N = 205$ women making HRT decisions, recruited from 26 general practices | Decisional conflict; perception of who made decision; treatment preference; anxiety; health services use | Decisional conflict was lower in decision aid group; physicians perceived more decisions by patients in decision aid group; no differences in treatment preference; no differences in anxiety; no differences in health services use. |
| O'Conner et al. (1998a) | None reported | One group pre- and post-test; audiotape and illustrated decision aid booklet with risk and benefit information and values clarification | $N = 94$ women at least 2 years post-menopausal, aged 50 to 60 from 6 family practices | Knowledge regarding HRT risks and benefits; decisional conflict | Improvement in all measures pre to post. |

| | Theoretical/ conceptual framework | Design | Sample | Measures | Results |
|---|---|---|---|---|---|
| O'Conner et al. (1998b) | None reported | RCT; (a) audiotape and illustrated decision aid booklet with risk and benefit information and values clarification or (b) general educational pamphlet developed by American College of Physicians | $N = 165$ women aged 50 to 69 not taking HRT and at least 1 year since last menses; recruited through health professionals, a variety of media, and a research assistant contact | Decisional conflict; personal expectations of HRT risks and benefits; general knowledge of risks, benefits, and side effects | Significant differences between groups for decisional conflict and expectations; no differences in knowledge; no differences in choice made. |
| O'Conner, Rostom, et al. (1999) | None reported | RCT; decision aid on options, risks, and benefits followed by graphic weigh scale exercise regarding risks, benefits, and summary of main risks and benefits | $N = 201$ women aged 50 to 69 who never used HRT | Perceived clarity of values; congruence between personal values and HRT choice | No differences by group for perceived clarity of values or congruence between personal values and HRT choice. |

(continued)

**Table 5.4  Studies on HRT Decisions** (*continued*)

| | Theoretical/ conceptual framework | Design | Sample | Measures | Results |
|---|---|---|---|---|---|
| Rothert et al. (1997) | None reported | RCT; (a) written information, (b) guided discussions, or (c) personalized decision exercise | $N = 379$ women aged 40 to 65, recruited from Midwestern community through print and media | Information/knowl edge of meno- pause; decisional conflicts; satisfac- tion with decision; behavior (exercise, calcium intake, HRT use) | All groups improved in knowledge with improvement greatest for the personalized decision exercise; all groups decreased deci- sional conflicts with no differences by group; no differences in satisfaction with decision; no differences in behavior. |

*Note: No theoretical models reported to guide studies are summarized here; models are discussed in chapter text.

about HRT constitute a daunting challenge for healthcare professionals who are not trained to present complex and imprecise risk information or elicit and weigh women's personal preferences.

Rothert et al. (1997) and Holmes-Rovner et al. (1999) published a pair of reports from a randomized trial to evaluate three intensities of a decision aid: (a) brochure, (b) lecture/discussion in a group format over three 90-minute sessions, or (c) a modified version of intervention B supplemented by activities to facilitate understanding and assess personal risks and values. The 1997 paper reported results from 379 participants; postdecision aid results were positive across the groups, with all three showing significant and sustained improvements in knowledge, decisional conflict, satisfaction with the healthcare provider, and self-efficacy. The differences among the groups were significant only for knowledge, which had the greatest increase among those in the personalized decision exercise group and least among those receiving only written information. Similarly, the 1999 report indicated that all three decision aid formats reduced uncertainty; none affected the likelihood to take HRT. However, the decisions of women in the brochure decision aid group were less congruent with individuals' expected utility of treatment than the decisions by members of the other two groups.

O'Connor et al. (1998a) developed a take-home decision aid comprised of a 32-page booklet, a 40-minute audiotape, and a personalized worksheet. The decision aid was distributed to 94 perimenopausal women from six family practice groups. From pre- to postintervention, women showed significant improvement in knowledge of HRT benefits, risks, and side effects and in decisional conflict (i.e., they felt more certain, informed, clear about their values, and supported in their HRT decision). In phase two of the study, O'Connor's team compared groups randomly assigned to receive the decision aid (an illustrated booklet, an audiotape, and a worksheet) or a general HRT education pamphlet. At follow-up, primary results (decisional conflict and personal expectations of HRT benefits and risks) were significantly more favorable among the decision aid recipients, but neither general HRT knowledge nor HRT choice differed by group. In a third report, O'Connor, Rostom, et al. (1999) assessed another variation on their HRT decision aid. In this study, all women received the booklet and audiotape. However, one group's audiotape ended with a guided values clarification weigh scale exercise, whereas the other group's audiotape simply summarized HRT's main risks and benefits. No significant differences between the groups were observed in the perceived clarity of values or congruence of values and HRT choice.

A group of British researchers conducted a randomized controlled trial among primary care patients making HRT decisions (Murray et al., 2001). One group used an interactive multimedia decision aid accompanied by a booklet and a printed summary; the others received usual care (no intervention). Decisional conflict was significantly lower in the decision aid group at 3 and 9 months postintervention, and physicians perceived that more HRT decisions were made "mainly or only" by the patients in the decision aid group. However, no differences between the groups took place in decisions on whether to use HRT, the anxiety levels, or the use of health services.

McBride et al. (2002) extended the technology of computer-tailored print materials (Skinner, Campbell, Rimer, Curry, & Prochaska, 1999) to decision aids by comparing, among a community sample of women, the effects of a tailored HRT decision aid versus no intervention. At both 1 and 9 months postintervention, the tailored decision aid group exhibited greater breast cancer risk accuracy and more confidence to understand HRT's risks and benefits. At the first follow-up only, the decision aid group was also more satisfied with HRT decisions.

## Genetic Testing

Genetic testing for cancer susceptibility is a relatively new phenomenon (Miki et al., 1994; Wells et al., 1994; Wells & Skinner 1998; Wooster et al., 1995). The benefits and risks associated with testing decisions involve medical, social, legal, and psychological factors, and are usually relevant not only to individuals considering testing, but also to their family members. Summaries of studies related to genetic testing are included in Table 5.3.

Due to differences in gene penetrance and the effectiveness of prophylactic measures, some susceptibility tests are more informative and lead to more straightforward choices than others. Testing for multiple endocrine neoplasia (MEN) is perhaps the most straightforward; physicians can tell individuals with identified mutations that they will certainly develop thyroid cancer, and if they undergo thyroidectomy, the cancer will be prevented (Skinner, DeBenedetti, Moley, Norton, & Wells, 1996; Skinner & Wells, 1997). This is very different from scenarios associated with breast, ovarian, or colon cancer susceptibility testing. For example, women with BRCA1 and BRCA2 mutations have an increased breast cancer risk of 33% to 50% by age 50 (Easton, Ford, & Bishop, 1995; Struewing et al., 1997). By age 70, a mutation carrier's risk of developing breast cancer is 56% to 87% (Ford, Easton, & Peto, 1995; Struewing et al., 1997) and her ovarian cancer risk is 28% to 44% (Ford, Easton, Bishop, Narod, & Goldgar, 1994). These are fairly wide risk ranges that leave even known mutation carriers wondering whether or when they will develop primary breast or ovarian cancer, or if a previous cancer will recur. To add to the uncertainty, whether or how much carriers' inherited breast and ovarian risk can be lowered through surgery, chemoprevention, or behavioral changes is unclear (Burke et al., 1997; Hartmann et al., 1999; Rebbeck et al., 1999; Schrag, Kuntz, Garber, & Weeks, 1997; Turner, Glazer, and Haffty, 1999). For most cancer-related genetic testing in the near future, there is no clear best choice.

Prior to the availability of BRCA1 testing, Lerman et al. (1997) randomized women who would be eligible for testing when it became available to receive no decision aid, receive a decision aid including an education session and take-home materials, or attend the education session and receive nondirective counseling. The groups did not differ in their intent to be tested or in donating blood samples for future testing. However, the education and counseling decision aid group increased more in knowledge regarding genetics and testing, whereas the education-only decision aid group had the greatest reduction in inflated perceived risks of carrying a mutation. Skinner et al. (2002) applied computer-tailoring technology to genetic testing decision aids. Postintervention, women who received tailored decision aids were more knowledgeable about breast cancer genetics and testing, and they more realistically estimated their risks of carrying a mutation. Anxiety, which was low across groups at baseline, did not differ at follow-up.

## Participation in Clinical Trials

Llewellyn-Thomas, McGreal, and Thiel (1995; see Table 5.2) compared two methods of providing information to patients considering clinical trial enrollment. Cancer patients with varied diagnoses undergoing radiotherapy were asked to imagine that they had to make a decision about participating in a phase III clinical trial that would assign them to standard care or adjuvant chemotherapy. Participants were randomized to a tape-recorded or interactive computerized decision aid. In the former group, participants listened to the tape while they followed a written copy. The same information was presented in an interactive, computerized format for the latter group, with a series of menus and submenus to select how often and in which order information was received. Participants who used the computerized format were more likely to say they would take part in the trial, but the groups did not differ in knowledge or satisfaction.

## SUMMARY OF THE REVIEWED STUDIES

Despite the high demand for decision aids from both patients and health-care providers, decision aids for cancer screening and treatment are a research area in its infancy. Only six controlled studies have been published evaluating decision aids for PSA screening and HRT decisions, which are decision problems faced by hundreds of thousands of individuals every year. Even fewer decision aid studies have been published for other sorts of decision problems. Of the studies conducted, great diversity is evident not only in delivery channels, which range from simple brochures to trained facilitators to interactive multimedia, but also in the results used to evaluate whether a decision aid has achieved its goal. Similar variability is evident in the types of comparison groups used in the trials reviewed. Some studies use usual-care groups, whereas others use some other form of decision aid. Inconsistent findings have been reported, even when studies addressed the same decision problem using similar samples, methods, and outcome variables. Although such diversity befits a young discipline attempting to winnow good methods from bad, the lack of unifying theoretical frameworks and methodologies combined with inconsistent patterns of results makes drawing generalizable conclusions difficult. Given the current state of research, little can be concluded about which features of decision aids will most likely facilitate good decisions.

However, the second point readily apparent from the preceding review is that decision aids work, at least at some level. Although the specifics concerning the active ingredients by which decision aids exert their effects are unclear, the vast majority of studies demonstrate positive results. Increased knowledge is one of the most common results of the use of decision aids, but a wide range of other variables also shows shifts in favorable directions, including decisional conflict, satisfaction, confidence, and quality of life. Given that many of the studies do not use usual-care comparison groups, but instead comparison groups exposed to an alternative decision aid, the beneficial effects of decision aids are probably even greater than suggested by the current literature.

Further, one feature of decision aids has been consistently associated with better results. In research that pitted more simple forms of decision aids against more complex versions, the more complex versions have produced superior results in all 17 studies. Decision aids that engaged multiple sensory modalities and/or were interactive have consistently exhibited more powerful effects. Written text decision aids (e.g., brochures) tend to produce better results compared to usual care, but videotapes or interactive media decision aids produce better results than brochures. However, it may also be true that increasing complexity beyond a certain point may result in diminishing returns, as suggested by several trials investigating decision aids for HRT.

The final point is that, although most decision aids affected such results as knowledge and decisional conflict, in only about half the studies a decision aid changed the decision alternative preferred or chosen by participants. That is, only about 50% of the time the decision aid group made decisions or stated preferences that differed on average from the comparison group.

A critical question is how to interpret studies whose results showed no differences. Should the lack of group differences be taken as evidence of an ineffective decision aid? From the classical decision-making perspective, the answer would be a qualified yes. A lack of change would tend to mean the decision aid is not affecting anything relevant. However, if participants' choices were already more or less consistent with their outcome preferences prior to the administration of the decision aid (i.e., participants were already leaning toward the correct decision alternative), then the lack of change would actually suggest a well-constructed decision aid (O'Connor, Rostom, et al., 1999). The fact that group differences (or lack thereof) varied as a function of the type of decision supports this second interpretation, at least for many of the studies reviewed in this chapter.

For example, PSA screening decision aids were among those most likely to change decisions; HRT decision aids were among those least likely. Because most women must contend with reproductive issues throughout their life span, they are probably better informed about issues relevant to HRT than men are about issues related to PSA screening. Following the use of a well-constructed decision aid, a healthcare provider would expect minimal changes in the former group, but greater changes in the latter; this pattern is exactly what occurred. Unfortunately, few studies have examined whether participants' outcome preferences are consistent with their decisions, either before or after the use of a decision aid. Without this information, judgments concerning the success or failure of a specific decision aid must be held in abeyance, at least from the perspective of classical decision theory.

From the social-cognitive perspective, a lack of change in the decision alternatives selected following the use of a decision aid is not problematic. Recall that the purpose of decision aids from this perspective is to place the decision maker in an optimal frame of mind and to facilitate the kind of decision-making that will mobilize coping and adaptational resources during the postdecision period. Whether decision aids change the actual decision is of minimal importance.

This perspective is probably best illustrated by the study conducted by Molenaar et al. (2001), who tested an interactive, multimedia computer decision aid designed to facilitate treatment decisions for women diagnosed with localized breast cancer. Women who used the program compared to women who were given a brochure to read did not differ in terms of the treatment they chose. However, women in the former group reported greater satisfaction and, most importantly, a higher quality of life at 3 and 9 months after treatment. Although alternative explanations are possible, the interactive decision aid used in this study probably exerted its beneficial effects through one or more of the psychosocial routes referred to earlier in the chapter. This perspective suggests that determining the success or failure of a specific decision aid requires the collection of quality of life or other data related to adaptation and coping. To date, few decision aid studies have employed these sorts of outcome measures, especially over the long term.

## GAPS IN THE LITERATURE AND FUTURE DIRECTIONS

The demand for decision aids is likely to continue to increase, especially as technological innovations expand the number of cancer-related screening and treatment alternatives. Perhaps most important for ensuring the long-term health of decision aid research is the formulation and use of appropriate theoretical frameworks. Currently, although most decision aids are based broadly on either the SEU or social-cognitive perspective, or both, little of the work done in this area appears to have been grounded in specific theory. Although this is to be expected in a relatively young field with an applied focus, the lack of theory-driven research makes it difficult to explain findings (or lack thereof), which in turn hinders the development of more effective decision aids. The lack of unifying theoretical frameworks also contributes to the methodological inconsistencies across studies, which further muddies the waters.

For example, it is currently unclear which outcome variables should be used to demonstrate the effectiveness of a decision aid. Whereas some investigators favor more proximal results such as decisional conflict, others prefer more distal results (such as quality of life). Whether and how proximal and distal results are related is currently unknown. A related issue is the lack of long-term follow-ups. Few studies have evaluated the downstream consequences of using a decision aid, which is critically important when assessing both effectiveness and cost effectiveness.

Finally, virtually no work has been done with minority or medically underserved populations. As these groups are often the ones most in need of assistance when making cancer-related decisions, the absence of decision aid research aimed at these populations is particularly unfortunate.

Although research addressing cancer-related decision aids suffers from several shortcomings, these are probably best characterized as the natural growing pains of an emerging field rather than insurmountable flaws. The studies reviewed in this chapter demonstrate the potential of decision aids to improve decision-making across a wide range of decision problems, using varied approaches and methods of delivery. Although the field has yet to achieve its potential, the increasing number and quality of studies appearing in the literature suggests that the integration of effective decision aids into clinical practice may occur in the not-too-distant future.

## REFERENCES

Albertsen, P. C., Fryback, D. G., Storer, B. E., Kolon, T. F., & Fine, J. (1995). Long-term survival among men with conservatively treated localized prostate cancer. *Journal of the American Medical Association, 274,* 626–631.

Bekker, H., Thornton, J. G., Airey, C. M., Connelly, J. B., Hewison, J., Robinson, M. B., et al. (1999). Informed decision making: An annotated bibliography and systematic review. *Health Technology Assessment, 3,* 1–156.

Burke, W., Petersen, G., Lynch, P., Botkin, J., Daly, M., Garber, J., et al. (1997). Recommendations for follow-up care of individuals with an inherited predisposition to cancer. I. Hereditary nonpolyposis colon cancer. Cancer Genetics studies consortium. *Journal of the American Medical Association, 277,* 915–919.

Cella, D. F. (1996). Quality of life outcomes: Measurement and validation. *Oncology, 10*(Suppl. 11), 233–246.

Chapman, G. B. (1996). Temporal discounting and utility for health and money. *Journal of Experimental Psychology: Learning, Memory, & Cognition, 22,* 771–791.

Chapman, G. B., Elstein, A. S., & Hughes, K. K. (1995). Effects of patient education on decisions about breast cancer treatments: A preliminary report. *Medical Decision Making, 15,* 231–239.

Coley, C. M., Barry, M. J., Fleming, C., & Mulley, A. G. (1997). Early detection of prostate cancer. Part I: Prior probability and effectiveness of tests. The American College of Physicians. *Annals of Internal Medicine, 126,* 394–406.

Cowen, M. E., Miles, B. J., Cahill, D. F., Giesler, R. B., Beck, J. R., & Kattan, M. W. (1998). The danger of applying group-level utilities in decision analyses of the treatment of localized prostate cancer in individual patients. *Medical Decision Making, 18,* 376–380.

Cramer, J. A., & Spilker, B. (1998). *Quality of life pharmacoeconomics: An introduction.* Philadelphia, Lippincott-Raven.

Davison, B. J., Kirk, P., Degner, L. F., & Hassard, T. H. (1999). Information and patient participation in screening for prostate cancer. *Patient Education and Counseling, 37,* 255–263.

Easton, D. F., Ford, D., & Bishop, D. T. (1995). Breast and ovarian cancer incidence in BRAC1-mutation carriers. Breast Cancer Linkage Consortium. *American Journal of Human Genetics, 56,* 265–271.

Feeny, D. H., & Torrance, G. W. (1989). Incorporating utility-based quality-of-life assessment measures in clinical trials. Two examples. *Medical Care, 27*(Suppl. 3), 190–204.

Flood, A. B., Wennberg, J. E., Nease, R. F., Fowler, F. J., Ding, J., & Hynes, L. M. (1996). The importance of patient preference in the decision to screen for prostate cancer. Prostate Patient Outcomes Research Team. *Journal of General Internal Medicine, 11,* 342–349.

Ford, D., Easton, D. F., Bishop, D. T., Narod, S. A., & Goldgar, D. E. (1994). Risk of cancer in BRCA1-mutation carriers. Breast cancer linkage consortium. *Lancet, 343,* 692–695.

Ford, D., Easton, D. F., & Peto, J. (1995). Estimates of the gene frequency of BRCA1 and its contribution to breast and ovarian cancer incidence. *American Journal of Human Genetics, 57,* 1457–1462.

Gerber, G. S., Thisted, R. A., Scardino, P. T., Frohmuller, H. G., Schroeder, F. H., & Paulson, D., et al. (1996). Results of radical prostatectomy in men with clinically localized prostate cancer. *Journal of the American Medical Association, 276,* 615–619.

Giesler, R. B. (2000). *Assessing the quality of life of patients with cancer.* St. Louis, MO: Mosby.

Giesler, R. B., Ashton, C. M., Brody, B., Byrne, M. M., Cook, K., Geraci, J. M., et al. (1999). Assessing the performance of utility techniques in the absence of a gold standard. *Medical Care, 37,* 580–588.

Gramlich, E. P., & Waitzfelder, B. E. (1998). Interactive video assists in clinical decision making. *Methods of Information in Medicine, 37,* 201–205.

Hartmann, L. C., Schaid, D. J., Woods, J. E., Crotty, T. P., Myers, J. L., Arnold, P. G., et al. (1999). Efficacy of bilateral prophylactic mastectomy in women with a family history of breast cancer. *New England Journal of Medicine, 340,* 77–84.

Holmes-Rovner, M., Kroll, J., Rovner, D. R., Schmitt, N., Rothert, M., Padonu, G., et al. (1999). Patient decision support intervention: Increased consistency with decision analytic models. *Medical Care, 37,* 270–284.

Hornberger, J. C., Redelmeier, D. A., & Petersen, J. (1992). Variability among methods to assess patients' well-being and consequent effect on a cost-effectiveness analysis. *Journal of Clinical Epidemiology, 45*, 505–512.

Hunt, S. (1998). Cross-cultural issues in the use of quality of life measures in randomized controlled trials. In M. Staquet, R. Hays, & P. Fayers (Eds.), *Quality of life assessment in clinical trials* (pp. 51–68). New York: Oxford University Press.

Kaplan, R. M., Feeny, D., & Revicki, D. A. (1993). Methods for assessing relative importance in preference based outcome measures. *Quality of Life Research, 2*, 467–475.

Kassirer, J. (1994). Incorporating patients' preferences into medical decisions. *New England Journal of Medicine, 330*, 1895–1896.

Kenemans, P., van Unnik, G. A., Mijatovic, V., & van der Mooren, M. J. (2001). Perspectives in hormone replacement therapy. *Maturitas, 38*(Suppl. 1), 41–82.

Kiebert, G. M., de Haes, J. C., & van de Velde, C. J. (1991). The impact of breast-conserving treatment and mastectomy on the quality of life of early-stage breast cancer patients: A review. *Journal of Clinical Oncology, 9*, 1059–1070.

Lerman, C., Biesecker, B., Benkendorf, J. L., Kerner, J., Gomez-Caminero, A., Hughes, C., et al. (1997). Controlled trial of pretest education approaches to enhance informed decision making for BRCA1 gene testing. *Journal of the National Cancer Institute, 89*, 148–157.

Llewellyn-Thomas, H. A., McGreal, M. J., & Thiel, E. C. (1995). Cancer patients' decision making and trial-entry preferences: The effects of "framing" information about short-term toxicity and long-term survival. *Medical Decision Making, 15*, 4–12.

Mandelson, M. T., Oestreicher, N., Porter, P. L., Taplin, S. H., & White, E. (2000). Breast density as a predictor of mammography detection: Comparison of interval- and screen-detected cancers. *Journal of the National Cancer Institute, 92*, 1081–1087.

Marks, G., Richardson, J. L., Graham, J. W., & Levine, A. M. (1986). Role of health locus of control beliefs and expectations of treatment efficacy in adjustment to cancer. *Journal of Personality and Social Psychology, 51*, 443–450.

McBride, C., Bastian, L., Halabi, S., Fish, L., Lipkus, I. M., Bosworth, H. B., et al. (2002). Efficacy of a tailored intervention to aid decision-making about hormone replacement therapy. *American Journal of Public Health, 92*, 1112–1114.

Miki, Y., Swensen, J., Shattuck-Eidens, D., Futreal, P. A., Harshman, K., Tavtigian, S., et al. (1994). A strong candidate for the breast and ovarian cancer susceptibility gene BRCA1. *Science, 266*, 66–71.

Molenaar, S., Sprangers, M. A., Rutgers, E. J., Luiten, E. J., Mulder, J., Bossuyt, P. M., et al. (2001). Decision support for patients with early-stage breast cancer: Effects of an interactive breast cancer CDROM on treatment decisions, satisfaction, and quality of life. *Journal of Clinical Oncology, 19*, 1676–1687.

Mulley, A. G., Jr. (1989). Assessing patients' utilities. Can the ends justify the means? *Medical Care, 27*(Suppl. 3), 269–281.

Murray, E., Davis, H., See Tai, S., Coulter, A., Gray, A., & Haines, A. (2001). Randomized controlled of an interactive multimedia decision aid on hormone replacement therapy in primary care. *British Medical Journal, 323*, 490.

National Cancer Institute. (1997). *Recommendations for women aged 40–49*. Rockville, MD: National Cancer Advisory Board.

Nixon, A. J., Troyan, S. L., & Harris, J. R. (1996). Options in the local management of invasive breast cancer. *Seminars in Oncology, 23,* 453–463.

O'Connor, A., Tugwell, P., Wells, G., Elmslie, T., Jolly, E., Hollingworth, G., McPherson, R., Bunn, H., et al. (1998a). A decision aid for women considering hormone therapy after menopause: Decision support framework and evaluation. *Patient Education and Counseling, 33,* 267–279.

O'Connor, A., Tugwell, P., Wells, G., Elmslie, T., Jolly, E., Hollingworth, G., McPherson, R., Drake, E., et al. (1998b). Randomized trial of a portable, self-administered decision aid for post-menopausal women considering long-term preventive hormone therapy. *Medical Decision Making, 18,* 295–303.

O'Connor, A. M., Drake, E. R., Fiset, V. J., Page, J., Curtin, D., & Llewellyn-Thomas, H. (1997). Annotated bibliography: Studies evaluating decision-support interventions for patients. *Canadian Journal of Nursing Research, 29,* 119–120.

O'Connor, A. M., Fiset, V., DeGrasse, C., Graham, I. D., Evans, W., Stacey, D., Laupacis, A., et al. (1999). Decision aids for patients considering options affecting cancer outcomes: Evidence of efficacy and policy implications. *Journal of the National Cancer Institute Monographs, 26,* 67–80.

O'Connor, A. M., Rostom, A., Fiset, V., Tetroe, J., Entwistle, V., Llewellyn-Thomas, H., et al. (1999). Decision aids for patients facing health treatment or screening decisions: systematic review. *British Medical Journal, 139,* 1475–1479.

Potosky, A. L., Miller, B. A., Albertsen, P. C., & Kramer, B. S. (1995). The role of increasing detection in the rising incidence of prostate cancer. *Journal of the American Medical Association, 273,* 548–552.

Read, J. (1993). The new era of quality of life assessment. In S. Walker & R. Rosser (Eds.), *Quality of life assessment: Key issues in the 1990s* (pp. 3–10). Boston: Kluwer Academic Publishers.

Rebbeck, T. R., Levin, A. M., Eisen, A., Snyder, C., Watson, P., & Cannon-Albright, L., et al. (1999). Breast cancer risk after bilateral prophylactic oophorectomey in BRAC1 mutation carriers. *Journal of the National Cancer Institutes, 91,* 1475–1491.

Rimer, B. K., Conaway, M., Lyna, P., Glassman, B., Yarnall, K. S. H., Lipkus, I., et al. (2000). The short-term impact of tailored mammography decision-making interventions. *Patient Education and Counseling, 1429,* 1–17.

Rothert, M. L., Holmes-Rovner, M., Rovner, D., Kroll, J., Breer, L., Talarczyk, G., et al. (1997). An educational intervention as decision support for menopausal women. *Research in Nursing & Health, 20,* 377–387.

Rutter, C. M., Mandelson, M. T., Laya, M. B., & Taplin, S. (2001). Changes in breast density associated with initiation, discontinuation, and continuing use of hormone replacement therapy. *Journal of the American Medical Association, 285,* 171–176.

Schapira, M. M., McAuliffe, T. L., & Nattinger, A. B. (2000). Underutilization of mammography in older breast cancer survivors. *Medical Care, 38,* 281–289.

Schrag, D., Kuntz, K. M., Garber, J. E., & Weeks, J. C. (1997). Decision analysis—effects of prophylactic mastectomy and oophorectomy on life expectancy among women with BRCA1 or BRCA2 mutations. *New England Journal of Medicine, 336*, 1465–1471.

Sebban, C., Browman, G., Gafni, A., Norman, G., Levine, M., Assouline, D., et al. (1995). Design and validation of a bedside decision instrument to elicit a patient's preference concerning allogenic bone marrow transplantation in chronic myeloid leukemia. *American Journal of Hematology, 48*, 221–227.

Sepucha, K. R., Belkora, J. K., Tripathy, D., & Esserman, L. J. (2000). Building bridges between physicians and patients: Results of a pilot study examining new tools for collaborative decision making in breast cancer. *Journal of Clinical Oncology, 18*, 1230–1238.

Skinner, C. S., Campbell, M. K., Rimer, B. K., Curry, S., & Prochaska, J. O. (1999). How effective is tailored print communication? *Annals of Behavioral Medicine, 21*, 290–298.

Skinner, C. S., Schildkraut, J., Berry, D., Calingaert, B., Marcom, P. K., Sugarman, J., et al. (2002). Pre-counseling education materials for BRCA testing: Does tailoring make a difference? *Genetic Testing, 6*, 93–105.

Skinner, M., & Wells, S. (1997). Medullary carcinoma of the thyroid gland and the MEN 2 syndromes. *Seminars in Pediatric Surgery, 6*, 134–140.

Skinner, M. A., DeBenedetti, M. K., Moley, J. F., Norton, J. A., & Wells, S. A. (1996). Medullary thyroid carcinoma in children with multiple endocrine neoplasia types 2A and 2B. *Journal of Pediatric Surgery, 31*, 177–181.

Street, R. L., Voigt, B., Geyer, C., Manning, T., & Swanson, G. P. (1995). Increasing patient involvement in choosing treatment for early breast cancer. *Cancer, 76*, 2275–2284.

Struewing, J. P., Hartge, P., Wacholder, S., Baker, S. M., Berlin, M., McAdams, M., et al. (1997). The risk of cancer associated with specific mutations of BRCA1 and BRCA2 among Ashkenazi Jews. *New England Journal of Medicine, 336*, 1401–1408.

Taylor, S. E., Lichtman, R. R., & Wood, J. V. (1984). Attributions, beliefs and control, and adjustment to breast cancer. *Journal of Personality and Social Psychology, 46*, 489–502.

Torrance, G. W. (1986). Measurement of health state utilities for economic appraisal. A review. *Journal of Health Economics, 5*, 1–30.

Turner, B. C., Glazer, P. M., & Haffty, B. G. (1999). BRCA1/BRCA2 in breast-conserving therapy. *Journal of Clinical Oncology, 17*, 3689.

Volk, R. J., Cass, A. R., & Spann, S. J. (1999). A randomized controlled trial of shared decision making for prostate cancer screening. *Archives of Family Medicine, 8*, 333–340.

Wells, S., & Skinner, M. (1998). Prophylactic thyroidectomy, based on direct genetic testing, in patients at risk for the multiple endocrine neoplasia type 2 syndromes. *Experimental and Clinical Endocrinology and Diabetes, 106*, 29–34.

Wells, S. A., Chi, D. D., Toshima, K., Dehner, L. P., Coffin, C. M., Dowton, S. B., et al. (1994). Predictive DNA testing and Prophylactic thyroidectomy in patients at risk for multiple endocrine neoplasia type 2A. *Annals of Surgery, 220*, 237–247.

Wennberg, J. E., Mulley, A. G., Hanley, D., Timothy, R. P., Fowler, F. J., Roos, N. P., et al. (1988). An assessment of prostatectomy for benign urinary tract obstruction. Geographic variations and the evaluation of medical care outcomes. *Journal of the American Medical Association, 259*, 3027–3030.

Wolf, A., & Schorling, J. (2000). Does informed consent alter elderly patients' preferences for colorectal cancer screening? Results of a randomized trial. *Journal of General Internal Medicine, 15*, 24–30.

Wolf, A. M., Nasser, J. F., Wolf, A. M., & Schorling, J. B. (1996). The impact of informed consent on patient interest in prostate-specific antigen screening. *Archives of Internal Medicine, 156*, 1333–1336.

Wooster, R., Bignell, G., Lancaster, J., Swift, S., Seal, S., Mangion, J., Collins, N., et al. (1995). Identification of the breast cancer susceptibility gene BRCA2. *Nature, 378*, 789–792.

Writing Group for the Women's Health Initiative Investigators. (2002). Risks and benefits of estrogen plus progestin in healthy postmenopausal women: Principal results from the Women's Health Initiative Randomized Controlled Trial. *Journal of the American Medical Association, 288*, 321–333.

Yang, F. E., Song, P. Y., Wayne, J., Vaida, F., & Vijayakumar, S. (1998). A new look at an old option in the treatment of early-stage prostate cancer: Hormone therapy as an alternative to watchful waiting. *Medical Hypotheses, 51*, 243–251.

# 6

## Psychological Interventions for Cancer Patients

### Barbara L. Andersen

T he adjustment process for cancer survivors may be burdensome and lengthy, and deteriorations in quality of life may go unrecognized if survivors also have adverse health effects. Gains in quality of life can be achieved with psychological interventions (Andersen, 1992). In this chapter, the accomplishments of the last decade to enhance biobehavioral outcomes through psychological interventions will be reviewed. Although few studies have assessed psychological, behavioral, and biologic mechanisms of change, this is a pathway for future research.

The biobehavioral model of cancer stress and disease course (Andersen, Kiecolt-Glaser, & Glaser, 1994) provides an organizational framework for this chapter. The model includes psychological (stress and quality of life), behavioral (health behaviors and compliance), and biologic (neuroendocrine and immune) factors, and it specifies the pathways by which health outcomes (e.g., disease endpoints, such as recurrence or a disease-free interval) might be affected (see Figure 6.1). Each component of the model will be briefly summarized prior to discussion of recent studies providing data on specific outcomes. The studies reviewed have been published since 1992 and come from a search of MEDLINE® and related sources. Only experimental studies are detailed, with data from quasi-experimental designs for emerging areas.

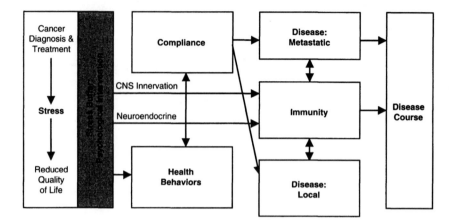

**FIGURE 6.1** A biobehavioral model of the psychological (stress and quality of life), behavioral (compliance and health behaviors), and biologic pathways from cancer stressors to disease course. Psychological interventions may moderate the effect of adverse psychological, behavioral, or biologic responses on disease outcomes. CNS = central nervous system (adapted from Figure 1 in Andersen, Kiecolt-Glaser, and Glaser, 1994; used with permission).

## STRESS AND QUALITY OF LIFE OUTCOMES

### Description and Effects of Stress

Severe, acute stress occurs at the time of cancer diagnosis (Andersen, Anderson, & deProsse, 1989; Maunsell, Brisson, & Deschenes, 1992). However, even after lengthy, difficult treatments have ended, individuals may still report disruptions in major life areas and some may report continued chronic stress (Cordova et al., 1995). If not remediated, both acute and chronic stress can contribute to emotional distress, life disruptions, and, in turn, to a lower quality of life for cancer patients. To prevent this chain of events, psychological interventions are considered; without them, many cancer survivors report continuing problems with emotional distress, fatigue, reduced energy, and loss of stamina (Andrykowski et al., 1996). Other permanent sequelae from cancer treatments have the potential to impact intimate relationships, alter social support, and even heighten emotional distress (Ey, Compas, Epping-Jordan, & Worsham, 1998; Ganz et al.,

1996; Hagedoorn et al., 2000; Spencer et al., 1999). Finally, a cancer diagnosis can also result in subsequent financial difficulties, jeopardize insurance coverage, and narrow employment options; 20% of cancer survivors report these chronic, stressful economic difficulties (Hewitt, Breen, & Devesa, 1999). In sum, when left untreated, stress and a lowered quality of life conspire to produce a difficult trajectory on the road to cancer survivorship (Green et al., 2000; Gotay & Muraoka, 1998).

## Review of Stress-related Studies

Five experimental studies have tested for effects on stress and/or quality of life outcomes (see Table 6.1); two employed a very brief intervention model. Larsson and Starrin (1992) examined the effectiveness of relaxation training for 64 breast cancer patients undergoing radiotherapy accrued and sequentially assigned to experimental (relaxation) or control (no treatment) groups. Those in the intervention condition were given 15 minutes of instruction, provided with an audiotape, and encouraged to practice progressive muscle relaxation at least four times per week. Women were assessed pretreatment, midtreatment (day 10), and end of treatment (day 20). Analyses revealed significant differential improvements for the relaxation group on measures of the lower frequency of daily hassles, more positive moods, and the appraisal of radiation therapy as less threatening and more benign and/or positive. No significant group differences were found in measures of daily uplifts, other treatment appraisal aspects, or cognitive coping strategies.

The second study, by McQuellon et al. (1998), examined the impact of a brief orientation to a medical oncology clinic on distress in a heterogeneous sample of cancer patients. The intervention was conducted prior to a patient's initial clinic visit. The 15- to 20-minute tour by a masters-level psychologist included reception, phlebotomy, nursing stations, and chemotherapy suites, etc.; written materials on clinic hours and procedures; and a question and answer session. Of 279 eligible patients, 180 (65%) were randomized, although only 150 (54%) completed both the pre- and postintervention (1 week later) assessments. The intervention group had significantly lower state anxiety (State Trait Anxiety Inventory [STAI]) and distress (Profile of Mood States [POMS]) than the control (no intervention) group. Fewer intervention patients reported depressive symptoms Center for Epidemiologic Depression Scale (CES-D). Additionally, intervention patients demonstrated significantly more knowledge of clinic procedures, greater

**TABLE 6.1  Stress, Quality of Life, and Compliance Outcomes**

| Stress and quality of life | Design | Sample | Measures | Results |
|---|---|---|---|---|
| Antoni et al. (2001) | Group treatment, 10 sessions (20 hours) Cognitive-behavioral Stress Management (CBSM) versus 1 session (6 hours) control (brief CBSM), follow-up at 6 and 12 months | N = 136 women, postsurgery, with stage I and II breast cancer | Positive benefits, POMS, Impact of Events Scale (IES) | 6 months: positive benefits* <br><br> 12 months: Positive benefits NS, (N only condition), GHQ-*, HADS-*, group x time NS |
| Fukui et al. (2000) | Group treatment, education and relaxation versus control, 6 sessions (9 hours), follow-up at 6 months | N = 50 women with stage II and III breast cancer | POMS, MAC, HADS | 6 and 12 months: POMS*, MAC NS, HADS NS |
| Helgeson, Cohen, Schulz, & Yasko (1999) | Group education (Ed; 8 sessions, 6 hours) versus peer discussion (PD; 8 sessions, 11 hours) versus Ed + PD (8 sessions, 17 hours) versus no treatment; follow-up at 6, 12, 24, and 36 months | N = 312 women with breast cancer | Positive affect, control, IES, SF-36 (physical) | 6 months: positive affect*, control*, IES*, SF-36 (physical)* <br><br> 12, 24, 36 months: SF-36 (vitality)*, SF-36 (physical functioning)*, SF-36 (physical) NS |

| Stress and quality of life | Design | Sample | Measures | Results |
| --- | --- | --- | --- | --- |
| Larsson & Starrin (1992) | Individual, relaxation versus no treatment, one 15-minute session plus audiotapes, follow-up after tenth and twentieth radiation treatments | N = 64 women with breast cancer | Daily hassles, mood daily uplifts, treatment appraisal, coping | Tenth Tx: Tx appraisal NS, coping NS<br><br>Twentieth Tx: Tx appraisal*, coping NS |
| McQuellon et al. (1998) | Brief clinic orientation versus no treatment, 20-minute clinic tour and question and answer session plus written material, follow-up at 1 week | N = 150, cancer stage not reported; 50% male | STAI, brief POMS, CES-D, clinic knowledge, care satisfaction | STAI*, brief POMS*, CESD*, clinic knowledge*, care satisfaction* |
| Rutter, Iconomou, & Quine (1996) | Physician communication training with patient handbook versus no training; follow-up after consult | N = 36 lung, breast, and other advanced disease patients; 50% male | Physician performance, BDI; satisfaction w/consult, personal control | Physician performance*; BDI*; satisfaction with consult*, personal control* |

(continued)

183

**TABLE 6.1  Stress, Quality of Life, and Compliance Outcomes** (*continued*)

| Stress and quality of life | Design | Sample | Measures | Results |
|---|---|---|---|---|
| COMPLIANCE | | | | |
| Richardson | Individual; education and shaping versus education and home visit versus education, shaping, and home visit versus no treatment; follow-up at 3 and 6 months | *N* = 92 patients accrued from large city medical center; 56% unemployed; 86% minority; multiple myeloma, leukemia, lymphoma, or Hodgkin's disease | Compliance with treatment, uncertainty about illness, satisfaction with medical care, knowledge of disease | Increased compliance among intervention groups, no differential effects between intervention groups, no significant differences in ratings of uncertainty, intervention patients reported significantly higher levels of satisfaction with medical care and knowledge of disease, intervention patients returned for significantly more follow-up visits |

*Note: $p \leq .05$

confidence in their physicians, higher levels of satisfaction, and higher levels of hope regarding their illness.

A related effort is the novel intervention of Rutter, Iconomou, and Quine (1996). A time-series design was used in which physician communication training was tested as a strategy to reduce patient distress. Patients were treated by physicians who had received communication training versus those who had received no communication training. Physicians in the experimental arm received approximately 75 minutes of communication training along with a handbook focused on improving the structure and style of their medical communications. Based on the work of Ley (1988), training included cognitive aids to understanding (e.g., simplification and repetition) and emotional aspects (e.g., conveying warmth, listening, and giving feedback). Also, physicians assigned to the intervention arm provided information booklets specific to a patient's adjuvant treatment (e.g., radiation and chemotherapy) to encourage patient participation and perceived control. Of 45 eligible patients, 36 (80%) participated. The majority of the patients had solid tumors, with 64% having advanced disease. Patients in both groups reported significant reductions in anxiety (STAI). More importantly, intervention patients reported significantly lower depression scores Beck Depression Inventory (BDI). Intervention patients also evaluated their physicians as more cognitively skilled, and they reported higher levels of satisfaction and personal control.

Group support with behavioral strategies was tested by two investigators. First, Fukui et al. (2000) attempted to replicate the intervention effects reported by Fawzy et al. (1990) with a sample of breast cancer patients. Women with stage II or III breast cancer who had completed their adjuvant chemotherapy were contacted by mail. Only women 65 years of age or less and those without psychiatric history were eligible. Fifty women (33%) were randomized to intervention or wait list control groups; participants were significantly older ($M = 53$ years) versus nonparticipants ($M = 50$ years). Consistent with Fawzy et al. (1990), intervention components included health education, coping skills training, stress management with progressive muscle relaxation and audiotapes, and group support. Groups of 6 to 10 patients met for 90 minutes weekly for 6 weeks (9 therapy hours). Assessments (POMS and Mental Adjustment to Cancer [MAC]) were administered at pre- and post-treatment and at 6 months. Analyses indicated significant effects for the group, however, no significant group $X$ time interactions.

Second, Antoni et al (2001) reported on the effects of a cognitive-behavioral stress management (CBSM) group intervention for women with breast cancer. Women with *in situ* disease or stage I or II breast cancer were randomized to 10 weekly group sessions of CBSM (20 therapy hours) or a control condition of abbreviated CBSM instruction (6 hours). The intervention included didactic and experiential exercises, which included making positive social comparisons for coping, using social support, emotional expression, assertion training, and progressive muscle relaxation. The control condition received similar information in an abbreviated (1-day) instructional format. Patients with evidence of prior psychiatric disorder were excluded for a final sample of 100 completed assessments postintervention and at 3 and 9 months. Analyses revealed main effects for time with overall reductions in distress, although no differential changes were found in the POMS, in depression (CES-D), or on the Impact of Events Scale (IES) for the intervention group. Follow-up analyses examined the CES-D scores; the number of women who scored higher than 16 at the initial assessment dropped significantly in the intervention condition in comparison to the control (6 compared to 11 at 9 months). In contrast to the distress measures, the analyses suggested significant differential gains for the intervention subjects in self-reports of optimism and immediate postintervention effects on emotional processing. Optimism was also examined as an individual difference variable, and analyses revealed that optimism moderated the effects of the intervention on an experimenter-derived measure of positive benefits of the cancer experience. That is, the greatest change in positive benefits was reported by the women in the intervention condition who were initially low in dispositional optimism.

Two investigators compared two interventions and tested for an additive effect of each. McArdle et al. (1996) compared the effects of supportive nursing care versus support from a cancer patient volunteer on reducing distress for a varied group of breast cancer patients. Four groups were compared: (a) nurse support, (b) cancer patient volunteer support, (c) combined nurse and cancer patient volunteer support, and (d) no treatment support (routine care). Nurse practitioner support consisted of the delivery of preoperative information (20 to 30 minutes) and follow-up postoperative visits as needed. In contrast, individuals assigned to volunteer support were visited postsurgery and provided written materials. Of 311 eligible patients, 272 (87%) were accrued. Assessments, occurring at the first postoperative visit and then at 3, 6, and 12 months, consisted of standardized self-report measures of general health (General Health Questionnaire [GHQ]) as well as anxiety and depression (Hospital Anxiety and Depression [HAD]). During the follow-up year, 26 (10%) women recurred and 9 (3%) died. Group comparisons were made with the follow-ups; analyses suggested improvements for the nurse care group only. In addition, levels of psychological morbidity for the two groups treated by volunteers were equivalent to, if not worse than, the morbidity levels for the no-treatment group.

The second factorial design was by Helgeson, Cohen, Schulz, and Yasko (1999), who compared the effects of education versus peer discussion on psychological adjustments for women with breast cancer. Women were randomized to one of four conditions: education only (ED), peer discussion only (PD), education plus peer discussion (ED/PD), or no treatment. The groups, facilitated by an oncology nurse and social worker, met for 8 consecutive weeks. The total duration of the therapy time differed across groups, with 11 hours for PD, 6 hours for ED, and 17 hours for ED/PD. The ED intervention provided information about the disease and treatment with strategies to manage treatment morbidity (e.g., nutrition, exercise, and body image) and to facilitate control. A lecture format was used and group discussion was discouraged. Patients were also taught relaxation and provided with an audiotape. Unlike the ED group, the PD group encouraged the expression of positive and negative feelings, and workbooks were provided to record feelings and thoughts.

Of 445 eligible patients, 312 (70%) women with stage I, II, or III breast cancer agreed to participate. Assessments were conducted pretreatment, post-treatment, and at 6 months. Psychological adjustment measures included standardized self-report measures of quality of life, positive and negative effects, intrusive thoughts of breast cancer, self-esteem, body image, perceived personal control, vicarious control, illness uncertainty, and positive versus negative comparisons of self with other group members. Women in the ED groups acquired more information about breast cancer and its treatment than women in the PD or control groups.

Education was the main effect at the post-treatment assessment, with significantly better mental health and physical scores (SF-36). Six-month follow-up findings were similar, with a main effect for education on a measure of positive effects and again on the physical component scores (SF-36). Additional analyses of the post-treatment data suggested that the ED condition resulted in higher levels of self-esteem, lower illness uncertainty, and more discussions about the illness, whereas the women in the PD groups reported more negative interactions with family members. Additional analyses of the 6-month data revealed that women in the ED conditions reported higher levels of control and fewer intrusive thoughts, whereas women in the PD conditions reported more avoidant thoughts. Post hoc analyses examined individual differences in outcomes (Helgeson et al., 2000). Contrasting women with high versus low levels of partner support, this variable interacted with the intervention condition; women with low levels of support responded similarly (positively) to both interventions, whereas women with high levels of support were unaffected by the ED intervention, but adversely affected by the PD groups.

## Summary of Stress and Quality of Life Interventions

Drawing general conclusions about the efficacy of psychological interventions is made difficult by the heterogeneity of the interventions represented. We appear to have "all of the above," including relaxation training alone (Larsson & Starrin, 1992); individual and group (Antoni et al., 2001; Moorey, Greer, Bliss, & Law, 1998) cognitive behavior therapy; replication efforts (Fukui et al., 2000); general clinic (McQuellon et al., 1998), disease, and treatment (Helgeson et al., 2000; McArdle et al., 1996) educational interventions; and indirect efforts to impact patient adjustment through physician training (Rutter et al., 1996). The factorial designs tested two different strategies of using peer support—group format (Helgeson, Cohen, Schulz, & Yasko, 1999) and individual counselors (McArdle et al., 1996) —but they produced null effects when compared with educational efforts.

The predominant disease group represented has been women with breast cancer, although three studies included samples heterogeneous in terms of site and extent of disease (McQuellon et al., 1998; Moorey et al., 1998; Rutter et al., 1996). Despite disease heterogeneity, significant effects emerged even with small sample sizes (e.g., $N = 36$ in Rutter et al., 1996). The samples from the U.S. remain primarily Caucasian, with minorities underrepresented among participants and/or overrepresented among refusers (e.g., McQuellon et al., 1998), although in Antoni et al. (2001) 26% of the subjects were minorities. An important indication of the universality of these issues for cancer patients is the international representation seen here with studies from the U.K. (McArdle et al., 1996; Moorey et al., 1998), Sweden (Larsson & Starrin, 1992), Greece (Rutter, Iconomou, & Quine, 1996), and Japan (Fukui et al., 2000).

Investigations began during the earliest days of the patients' cancer experiences, the first clinic visits, or very early in the treatment process; as such, stress is likely to be at its highest level, but if untreated it will dissipate rapidly for the majority (e.g., Antoni et al., 2001). When patients are accrued months after therapy has ended, intervention effects may be difficult to achieve (e.g., Fukui et al., 2000). Reductions in anxiety and/or depression may be transitory, and intervention and control conditions are often equivalent at follow-up. Repeated measure designs require *more* power to detect intervention effects at later follow-up assessments. This is a challenge in longitudinal cancer studies, as sources of attrition (e.g., death, disease progression, and dropout; Moorey et al., 1998) are varied and can be common.

## COMPLIANCE WITH CANCER THERAPIES

### Description of Compliance with Cancer Therapies

The biobehavioral model suggests that one plausible behavioral route to impact disease outcome is compliance with cancer therapies (see Figure 6.1). Compliance might be improved directly, such as including a patient education component so that patients have greater knowledge and the ability to be compliant. Or compliance might be influenced indirectly, such as when psychological interventions improve patients' moods or reduce the occurrence and/or severity of treatment-related side effects (e.g., nausea or vomiting), so that cancer patients are more accepting or tolerant of toxic cancer treatment regimens (Redd, Montgomery, & DuHamel, 2001). Compliance can be considered in the context of the receipt of chemotherapy and related therapies (e.g., hormonal and radiation therapy).

### Review and Summary of Compliance-related Studies

A search of the literature revealed no studies of the factors governing treatment refusals, premature terminations, or the receipt of fewer radiation sessions than prescribed, although these circumstances do, indeed, occur. The absence of data is somewhat surprising in that certain regimens for some disease sites (e.g., vulvar cancer or head/neck cancers) include high doses to sensitive tissues, combine radiotherapy with chemotherapy, and incur considerable toxicity (e.g., skin reactions including burning and/or pain). Refusal of therapy, which can directly impact local as well as distant control of the disease, has been noted in some clinical trials (Vokes et al., 2000).

Considering chemotherapy, Budman et al. (1998) reported that women who received a high or moderate intensity dose of a standard chemotherapy regimen (i.e., cyclophosphamide, doxorubicin, and 5-fluorouracil) for stage II breast cancer had a 77% to 79% likelihood of 5-year survival versus only a 66% 5-year survival for women receiving a low-dose intensity. Similar studies were reported earlier (Bonadonna & Valagussa, 1981).

Noncompliance in clinical trials can invalidate data. Despite the thousands of cancer patients entered in chemotherapy trials (and the hundreds of thousands of patients treated off protocol) each year, few reports are made of the interaction of quality of life variables and the feasibility, acceptability, or compliance with cancer therapies. Some chemotherapy pilot studies have examined these variables, but subject samples have been equivalent or even smaller in size than the number of variables studied (e.g., 79 patients in Macquart-Moulin et al., 2000; 19 patients in Swain, Roland, King, & Spertur, 1996). Surprisingly, investigators have concluded that toxicity is "tolerable" or "manageable" even when 50% or more of the patients reported moderate to severe disruption in their personal relationships and work-related problems (Swain et al., 1996). In such a context, data on compliance would seem of paramount importance, as these same psychological and behavioral variables—disruption of social function, work-related difficulties, and significant emotional distress—have been correlated with low rates of compliance (Lebovitz, Strain, Schleifer, Tanaka, Bhardwaj, & Messe, 1990; McDonough, Boyd, Varvares, & Maves, 1996) as well as refusal of chemotherapy (Levin, Mermelstein, & Rigberg, 1999).

Despite the plausibility and importance of psychological or behavioral routes to enhanced compliance and, in turn, improved disease outcomes, there has been minimal investigation of compliance with cancer therapies. The notable exception is an important study by Richardson et al. (1987), who compared medication shaping to a home visit to enhance supportive medication and chemotherapy for hematologic malignancies. Of the 115 patients eligible, 92 (80%) were accrued from a large city medical center. Importantly, the sample was comprised of unemployed (56%), minority (86%), and low-income individuals with one of the following hematologic malignancies: multiple myeloma, leukemia, lymphoma, or Hodgkin's disease. Heterogeneity of disease severity was also present, with subjects having high (26%) or moderate disease severity (31%), and some having relatively indolent diseases (43%). In addition to the target drugs, many patients received multiple other chemotherapies, with 31% of the regimens rated as "easy" and 69% as "complex."

Patients were assigned in randomized blocks to one of four conditions: (a) no-treatment control; (b) education and shaping; (c) education and home visit; or (d) education, shaping, and home visit. The education provided to all intervention patients consisted of providing disease and treatment information and emphasizing patient responsibilities to be compliant. The home visit was by a project nurse, who, with the patient, attempted to develop a "cue" system for pill taking (e.g., a reminder sign next to the home coffeepot). The shaping intervention was conducted while patients were hospitalized and shifted from nurse-administered medication to patient-initiated requests for medication under nurse supervision. Patients were followed for 3- and 6-month assessments, and self-reports of compliance were supplemented with serum samples for analysis of the drugs and their metabolites.

Analyses indicated significant increases in compliance for all intervention groups when compared with no treatment but no differential effects between them. Intervention patients were more compliant with Allopurinol (50% versus 23% for control), though no compliance group differences took place with prednisone (approximately 35% compliance). Attitudinal measures were also obtained; the groups did not differ significantly in their ratings of uncertainty about their illnesses, although intervention patients reported significantly higher levels of satisfaction with medical care and knowledge of their disease than control patients. Finally, compliance with follow-up clinic visits was also recorded, and the intervention patients returned for significantly more of their follow-up visits (approximately 85% of the time) compared to the control patients (61% return rate). Follow-up analyses examined variables predictive of compliance. Satisfaction with treatment was predictive of appointment keeping, though not predictive of medication compliance. Also, compliance with appointments also decreased as difficulty in tolerating side effects (e.g., hair loss, nausea, and anorexia) increased and as the level of interference of the side effects with daily activities increased.

Although dated, the Richardson et al. (1987) study had multiple strengths (e.g., the inclusion of an underrepresented, sociodemographically varied sample) and a similar comprehensive effort has yet to be conducted. It is likely that the difficulty in comparing the treatment alternatives (shaping versus home visits) was limited by two factors: the inclusion of an important educational component that might have "leveled" the group differences and the small sample sizes. However, the study provides an important basis for generating hypotheses for future efforts.

## HEALTH BEHAVIORS

### Description of Health Behaviors

The biobehavioral model suggests important health behavior sequelae (see arrow from stress to reduced quality of life to health behaviors in Figure 6.1), and interest in these variables in the context of cancer has expanded (see Pinto, Eakin, & Maruyama, 2000 for a review), including both negative and positive health behaviors. Many manifestations of negative health behaviors arise in the context of cancer diagnosis and treatment. For example, distressed individuals often have appetite disturbances or experience dietary changes, such as eating less often or eating meals of lower nutritional value (Grunberg & Straub, 1992). If eating habits are changed due to cancer treatments (e.g., food restriction with nausea or taste aversions from chemotherapy; Broeckel, Jacobsen, & Hann, 2000; Jacobsen et al., 1995), vulnerability may be heightened (Wellisch, Wolcutt, Pasnau, Fawzy, & Landsverk, 1989). In contrast, some cancer patients, particularly those with breast disease who have received adjuvant chemotherapy, are at risk for weight gain (Camoriano et al., 1990), perhaps due to changed metabolic requirements (Denmark-Wahnefried et al., 1997). Distressed individuals may report sleep disturbances, such as early morning awakening or insomnia (Lacks & Morin, 1992).

Positive health behaviors, such as regular physical exercise, may be abandoned, as many patients feel they have neither the time nor the energy to begin or resume an exercise program as they undergo or recover from cancer treatments. These are among the complex circumstances posed when conducting health behavior interventions with cancer patients. For each of the following three areas reviewed, important reasons for considering their use with selected cancer groups are related to quality of life and health outcomes.

### Summary of Health Behavior Studies

Health behavior interventions are included in the biobehavioral model as they potentially have important implications for affect regulation and disease progression (see arrow to Disease: Metastatic in Figure 6.1) for selected disease sites. The empirical case for dietary and exercise interventions is easily made for breast cancer patients. Considering exercise, the results are also quite positive. Although lengthy follow-ups have not been conducted to test if disease outcomes differ following either dietary or exercise interventions, the two literatures are sufficiently encouraging that second-generation trials appear to be an important next step for research with breast cancer patients (Stoll, 1996). See Chapter 2 "Behavioral Interventions for Cancer Prevention: Dietary Intake and Physical Activity," and Chapter 8, "Cancer-Related Fatigue," for detailed discussions of diet and exercise-related studies.

In contrast, smoking cessation gains have been difficult to achieve. Also, important health behavior intervention targets have been established for this cancer group, and future research efforts are needed in these areas along with the focus on smoking cessation. Table 6.2 summarizes smoking-related studies (Griebel, Wewers, & Baker, 1998; Gritz et al., 1993; Stanislaw & Wewers, 1994; Wewers, Bowen, Stanislaw, & Desimone, 1994); also see Chapter 4, "Smoking Cessation in Cancer Patients: Never Too Late to Quit," for a detailed discussion of smoking-related studies.

## BIOLOGIC RESPONSES

### Description of Biologic Responses

Focus on the health behaviors discussed earlier is important due to their relationship to biological responses. Compelling evidence exists to focus intervention efforts on changing health behaviors for exercise, physical activity, and smoking. The biobehavioral model suggests that stress triggers important biological effects involving the autonomic, endocrine, and immune systems (see Figure 6.1). Stress may be routed to the immune system by the central nervous system via activation of the sympathetic nervous system (e.g., Felten, Ackerman, Wiegand, & Felten, 1987) or through neuroendocrine-immune pathways (i.e., the release of steroid hormones, glucocorticoids). Few neuroendocrine studies of cancer patients exist, but studies suggest that cancer patients may exhibit dysregulations similar to those observed in depressed patients without cancer (Evans et al., 1986; Joffe, Rubinow, Denicoff, Maher, & Sindelar, 1986; McDaniel, Musselman, Porter, Reed, & Nemeroff, 1995). Also, hormones released under stress have been implicated in immune modulation (see Maier, Watkins, & Fleshner, 1994 for a discussion; Rabin, Cohen, Ganguli, Lysle, & Cunnick, 1989; Sabharwal et al., 1992). Epinephrine and norepinephrine, for example, regulate lymphocyte levels that can, in turn, alter immune responses (Madden & Livnat, 1991). Immunologic responses can affect

**TABLE 6.2  Health Behaviors, Smoking Experimental Study Outcomes**

| | Design | Sample | Measures | Results |
|---|---|---|---|---|
| Griebel, Wewers, & Baker (1998) | Individual; nurse-delivered minimal smoking cessation program versus no treatment; one 20-minute session, five 10-minute weekly phone calls, booklet, and relaxation exercises; follow-up at 6 weeks | N = 28 gynecological and breast cancer patients; 57 percent female | Abstinence; cotinine levels | Abstinence NS; cotinine levels NS |
| Gritz et al. (1993) | Individual; physician-delivered smoking cessation advice versus no treatment; 7 sessions, 6 monthly booster sessions, and written materials; follow-up at 1, 6, and 12 months | N = 186 head and neck, and breast cancer patients; 74% male | Abstinence; cotinine levels | Cotinine levels NS, abstinence NS |

| | Design | Sample | Measures | Results |
|---|---|---|---|---|
| Stanislaw & Wewers (1994) | Individual; nurse-delivered structured smoking cessation program versus no treatment; three 20- to 30-minute sessions, 5 weekly phone calls, booklet, audiotape, and relaxation exercises; follow-up at 6 weeks | $N = 26$ head and neck cancer patients, stages II-IV; 73% female | Abstinence; cotinine levels | Abstinence*; cotinine levels* |
| Wewers, Bowen, Stanislaw, & Desimone (1994) | Individual; nurse-delivered structured smoking cessation program versus no treatment; three 20- to 30-minute sessions, 5 weekly phone calls, booklet, audiotape, and relaxation exercises; follow-up at 6 weeks | $N = 80$; $n = 30$ oncology patients; head and neck, and breast cancer; 66% female | Abstinence; cotinine levels | Abstinence*; cotinine levels NS |

*Note: $p \leq .05$

susceptibility to infectious pathogens requiring a cellular response (Clerici et al., 1997). Table 6.3 summarizes biologic response studies.

## Review of Biologic Responses Studies

BIOLOGIC RESPONSES STUDIES: ENDOCRINE

A single randomized study examined endocrine outcomes; Cruess et al. (2000) conducted a small-sample randomized design examining the effect of cognitive-behavioral stress management in a group treatment for women with stage I or II breast cancer. The intervention consisted of 10 weekly meetings of 120 minutes (20 therapy hours) including cognitive restructuring, coping skills, assertive and anger management training, social support, and relaxation training (a combination of progressive muscle, meditation, breathing, and guided imagery). The control condition was described as a wait list. Thirty-four women (24 intervention, 10 control), part of a larger clinical trial, participated. Assessments were conducted pre- and post-treatment. Analyses of Covariance indicated a significant reduction in cortisol and significant increases in an experimenter-derived measure of the positive benefits from cancer. No significant differences were found between groups in emotional distress (POMS). Investigators provided path analysis data suggesting that changes in the positive benefits from cancer measure mediated the effects of the intervention on cortisol reduction.

BIOLOGIC RESPONSES STUDIES: IMMUNE

Two studies have reported immune outcomes. Elsesser, van Berkel, Sartory, Biermann-Gocke, and Ohl (1994) conducted a small randomized study comparing anxiety-management training with a wait list control for a heterogeneous sample of German cancer patients. The treatment consisted of instruction in progressive muscle relaxation training and cognitive restructuring for anxiety-provoking cognitions and was administered in eight individual sessions during a 6-week period. The predominantly female sample (85%) of 20 (intervention, $n = 10$; wait list, $n = 10$) had stage I cancer but represented six different disease sites. The sample was self-selected; individuals were recruited, having completed their medical therapy, from existing self-help groups. Psychological measures of anxiety, depression, and quality of life were administered, and a blood sample was drawn for cell counts at pre-, mid-, and post-treatment intervals. Analyses indicated significant reductions in both state and trait anxiety (STAI); however, no

**TABLE 6.3  Biologic (Endocrine, Immune, and Combined) Experimental Study Outcomes**

| | Theoretical/conceptual framework | Design | Sample | Measures | Results |
|---|---|---|---|---|---|
| **Endocrine** | | | | | |
| Cruess et al. (2000) | Cognitive-behavioral stress management | Group treatment; 10 sessions (20 hours); CBSM versus 1 session (6 hours) control (1 session CBSM); follow-up at 10 weeks | *N* = 34 women with stage I and II breast cancer | Plasma cortisol | 10 weeks postsurgery: plasma cortisol NS |
| **Immune** | | | | | |
| Elsesser, van Berkel, Sartory, Biermann-Gocke, & Ohl (1994) | None reported | Individual; anxiety management and stress inoculation training versus control; 8 sessions over 6 weeks; follow-up at 6 weeks | *N* = 20, 40% were women with breast cancer; stage not reported; 85% female | Bodily complaints; cell counts | 6 weeks: bodily complaints NS; cell counts NS |

*(continued)*

**TABLE 6.3  Biologic (Endocrine, Immune, and Combined) Experimental Study Outcomes** (*continued*)

| | Theoretical/ conceptual framework | Design | Sample | Measures | Results |
|---|---|---|---|---|---|
| Larson, Duberstein, Talbot, Caldwell, & Moynihan (2000) | None reported | Individual or small groups; presurgery psychosocial intervention versus no treatment; two 90-minute sessions and audiotape; follow-up 1 week postsurgery | $N = 41$ women with breast cancer, 90% stage I and II | Natural killer (NK) cell activity; IFN | 1 week postsurgery: NK cell activity NS; IFN NS |
| **Combined** | | | | | |
| Gruber et al. (1993) | None reported | Group relaxation, guided imagery, and biofeedback versus control; 9 weekly sessions, 3 monthly sessions, and audiotapes; follow-up 1 through 9 weeks | $N = 13$ women with breast cancer; stage not reported | Plasma cortisol; PBL; WBC; Con-A; NK cell activity | Plasma cortisol*; PBL*; WBC*; Con-A*; NK cell activity NS |

| | Theoretical/ conceptual framework | Design | Sample | Measures | Results |
|---|---|---|---|---|---|
| Richardson et al. (1997) | None reported | Group support versus imagery/ relaxation versus no treatment; 6 weekly sessions; follow-up at 6 weeks | $N = 47$ women with breast cancer, stages I-III; 73% female | Beta endorphins; NK activity; cytokines | Beta endorphins NS; NK activity NS; cytokines NS |
| Van der Pompe, Duivenoorden, Antoni, Visser, and Heijnen (1997) | None reported | Group; experiential-existential group psychotherapy (EEGP) versus control; 13 2.5-hour weekly sessions; follow-up at 13 weeks | $N = 31$ women with breast cancer, 74% stages II and III, 26% stage IV | Plasma cortisol; prolactin; PBL; NK cell activity; PHA | Plasma cortisol NS; prolactin NS; PBL NS; NK cell activity NS; PHA NS |

*Note: $p \leq .05$

significant differences existed in the remaining psychological measures or cell counts of total lymphocytes or T or B cells.

Larson, Duberstein, Talbot, Caldwell, and Moynihan (2000) reported on a randomized study comparing an intervention designed to reduce presurgical anxiety with no treatment (standard care) control for newly diagnosed breast cancer patients. The intervention consisted of two 90-minute (3 therapy hours) sessions that included information on common somatic and psychological reactions to stress, individualized active problem-solving strategies, support, and progressive muscle relaxation training (with an audiotape and instructions to practice). The sessions occurred at least one day prior to surgery, and depending on accrual rates, some intervention sessions were conducted individually while others were conducted with two to three patients. Procedures for accrual were not described; however, 41 women were randomized: 23 to the intervention group and 18 to the control. A heterogeneous group (stages I through IV) of breast cancer patients was included. Assessments included psychological measures of depression symptoms, traumatic stress, quality of life, and optimism, as well as immunologic assays for NK cell lysis and IFNg production. Assessments were completed pre- and postintervention (1 to 3 days prior to surgery) and one week following surgery. Data loss was substantial following the initial assessment, and repeated measures ANOVA revealed no significant group differences for either the psychological or immunologic measures.

BIOLOGIC RESPONSES STUDIES: ENDOCRINE AND IMMUNE

Three studies provided biologic outcomes for endocrine and immune interventions. Gruber et al. (1993) reported a randomized study comparing "enhanced" relaxation with a wait list control in a small group of women with stage I breast cancer. Progressive muscle relaxation was enhanced with guided imagery exercises and EMG biofeedback assistance. Treatment was administered in nine consecutive weekly sessions, followed by monthly sessions for 3 months. Thirteen women treated with surgery only (no adjuvant therapy) were randomized: seven to immediate treatment, six to the wait list. Psychological measures of mood, social support, and quality of life were completed pre- and post-treatment for both groups, but blood samples were drawn on a weekly basis. Analyses revealed no significant group differences on the psychological measures but showed significantly higher cell counts and blastogenesis with significantly lower levels of cortisol for the intervention group in comparison to the wait list. No group differences existed in the NK cell counts or the antibody assay.

Richardson et al. (1997) reported on a small sample randomized study comparing two group treatments—support versus imagery/relaxation—with a no-treatment control for stage I through III breast cancer patients. The support intervention focused on reducing stress, minimizing feelings of isolation, and enhancing self-esteem with six weekly sessions (duration not specified). The imagery intervention, also six sessions, provided instructions in relaxation, imaging ability, and breathing. In particular, the intervention attempted to use imagery to enhance the body's healing and stimulate immune functions. A sample was screened and 47 women (30%) accrued; they were assigned to support ($n = 16$), imagery/relaxation ($n = 16$), or control ($n = 15$) groups. Unfortunately, the groups differed significantly in the stage of disease (fewer stage II in the control group) as well as the receipt of adjuvant therapy (fewer in the control group). Analyses found no differences between groups in mood (POMS), quality of life (Functional Assessment of Cancer Therapy–Breast [FACT–B]), or any biologic variable. The only group differences were found in the measure of coping (ways of coping), which indicated that both intervention groups sought more support from others than did women in the control group. Also, women in the imagery group indicated use of positive coping strategies, whereas women in the support group reported trying to distance themselves from the stressor.

Van der Pompe, Duivenoorden, Antoni, Visser, and Heijnen (1997) conducted a randomized study comparing experiential-existential group psychotherapy with a wait list control for a small group of breast cancer patients. The treatment included expressing emotions through self-disclosure, body awareness exercises and relaxation, social support, and conflict resolution skills. Study participants were women with stage II, III, or recurrent breast cancer; no information was provided on accrual procedures. The intervention group included 15 women, and the wait list included 16 women; with attrition, however, data was analyzed from 11 intervention and 12 wait list subjects. Comparisons were also made with data from a sample of 15 age-matched healthy women from the community. Regression analyses suggested that there was no intervention effect on the endocrine or immune outcomes. Moreover, no significant correlations took place between changes in endocrine levels and psychological measures, and some immune findings were in the opposite direction (e.g., higher NK percent scores for the wait list group than the intervention group at post-treatment).

## Summary of Biologic Responses Studies

Since the research of Fawzy et al. (1990), psychoneuroimmunology studies with cancer patients have been conducted and collectively they illustrate the difficulties inherent in intervention research and the added challenge of including biologic measures. Some consistencies have emerged. First, three correlational reports (Sachs et al., 1995; Van der Pompe et al., 1997; Vitaliano et al., 1998) replicate the finding of "lower" immune responses for cancer patients versus healthy comparisons. Second, within the cancer samples, contrasting individuals who differ in their levels of stress and distress yield conceptually consistent effects, that is, "lower" immune/higher stress hormone (cortisol) responses for a high-stress group versus "higher" immune/lower stress hormone responses for the low-stress group (Andersen et al., 1998; Sachs et al., 1995; Vitaliano et al., 1998).

In contrast, data from experimental studies are less positive. Data analyses were hampered by the small sample sizes (e.g., numbers from 13 to 47), resulting in large within-group variability and/or insufficient power. Generalization can be further limited due to the selectivity of the samples and often high attrition. Thus, it is not surprising that analyses of intervention effects yielded null findings, with the exception of the cortisol data in the Cruess et al. (2000) report. Nevertheless, these reports are resources for investigators wanting to meet the methodological challenges faced in these pioneering efforts.

## DISEASE OUTCOMES AND MORTALITY

### Description of Disease Outcomes

Considerable interest exists in linking psychological interventions to disease course (see Figure 6.1). Early studies were not designed *a priori* to test disease endpoints (Sampson, 1997). However, the most comprehensive of them was by Fawzy et al. (1990). For patients with melanoma randomized to a psychoeducational intervention, differences in survival were reported, with 29% of controls but only 9% of experimental subjects dying after a 6-year follow-up (Fawzy et al., 1993). Also, Richardson, Zarnegar, Bisno, and Levine (1990) reported higher survival rates for intervention patients beyond the gains achieved with improved treatment compliance.

Two other studies provided data from patients with a poor prognosis. Spiegel, Bloom, et al. (Spiegel, Bloom, & Yalom, 1981; Spiegel & Bloom,

1983) randomized women to a supportive–expressive therapy intervention, and a 10-year follow-up indicated a significant survival time difference: 18.9 months for the control subjects and 36.6 months for the intervention subjects (Spiegel, Bloom, Kraemer, & Gottheil, 1989). However, a reanalysis of data suggests that the control group may have had more progressive disease, with more bone ($p = .07$) and lung metastases ($p = .09$), and receipt of more radical treatment (i.e., adrenalectomy, $p = .08$; Kogon, Biswas, Pearl, Carson, & Spiegel, 1997). In contrast, Linn, Linn, and Harris (1982) offered a supportive death and dying intervention to male cancer patients (46% had lung cancer) and found no survival advantage despite favorable quality of life outcomes. This is the context in which we consider the investigations of the last decade.

## Review of Disease Outcome Studies

Two experiments have been conducted (see Table 6.4): Cunningham et al. (Cunningham et al., 1998; Edmonds, Lockwood, & Cunningham, 1999) reported outcomes for a randomized study of a psychological intervention versus control (the provision of information only) for Canadian women with metastatic breast cancer. The intervention was designed to incorporate supportive–expressive elements (Spiegel et al., 1981), cognitive techniques (e.g., thought monitoring, goal setting, mental imaging, and homework exercises), and relaxation training. Treatment was conducted in a group format (5 to 8 patients with two therapists) of 35 weekly sessions of 2 hours each (70 therapy hours). An additional weekend-long session was also offered for coping skills training, with accompanying written materials. The control subjects received the written materials, two relaxation training audiotapes, and telephone calls at 2, 4, 6, 10, and 12 months to offer support and assist in study retention. Hospital records identified 246 female metastatic breast cancer patients, with 66 women (27%) eventually accrued and randomized: 30 to the intervention arm and 36 to the control arm.

Importantly, age (less than 50 years versus 50 or older) and presence and/or absence of visceral metastases were used as strata in randomization. Assessments were conducted at baseline and at 4, 8, and 14 months, with significant attrition for the latter assessments. Data on compliance with the intervention indicated that the intervention subjects attended 22 of 35 intervention sessions and completed, on average, 8 of 20 homework assignments. Baselines to follow-up change scores were calculated for the majority of the analyses and suggested no differential improvements or

**TABLE 6.4  Disease (Survival) Experimental Study Outcomes**

| | Theoretical/ conceptual framework | Design | Sample | Measures | Results |
|---|---|---|---|---|---|
| Cunningham et al. (1998) | Cognitive-behavioral therapy | Group support plus cognitive-behavioral therapy (SCBT; 35 2-hour weekly sessions, workbook, and audiotapes) versus control (written materials, audio-tapes, and 5 phone calls over 12 months); follow-up at 5 years | $N = 66$ women with metastatic breast cancer | Survival | Survival NS |
| Edelman, Bell, & Kidman (1999) | Cognitive-behavioral therapy | Group cognitive-behavioral therapy versus no treat-ment; 12 2-hour sessions and writ-ten materials; follow-up at 5 years | $N = 92$ women with metastatic breast cancer | Performance status; survival | Performance status NS; survival NS |

*Note: $p \leq .05$

reductions in distress (POMS), quality of life (Functional Living Index for Cancer, [FLIC]), mental adjustment to cancer, or social support. Moreover, Kaplan-Meier survival plots revealed no significant differences between the groups in 5 years of follow-up, with a median survival of 28 months for the intervention group and 24 months for the control group. Post hoc analyses examined several variables, with two being significant: Individuals reporting higher rates of physical exercise and those participating in an additional support group survived significantly longer.

Edelman et al. (Edelman, Bell, & Kidman, 1999; Edelman & Kidman, 1999; Edelman, Lemon, Bell, & Kidman, 1999) described the comparison of cognitive-behavioral therapy versus no treatment for Australian women with metastatic breast cancer. The intervention consisted of 12 sessions of 2 hours each (24 therapy hours) in a group format that included identifying and challenging maladaptive cognitions, problem solving, goal setting, assertive communication, homework exercises, relaxation training, and group support. Of 200 women approached for participation, 121 (61%) were accrued. Subjects were randomized by blocks of 10 to the two study arms, with 60 in the intervention group and 61 in the no-treatment group. Twenty-nine patients (24%), half of whom died of their disease, dropped out following the initial assessment. Analyses indicated that dropouts reported significantly higher levels of emotional distress, lower levels of self-esteem, more advanced disease, and lower performance status. Standardized self-report measures and physical performance status evaluations were completed at pre- and post-treatment and at 3- and 6-month follow-ups. Analyses indicated significant improvements for the intervention group in terms of significantly lower emotional distress (POMS) and higher self-esteem at the post-treatment assessment; however, differences were absent at the 3- and 6-month follow-ups. No changes existed in the performance status evaluations. Two years following completion of the trial, survival analyses were conducted with the entire sample ($N = 121$), at which time 85 individuals (70%) were deceased. Using a Cox regression model, only disease variables predicted survival, whereas the study arm did not.

## Summary of Disease Outcome Studies

Several efforts have been made to examine disease outcomes in recent years. The nonexperimental studies included breast (Gellert, Maxwell, & Siegel, 1993; Shrock, Palmer, & Taylor, 1999), prostate (Shrock et al., 1999), or a mixed-disease site sample (DeVries et al., 1997), with sample sizes ranging from 35 to 136 and follow-up intervals ranging from 4 to 10 years. All studies reported null effects. Of the experimental studies, both accrued women with recurrent breast cancer (Cunningham et al., 1998; Edelman, Bell, & Kidman, 1999; Edelman & Kidman, 1999; Edelman, Lemon, Bell, & Kidman, 1999). Sample sizes ranged from 66 to 127 and follow-ups were from 2 to 11 years. These studies also reported null effects. These are difficult studies to conduct, and maintaining accrual and retention goals are challenging as selective study samples, high rates of attrition, and weak and/or nonexistent intervention effects make testing the survival hypothesis all the more difficult.

## FUTURE DIRECTIONS FOR BIOBEHAVIORAL INTERVENTIONS

The previous summaries provide outcome-specific commentaries for methodological issues and areas of needed emphasis. Here cross-cutting methodological issues and research directions are discussed.

Three classes of variables—sociodemographic characteristics, premorbid status, and individual differences—are important issues to consider. Considering the first, study samples are not heterogeneous, as the young (e.g., 20 to 40 years), the old (65+ years), the non-Caucasian, the males, and the lower education and income groups remain understudied. Intervention study samples need to be more diverse; otherwise, the field is at risk of characterizing intervention outcomes for only middle-aged, middle-class women with cancer.

Concerning the second class of variables, premorbid status refers to both physical and mental health conditions that predate the onset of cancer. Most investigators screen out individuals with one or both conditions in a likely attempt to decrease heterogeneity. Screening, however, may adversely affect the likelihood of finding intervention effects, as either condition adds to the risk of adjustment difficulties (e.g., Satariano, 1992; Wells et al., 1989). In some studies, intervention effects were weak to nonexistent. Post hoc analyses often reveal interaction effects with individual differences, such that positive intervention effects are found only in patients with initial high distress rather than low distress (Antoni et al., 2001) or initial low rather than high levels of support (Helgeson et al., 2000). Moreover, the Helgeson et al. (2000) data suggest that a peer support intervention had a *negative* effect on the outcomes for women who began the study with high levels of support. Thus, investigators should reconsider and include individuals with histories of significant distress, such as depressive or anxiety disorders, and consider using screening measures and excluding those with initial levels of low distress.

Concerning the third class of variables, meta-analytic data have suggested that intervention effects on anxiety and perhaps depression are reliable (e.g., Sheard & Maguire, 1999). Some researchers with longitudinal data sets are attempting to characterize the post-treatment trajectory for individuals with differential levels of distress at diagnosis, and additional reports would be informative. Data from Epping-Jordan et al. (1999), for example, suggest that upwards of 80% of patients report low distress as they cope with cancer treatments and recover. Research must consider criteria that include rather than exclude patients with premorbid conditions as well as include only those of moderate to high levels of distress.

Research on individual differences can proceed in at least two salient directions. One avenue includes identifying psychological factors (aside from premorbid or overall stress levels) that place patients at risk for poorer psychological and behavioral outcomes. Some researchers have proposed models for predicting risk (e.g., such as Andersen, 1994), and other testable conceptualizations are needed. Thus far, empirical analyses have been based on social-cognitive factors, including attributions (e.g., self-blame in Glinder & Compas, 1999, and control in Astin et al., 1999) and social comparison processes (Stanton, Danoff-Burg, Snider, Cameron, & Kirk, 1999). They have also included the differential use of coping strategies (e.g., avoidant coping in McCall, Sandgren, King, O'Donnell, Branstetter, & Foreman, 1999 and emotion-focused disengagement in Epping-Jordan et al., 1999 and Livneh, 2000) as well as a study of individual difference variables (e.g., sexual self-schemas for sexual morbidity in Yurek, Farrar, & Andersen, 2000). A related direction is the analysis of positive, in contrast to negative, factors. This includes individual difference factors such as optimism (Epping-Jordan et al., 1999), but positive coping (Andrykowski et al., 1996), positive meaning, and perspective taking (Antoni et al., 2001) are other examples. Positive factors may take on added relevance if studies oversample the moderately to severely distressed, as these factors often vary with distress. These two directions would be important for future intervention studies as well as descriptive efforts.

Investigators have become more alert to the importance of fully describing the relevant characteristics (e.g., the site, stage, the time since diagnosis, and treatments received) of study samples, though continued vigilance is in order. An adequate description takes on added importance as the heterogeneity of study samples increases. The larger issue regarding cancer variables is the pattern of patient selection that has evolved. That is, study samples in the intervention studies are homogeneous, with an over-sampling of women, primarily women with breast cancer. The generalizability of our findings to both research and clinical contexts will be constrained if research does not have more diverse samples.

The interventions testing for psychological/behavioral, biologic, and/or disease outcomes were multimodal and included components consisting of stress reduction (usually progressive muscle relaxation training), disease and treatment information, cognitive-behavioral coping strategies, and social support, as was previously the case (Andersen, 1992). In an examination of treatment components, the factorial designs suggest that volunteers or peers may not be effective in a "support-only" context (Helgesen et al., 1999; McArdle et al., 1996), whereas peers or volunteers may be quite effective when asked to deliver a content-specific treatment, such as dietary counseling (e.g., Kristal et al., 1997). Aside from peers, other interventions were conducted by a range of professionals (e.g., psychologist, psychiatrist, nurse, and social worker) who performed similar tasks (e.g., relaxation or cognitive-behavioral interventions). The data do not show any differential outcomes among professionals.

The most novel intervention reviewed was the cost-effective physician communication training intervention of Rutter et al. (1996), with the also noteworthy clinic orientation of McQuellon et al. (1998). Both produced positive, immediate outcomes on measures of anxiety and depression. These interventions, as well as relaxation therapy alone (Larsson & Starrin, 1992), are the types of efforts that could be implemented widely for all cancer patients with more intensive efforts, such as group or individual interventions, reserved for moderate-to-high risk and/or high-distress patients. Moreover, with the latter patients, pharmacological therapy in combination with psychological/behavioral interventions might be considered (Heimberg et al., 1998).

Interventions for compliance and health behaviors have included strong educational components and behavioral strategies for change and maintenance. For health behavior interventions, it is unclear if the diet, exercise, and smoking cessation studies with cancer patients have benefited sufficiently from the basic research and intervention developments within these respective content areas (see Chapters 2, 3, and 8; Dubbert, 2002; Niaura & Abrams, 2002; Wadden, Brownell, & Foster, 2002). It is important to incorporate advances in the respective content areas as these behaviors have important health implications, and the early intervention efforts are encouraging, particularly for diet and exercise. Finally, interventions for compliance have been largely ignored. Descriptive studies with large samples of common drug regimens, combination regimes with high toxicity (e.g., chemo/radiation), and newer, promising therapies (e.g., Herceptin or Taxotere) are needed. Moreover, individuals at the highest risk for compliance problems (e.g., those with complex and/or high toxicity regimens or those with limited economic resources) need special attention, as was illustrated by Richardson et al. (1987).

Significant progress has been made in the domain of assessment. It would appear that general strategies have emerged for assessing self-reports of mood (e.g., POMS), depressive symptoms (e.g., CES-D), quality of life (e.g., SF-36), stress (e.g., impact of events or perceived stress scale), and related concepts. Measures such as these are sensitive to differences between groups and to change across time. However, if patients with premorbid difficulties and/or higher distress are included and/or oversampled, formal assessments of psychopathology and psychiatric history (e.g., diagnostic interviews) will likely become necessary.

Beyond stress and quality of life outcomes, the assessment of behavioral and biologic outcomes for the compliance, exercise, diet, and smoking cessation areas is important. Importantly, investigators have sampled from the assessment developments in the respective areas. For example, Richardson et al. (1987) took blood samples to document drug metabolites; Dimeo, Fetscher, Lange, Mertelsmann, and Keul (1997) assessed cardiac indices and functional status; Pierce et al. (1997) assessed biomarkers; and Wewers (e.g., Stanislaw & Wewers, 1994) used saliva cotinine samples to document nicotine intake. Despite the logistic difficulties and costs of these efforts, they are important as they confirm that behavioral interventions have the predicted effects on physical and/or biologic indicators.

Regarding endocrine and immune measures, the interventions used thus far are common to the stress and psychoneuroimmunology literatures (e.g., Miller & Cohen, 2001), although many have no particular relevance to cancer per se. The case can be made for selective ones, some hormonal responses (Gatti et al., 1993), or NK cell lysis or NK cell responses to cytokines, for example, where it is more difficult for others (e.g., cell proliferation or salivary IgA). Although assays of this sort are familiar and easy to perform, they have their drawbacks, as they are nonspecific and not enough data exist to show that changes in nonspecific immune responses are paralleled by changes in specific immune responses. For example, NK cell function may improve with an intervention in the hope that the disease outcome may change as well. However, if no tumor-specific T lymphocytes or antibodies can fight the tumor(s), the relevant disease outcomes will not improve.

In summary, intervention studies with cancer patients have been conducted more rapidly than ever, findings are disseminated, and replications and extensions are under way. The need for progress in addressing the behavioral issues of cancer is great, but we need to widen our accrual bases so that study participants represent the diversity of cancer, as the disease spares no race, gender, age, or ethnic group. The same is also true when considering issues of cancer survivorship. Finally, increasing the numbers of new behavioral scientists entering the area and training them with interdisciplinary mentors who can offer biobehavioral perspectives on the cancer problem are important tasks. These are the issues of a maturing discipline, and it is all the more exciting that psychological research in cancer has reached this milestone.

## ACKNOWLEDGMENT

This research was supported by the U.S. Army Medical Research Acquisition Activity Grants (DAMD17-94-J-4165 and DAMD17-96-1-6294) and the National Institutes of Mental Health (1 RO1 MH51487).

## REFERENCES

Andersen, B. L. (1992). Psychological interventions for cancer patients to enhance the quality of life. *Journal of Consulting and Clinical Psychology, 60,* 552–568.

Andersen, B. L. (1994). Surviving cancer. *Cancer, 74,* 1484–1495.

Andersen, B. L., Anderson, B., & deProsse, C. (1989). Controlled prospective longitudinal study of women with cancer: II. Psychological outcomes. *Journal of Consulting and Clinical Psychology, 57,* 692–697.

Andersen, B. L., Farrar, W. B., Golden-Kreutz, D., Kutz, L. A., MacCallum, R., Courtney, M. E, .et al. (1998). Stress and immune responses after surgical treatment for regional breast cancer. *Journal of the National Cancer Institute, 90,* 30–36.

Andersen, B. A., Kiecolt-Glaser, J. K., & Glaser, R. (1994). A biobehavioral model of cancer stress and disease course. *American Psychologist, 49*(3), 1–16.

Andrykowski, M. A., Curran, S. L., Studts, J. L., Cunningham, L., Carpenter, J. S., McGrath, P. C., et al. (1996). Psychosocial adjustment and quality of life in women with breast cancer and benign breast problems: A controlled comparison. *Journal of Clinical Epidemiology, 49,* 827–834.

Antoni, M. H., Lehman, J. M., Kilbourn, K. M., Boyers, A. E., Culver, J. L., Alferi, S. M., et al. (2001). Cognitive-behavioral stress management intervention decreases the prevalence of depression and enhances benefit finding among women under treatment for early-stage breast cancer. *Health Psychology, 20,* 20–32.

Astin, J. A., Anton-Culver, H., Schwartz, C. E., Shapiro, D. H., McQuade, J., Breuert, A. M., et al. (1999). Sense of control and adjustment to breast cancer: The importance of control coping styles. *Behavioral Medicine, 25,* 101–109.

Baquet, C. R., Horm, J. W., Gibbs, T., & Greenwald, P. (1991). Socioeconomic factors and cancer incidence among Blacks and Whites. *Journal of the National Cancer Institute, 83,* 551–557.

Bonadonna, G., & Valagussa, P. (1981). Dose-response effect of adjuvant chemotherapy in breast cancer. *New England Journal of Medicine, 304,* 10–15.

Broadhead, W. E., Gehlback, S. H., DeGruy, F. V., & Kaplan, B. H. (1988). The Duke-UNC Functional Social Support Questionnaire: Measurement of social support in family medicine patients. *Medical Care, 26,* 709–723.

Broeckel, J. A., Jacobsen, P. B., & Hann, D. M. (2000). Quality of life after adjuvant chemotherapy for breast cancer. *Breast Cancer Research and Treatment, 62,* 141–150.

Budman, D. R., Berry, D. A., Cirrincione, C. T., Henderson, I. C., Wood, W. C., Weiss, R. B., et al. (1998). Dose and dose intensity as determinants of outcome in the adjuvant treatment of breast cancer. *Journal of the National Cancer Institute, 90,* 1205–1211.

Camoriano, J. K., Loprinzi, C. L., Ingle, J. N., Therneau, T. M., Krook, J. E., & Veeder, M. H. (1990). Weight change in women treated with adjuvant therapy or observed following mastectomy for node-positive breast cancer. *Journal of Clinical Oncology, 8,* 1327–1334.

Clerici, M., Merola, M., Ferrario, E., Trabattoni, D., Villa, M. L., Stefanon, B., et al. (1997). Cytokine production patterns in cervical intraepithelial neoplasia: Association with human papillomavirus infection. *Journal of the National Cancer Institute, 89,* 245–250.

Cordova, M. J., Andrykowski, M. A., Kenady, D. E., McGrath, P. C., Sloan, D. A., & Redd, W. H. (1995). Frequency and correlates of PTSD-like symptoms following treatment for breast cancer. *Journal of Consulting and Clinical Psychology, 63,* 981–986.

Cruess, D. G., Antoni, M. H., McGregor, B. A., Kilbourn, K. M., Boyers, A. E., Alferi, S. M., et al. (2000). Cognitive-behavioral stress management reduces serum cortisol by enhancing benefit finding among women being treated for early stage breast cancer. *Psychosomatic Medicine, 62,* 304–308.

Cunningham, A. J., Edmonds, C. V. I., Jenkins, G. P., Pollack, H., Lockwood, G. A., & Warr, D. (1998). A randomized controlled trial of the effects of group psychological therapy on survival in women with metastatic breast cancer. *Psycho-oncology, 7,* 508–517.

Denmark-Wahnefried, W., Hars, V., Conaway, M. R., Havlin, K., Rimer, B. K., McElveen, G., et al. 1997. Reduced rates of metabolism and decreased physical activity in breast cancer patients receiving adjuvant chemotherapy. *American Journal of Clinical Nutrition, 65,* 1495–1501.

DeVries, M. J., Schilder, J., Mulder, C., Vrancken, A. M. E., Remie, M. E., & Garssen, B. (1997). Phase II study of psychotherapeutic intervention in advanced cancer. *Psycho-oncology, 6,* 129–137.

Dimeo, F., Fetscher, S., Lange, W., Mertelsmann, R., & Keul, J. (1997). Effects of aerobic exercise on the physical performance and incidence of treatment-related complications after high-dose chemotherapy. *Blood, 90,* 3390–3394.

Dubbert, P. (in press.) Exercise. *Journal of Consulting and Clinical Psychology, 70.*

Edelman, S., Bell, D. R., & Kidman, A. D. (1999). A group cognitive behavior therapy programme with metastatic breast cancer patients. *Psycho-oncology, 8,* 295–305.

Edelman, S., & Kidman, A. D. (1999). Description of a group cognitive behavior therapy programme with cancer patients. *Psycho-oncology, 8,* 306–314.

Edelman, S., Lemon, J., Bell, D. R., & Kidman, A. D. (1999). Effects of group CBT on the survival time of patients with metastatic breast cancer. *Psycho-oncology, 8,* 474–481.

Edmonds, C. V. I., Lockwood, G. A., & Cunningham, A. J. (1999). Psychological response to long term group therapy: A randomized trial with women with metastatic breast cancer patients. *Psycho-oncology, 8,* 74–91.

Elsesser, K., van Berkel, M., Sartory, G., Biermann-Gocke, W., & Ohl, S. (1994). The effects of anxiety management training on psychological variables and immune parameters in cancer patients: A pilot study. *Behavioral and Cognitive Psychotherapy, 22,* 13–23.

Emmons, K. M., Goldstein, M. G., Roberts, M., Cargill, B., Sherman, C. B., Millman, R., et al. (2000). The use of nicotine replacement therapy during hospitalization. *Annuals of Behavioral Medicine, 22,* 325–329.

Epping-Jordan, J. E., Compas, B. E., Osowiecki, D. M., Oppedisano, G., Gerhardt, C., Primo, K., et al. (1999). Psychological adjustment in breast cancer: Processes of emotional distress. *Health Psychology, 18,* 315–326.

Evans, D. L., McCartney, C. F., Nemeroff, C. B., Raft, D., Quade, D., Golden, R. N., et al. (1986). Depression in women treated for gynecological cancer: Clinical and neuroendocrine assessment. *American Journal of Psychiatry, 143,* 447–452.

Ey, S., Compas, B. E., Epping-Jordan, J. E., & Worsham, N. (1998). Stress responses and psychological adjustment in patients with cancer and their spouses. *Journal of Psychosocial Oncology, 16,* 59–77.

Fawzy, F. I., Cousins, N., Fawzy, N. W., Kemeny, M. E., Elashoff, R., & Morton, D. (1990). A structured psychiatric intervention for cancer patients: I. Changes over time in immunological measures. *Archives of General Psychiatry, 47,* 729–735.

Fawzy, F. I., Fawzy, N. W., Hyun, C. S., Elashoff, R., Guthrie, D., Fahey, J. L., et al. (1993). Malignant melanoma: Effects of a structured psychiatric intervention, coping, affective state, and immune parameters on recurrence and survival 6 years later. *Archives of General Psychiatry, 50,* 681–689.

Felten, D. L., Ackerman, K. D., Wiegand, S. J., & Felten, S. Y. (1987). Noradrenergic sympathetic innervation of the spleen: I. Nerve fibers associate with lymphocytes and macrophages in specific compartments of the splenic white pulp. *Journal of Neuroscience Research, 18,* 28–36.

Fukui, S., Kugaya, A., Okamure, H., Kamiya, M., Koike, M., Nakanishi, T., et al. (2000). A psychosocial group intervention for Japanese women with primary breast carcinoma. *Cancer, 89*, 1026–1036.

Ganz, P. A., Coscarelli, A., Fred, C., Kahn, B., Polinsky, M. L., & Petersen, L. (1996). Breast cancer survivors: Psychosocial concerns and quality of life. *Breast Cancer Research and Treatment, 38*, 183–199.

Gatti, G., Masera, R. G., Pallavinini, L., Sartori, M. L., Staurenghi, A., & Orlandi, F. (1993). Interplay in vitro between ACTH, beta-endorphin, and glucocorticoid in the modulation of spontaneous and lymphokine-inducible human natural killer (NK) cell activity. *Brain, Behavior, and Immunity, 7*, 16–28.

Gellert, G. A., Maxwell, R. M., & Siegel, B. S. (1993). Survival of breast cancer patients receiving adjunctive psychosocial support therapy: A 10-year follow-up study. *Journal of Clinical Oncology, 11*, 66–69.

Glinder, J. G., & Compas, B. E. (1999). Self-blame attributions in women with newly diagnosed breast cancer: A prospective study of psychological adjustment. *Health Psychology, 18*, 475–481.

Gotay, C. C., & Muraoka, M. Y. (1998). Quality of life in long-term survivors of adult-onset cancers. *Journal of the National Cancer Institute, 90*, 656–667.

Green, B. L., Krupnick, J. L., Rowland, J. H., Epstein, S. A., Stockton, P., Spertus, I., et al. (2000). Trauma history as a predictor of psychologic symptoms in women with breast cancer. *Journal of Clinical Oncology, 18*, 1084–1093.

Griebel, B., Wewers, M. E., & Baker, C. A. (1998). The effectiveness of a nurse-managed minimal smoking-cessation intervention among hospitalized patients with cancer. *Oncology Nursing Forum, 25*, 897–902.

Gritz, E. R., Carr, C. R., Rapkin, D., Abemayor, E., Chang, L. C., Wong, W., et al. (1993). Predictors of long-term smoking cessation in head and neck cancer patients. *Cancer Epidemiology Biomarkers & Prevention, 2*, 261–270.

Gruber, B. L., Hersh, S. P., Hall, N. R. S., Waletzky, L. R., Kunz, J. F., Carpenter, J. K., et al. (1993). Immunological responses of breast cancer patients to behavioral interventions. *Biofeedback and Self-Regulation, 18*, 1–22.

Grunberg, N. E., & Straub, R. O. (1992). The role of gender and taste class in the effects of stress on eating. *Health Psychology, 11*, 97–100.

Hagedoorn, M., Kuijer, R. G., Buunk, B. P., DeJohng, G. M., Wobbes, T., & Sanderman, R. (2000). Marital satisfaction in patients with cancer: Does support from intimate partners benefit those who need it the most? *Health Psychology, 19*, 274–282.

Heimberg, R. G., Liebowitz, M. R., Hope, D. A., Schneider, F. R., Holt, C. S., Weolkowitz, L., et al. (1998). Cognitive-behavioral group therapy versus phenelzine in social phobia: 12 week outcome. *Archives of General Psychiatry, 55*, 1133–1141.

Helgeson, V. S., Cohen, S., Schulz, R., & Yasko, J. (1999). Education and peer discussion group interventions and adjustment to breast cancer. *Archives of General Psychiatry, 56*, 340–347.

Helgeson, V. S., Cohen, S., Schulz, R., & Yasko, J. (2000). Group support interventions for women with breast cancer: Who benefits from what? *Health Psychology, 19*, 107–114.

Hewitt, M., Breen, N., & Devesa, S. (1999). Cancer prevalence and survivorship issues: Analyses of the 1992 National Health Interview Survey. *Journal of the National Cancer Institute, 91*, 1480–1486.

Jacobsen, P. B., Bovberg, D. H., Schwartz, M. D., Hudis, C. A., Gilewski, T. A., & Norton, L. (1995). Conditioned emotional distress in women receiving chemotherapy for breast cancer. *Journal of Consulting and Clinical Psychology, 63*, 108–114.

Joffe, R. T., Rubinow, D. R., Denicoff, K. D., Maher, M., & Sindelar, W. F. (1986). Depression and carcinoma of the pancreas. *General Hospital Psychiatry, 8*, 241–245.

Kogon, M. M., Biswas, A., Pearl, D., W. Carson, R., & Spiegel, D. (1997). Effects of medical and psychotherapeutic treatment on the survival of women with metastatic breast carcinoma. *Cancer, 80*, 225–230.

Kristal, A. R., Shattuck, A. L., Bowen, D. J., Sponzo, R. W., & Nixon, D. W. (1997). Feasibility of using volunteer research staff to deliver and evaluate a low-fat dietary intervention: The American Cancer Society Breast Cancer Dietary Intervention Project. *Cancer Epidemiology, Biomarkers & Prevention, 6*, 459–467.

Lacks, P., & Morin, C. M. (1992). Recent advances in the assessment and treatment of insomnia. *Journal of Consulting and Clinical Psychology, 60*, 586–594.

Larson, M. R., Duberstein, P. R., Talbot, N. L., Caldwell, C., & Moynihan, J. A. (2000). A presurgical psychosocial intervention for breast cancer patients: Psychological distress and the immune response. *Journal of Psychosomatic Research, 48*, 187–194.

Larsson, G., & Starrin, B. (1992). Relaxation training as an integral part of caring activities for cancer patients: Effects on well-being. *Scandinavian Journal of Caring Sciences, 6*, 179–186.

Lebovits, A. H., Strain, J. J., Schleifer, S. J., Tanaka, J. S., Bhardwaj, S., & Messe, M. R. (1990). Patient noncompliance with self-administered chemotherapy. *Cancer, 65*, 17–22.

Levin, M., Mermelstein, H., & Rigberg, C. (1999). Factors associated with acceptance or rejection of recommendation for chemotherapy in a community cancer center. *Cancer Nursing, 22*, 246–250.

Ley, P. (1988). *Communicating with patients.* London: Chapman & Hall.

Linn, M. W., Linn, B. S., & Harris, R. (1982). Effects of counseling for late stage cancer patients. *Cancer, 49*, 1048–1055.

Livneh, H. (2000). Psychosocial adaptation to cancer: The role of coping strategies. *Journal of Rehabilitation, 66*, 40–49.

Macquart-Moulin, G., Viens, P., Palangie, T., Bouscary, M. L., Delozier, T., Roche, H., et al. (2000). High-dose sequential chemotherapy with recombinant granulocyte colony-stimulating factor and repeated stem-cell support for inflammatory breast cancer patients: Does impact on quality of life jeopardize feasibility and acceptability of treatment? *Journal of Clinical Oncology, 18*, 754–764.

Madden, K. S., & Livnat, S. (1991). Catecholamine action and immunologic reactivity. In R. Ader, D. L. Felten, & N. Cohen (Eds.), *Psychoneuroimmunology* (2nd ed., pp. 283–310). San Diego, CA: Academic Press, Inc.

Maier, S. F., Watkins, L. R., & Fleshner, M. (1994). Psychoneuroimmunology: The interface between behavior, brain, and immunity. *American Psychologist, 49*, 1004–1017.

Maunsell, E., Brisson, J., & Deschenes, L. (1992). Psychological distress after initial treatment of breast cancer. *Cancer, 70*, 120–125.

McArdle, J. M. C., George, W. D., McArdle, C. S., Smith, D. C., Moodie, A. R., Hughson, A. V. M., et al. (1996). Psychological support for patients undergoing breast cancer surgery: A randomized study. *British Medical Journal, 312*, 813–816.

McDaniel, J. S., Musselman, D. L., Porter, M. R., Reed, D. A., & Nemeroff, C. B. (1995). Depression in patients with cancer: Diagnosis, biology, and treatment. *Archives of General Psychiatry, 52*, 89–99.

McDonough, E. J., Boyd, J. H., Varvares, M. A., & Maves, M. D. (1996). Relationship between psychological status and compliance in a sample of patients treated for cancer of the head and neck. *Head & Neck, 18*, 269–276.

McQuellon, R. P., Wells, M., Hoffman, S., Craven, K. B., Russell, K. G., Cruz, J., et al. (1998). Reducing distress in cancer patients with an orientation program. *Psychooncology, 7*, 207–217.

Miller, G. E., & Cohen, S. (2001). Psychological interventions and the immune system: A meta-analytic review and critique. *Health Psychology, 20*, 47–63.

Moorey, S., Greer, S., Bliss, J., & Law, M. (1998). A comparison of adjuvant psychological therapy and supportive counseling in patients with cancer. *Psychooncology, 7*, 218–228.

National Cancer Institute. (2000). SEER Cancer Statistics Review, 1973–1997. Retrieved January 18, 2002, from http://seer.cancer.gov/.

Niaura, R., & Abrams, D. (in press). Smoking Cessation. *Journal of Consulting and Clinical Psychology, 70*.

Pierce, J. P., Faerber, S., Wright, F. A., Newman, V., Flatt, S. W., Kealey, S., et al. (1997). Feasibility of a randomized trial of a high vegetable diet to prevent breast cancer recurrence. *Nutrition and Cancer, 28*, 282–288.

Pinto, B. M., Eakin, E., & Maruyama, N. C. (2000). Health behavior changes after a cancer diagnosis: What do we know and where do we go from here? *Annals of Behavioral Medicine, 22*, 38–52.

Rabin, B. S., Cohen, S., Ganguli, R., Lysle, D. T., & Cunnick, J. E. (1989). Bidirectional interaction between the central nervous system and the immune system. *Critical Reviews in Immunology, 9*, 279–312.

Redd, W. J., Montgomery, G. H., & DuHamel, K. N. (2001). Behavioral intervention for cancer treatment side effects. *Journal of the National Cancer Institute, 93*, 810–823.

Richardson, J. L., Marks, G., Johnson, C. A., Graham, J. W., Chan, K. K., Selser, J. N., et al. (1987). Path model of multidimensional compliance with cancer therapy. *Health Psychology, 6*, 183–207.

Richardson, J. L., Marks, G., & Levine, A. M. (1988). The influence of symptoms of disease and side effects of treatment on compliance with cancer therapy. *Journal of Clinical Oncology, 6*, 1746–1752.

Richardson, J. L., Zarnegar, Z., Bisno, B., & Levine, A. (1990). Psychosocial status at initiation of cancer treatment and survival. *Journal of Psychosomatic Research, 34,* 189–201.

Richardson, M. A., Post-White, J., Grimm, E. A., Moye, L. A., Singletary, S. E., & Justice, B. (1997). Coping, life attitudes, and immune responses to imagery and group support after breast cancer treatment. *Alternative Therapies, 3,* 62–70.

Roth, A. J., & Massie, M. J. (2001). Psychiatric complications in cancer patients. In R. E. Lenhard, R. T. Osteem, & T. Tansler (Eds.), *ACS's clinical oncology* (pp. 837–851). Atlanta, GA: American Cancer Society.

Rutter, D. R., Iconomou, G., & Quine, L. (1996). Doctor-patient communication and outcome in cancer patients: An intervention. *Psychology and Health, 12,* 57–71.

Sabharwal, P. J., Glaser, R., Lafuse, W., Liu, Q., Arkins, S., Koojiman, R., et al. (1992). Prolactic synthesis and secretion by human peripheral blood mononuclear cells: An autocrine growth factor for lymphoproliferation. *Proceedings of the National Academy of Science, 89,* 7713–7716.

Sachs, G., Rasoul-Rockenschaub, S., Aschauer, H., Spiess, K., Gober, I., Staffen, A., et al. (1995). Lytic effector cell activity and major depressive disorder in patients with breast cancer: A prospective study. *Journal of Neuroimmunology, 59,* 83–89.

Sampson, W. L. (1997). Studies of counselings' impact on survival challenged: AAAS meeting. *Oncology News, 6*(6), 1–2.

Satariano, W. A. (1992). Comorbidity and functional status in older women with breast cancer: Implications for screening, treatment, and prognosis. *The Journals of Gerontology, 47,* 24–31.

Scheier, M., Carver, C. S., & Bridges, M. (1994). Distinguishing optimism from neuroticism (and trait anxiety, self-mastery, and self-esteem): A re-evaluation of the Life Orientation Test. *Journal of Personality and Social Psychology, 67,* 1063–1078.

Sheard, T., & Maguir, P. (1999). The effect of psychological interventions on anxiety and depression in cancer patients: Results of two meta-analyses. *British Journal of Cancer, 80,* 1770–1780.

Shrock, D., Palmer, R. F., & Taylor, B. (1999). Effects of a psychosocial intervention on survival among patients with stage I breast and prostate cancer: A matched case-control study. *Alternative Therapies and Health Medicine, 5,* 49–55.

Spencer, S. M., Lehman, J. M., Wynings, C., Arena, P., Carver, C. S., Antoni, M. H., et al. (1999). Concerns about breast cancer and relations to psychosocial well-being in a multiethnic sample of early stage patients. *Health Psychology, 18,* 159–168.

Spiegel, D., & Bloom, J. R. (1983). Group therapy and hypnosis reduce metastatic breast carcinoma pain. *Psychosomatic Medicine, 45,* 333–339.

Spiegel, D., Bloom, J. R., Kraemer, H. C., & Gottheil, E. (1989). Effect of psychosocial treatment on survival of patients with metastatic breast cancer. *Lancet, 2,* 888–901.

Spiegel, D., Bloom, J. R., & Yalom, I. (1981). Group support for patients with metastatic cancer: A randomized outcome study. *Archives of General Psychiatry, 38,* 527–533.

Stanislaw, A. W., & Wewers, M. E. (1994). A smoking cessation intervention with hospitalized surgical cancer patients: A pilot study. *Cancer Nursing, 17*, 81–86.

Stanton, A. L., Danoff-Burg, S., Snider, P. R., Cameron, C. L., & Kirk, S. B. (1999). Social comparison and adjustment to breast cancer: An experimental examination of upward affiliation and downward evaluation. *Health Psychology, 18*, 151–158.

Stanton, A. L., Kirk, S. B., Cameron, C. L., & Danoff-Burg, S. (2000). Coping through emotional approach: Scale construction and validation. *Journal of Personality and Social Psychology, 78*, 1150–1169.

Stat bite. (1998). *Journal of the National Cancer Institute, 90*, 565.

Stoll, B. A. (1996). Diet and exercise regimens to improve breast carcinoma prognosis. *Cancer, 78*, 2465–2470.

Swain, S. M., Rowland, J., Weinfurt, K., Berg, C., Lippman, M. E., Walton, L., et al. (1996). Intensive outpatient adjuvant therapy for breast cancer: Results of dose escalation and quality of life. *Journal of Clinical Oncology, 14*, 1565–1572.

Van der Pompe, G., Duivenoorden, H. J., Antoni, M. H., Visser, A., & Heijnen, C. J. (1997). Effectiveness of a short-term group psychotherapy program on endocrine and immune function in breast cancer patients: An exploratory study. *Journal of Psychosomatic Research, 42*, 453–466.

Vitaliano, P. P., Scanlan, J. M., Ochs, H. D., Syrjala, K., Siegler, I. C., & Snyder, E. A. (1998). Psychosocial stress moderates the relationship of cancer history with natural killer cell activity. *Annals of Behavioral Medicine, 20*, 199–203.

Vokes, E. E., Haraf, D. J., Stenson, K., List, M., Humerickhouse, R., Dolan, M. E., et al. (2000). Concomitant chemoradiotherapy as primary therapy for loco-regionally advanced head and neck cancer. *Journal of Clinical Oncology, 18*, 1652–1661.

Wadden, T. A., Brownell, K. D., & Foster, G. D. Obesity. (in press.) *Journal of Consulting and Clinical Psychology, 70*.

Wellish, D. K., Wolcott, D., Pasnau, R., Fawzy, F., & Landsverk, J. (1989). An evaluation of the psychosocial problems of the homebound cancer patient: Relationship of patient adjustment to family problems. *Journal of Psychosocial Research, 7*, 55–76.

Wells, K. B., Steward, A., Hays, R. D., Burnam, A., Rogers, W., Daniels, M., et al. (1989). The functioning and well-being of depressed patients: Results from the Medical Outcomes Study. *Journal of the American Medical Association, 262*, 914–919.

Wewers, M. E., Bowen, J. M., Stanislaw, A. E., & Desimone, V. B. (1994). A nurse-delivered smoking cessation intervention among hospitalized postoperative patients—influence of a smoking-related diagnosis: A pilot study. *Heart & Lung, 23*, 151–156.

Woods, J. A., Davis, J. M., Smith, J. A., & Nieman, D. C. (1999). Exercise and cellular innate immune function. *Medicine and Science in Sports and Exercise, 31*, 57–66.

Yurek, D., Farrar, W., & Andersen, B. L. (2000). Breast cancer surgery: Comparing surgical groups and determining individual differences in post operative sexuality and body change stress. *Journal of Consulting and Clinical Psychology, 68*, 697–709.

# 7

---
---

# The PRO-SELF© Program:
# A Self-Care Intervention Program

---
---

## Marylin J. Dodd
## Christine Miaskowski

Patients usually do better, physiologically and psychologically, when the symptoms associated with cancer treatment (e.g., nausea, fatigue, or hair loss) are either prevented or, at the very least, managed effectively. Most importantly, during treatment protocols, patients want their symptoms managed effectively so that they can maintain their treatment protocols, obtain the best clinical outcome, and have the best possible quality of life during treatment (Griffiths & Leek, 1995).

Most of the materials and approaches used to assist oncology patients with managing their symptoms lack empiric testing. As a result, most symptom-management strategies are not evidenced based, are quite variable in terms of the information and the skills training they provide to the patient to monitor and manage anticipated symptoms, are inconsistent in their approaches, and are unclear as to what results are to be achieved due to implementing the symptom-management strategy. Further, now that the majority of oncology patients receive their treatment on an outpatient basis and must manage their treatment-related symptoms at home, it is even more imperative that patients have the essential information, skills, and support to carry out effective self-care symptom management without the direct supervision of a healthcare provider.

Symptom management using the PRO-SELF Program is the focus of this chapter. It discusses the clinical trials conducted over the past decade that have focused on facilitating patient and family symptom control during the treatment of cancer, HIV/AIDS, and Parkinson's disease. A discussion of the self-care framework is included. Interventions and results for a variety of symptoms are discussed and detailed. The implications for further research are presented in the final section. Table 7.1 summarizes the PRO-SELF Program series of studies.

The PRO-SELF Program is designed to provide adult patients undergoing cancer treatment with the information, skills, and support needed to engage effectively and consistently in prescribed self-care symptom management. PRO-SELF simply means "For You." The aim of the Program is to enhance patients' self-care abilities and thereby prevent or reduce the severity and duration of the symptoms associated with their disease and treatment. The PRO-SELF Program is based on Orem's theory of self-care. The purpose of this chapter is to describe the development, testing, and refinement of the PRO-SELF Program, a self-care intervention used in randomized clinical trials. The PRO-SELF Program has made an important contribution in enhancing patients' self-care and reducing morbidity. It is believed to be highly generalizable to children and adolescents who have cancer and to their families.

## BACKGROUND

Interventions focused on assisting patients with the cancer treatment experience have been reported in the oncology literature for over 20 years. Studies have tested the effects of psychoeducational, psychosocial, and symptom-management strategies. The targeted results have ranged from decreasing mood disturbances to prolonging the patient's life (Devine & Westlake, 1995; Fawzy, Fawzy, Arndt, & Pasnau, 1995; Griffiths & Leek, 1995; Meyer & Mark, 1995; Smith, Holcombe, & Stullenbarger, 1994; Spiegel, 1995). In almost every instance, results from these studies indicate that patients who received specific interventions generally did better than patients who served as controls. This generalization holds true, regardless of the approach. However, these studies typically had small numbers of patients, used a wide variety of approaches to improve symptom management, and focused most outcome measurement on the psychosocial dimensions of care. A review of the published literature indicates that very few of these studies were replicated and, if replicated, did not always corroborate earlier findings. This work, although important in determining potentially useful approaches for improving symptom management, does not provide clinicians with clear empiric evidence of the best approach to use.

**TABLE 7.1  PRO-SELF Program Intervention**

| | Theoretical/ conceptual framework | Design | Sample | Measures | Results |
|---|---|---|---|---|---|
| Dodd et al. (1992) | Physiology/ pathophysiology, pharmacology, self-care, Adult Learning Theory | Randomized control trial (RCT), 2-group design; self-care intervention targeted nausea, vomiting, mucositis, and infection | N = 127 with mixed cancers, initiating chemotherapy | Reduce chemotherapy morbidity. | Not significant |
| Dodd et al. (1996) | Physiology/ pathophysiology, pharmacology, self-care, Adult Learning Theory | RCT, 2-group design; self-care intervention targeted prevention of chemotherapy-induced mucositis | N = 222 with mixed cancers, receiving mucositis-inducing chemotherapy | Reduce incidence of mucositis. | Not significant |
| Dodd et al. (2000) | Physiology/ pathophysiology, pharmacology, self-care, Adult Learning Theory | RCT, 3-group design; self-care intervention targeted treatment of chemotherapy-induced mucositis | N = 204 with mixed cancers, developed chemotherapy-induced mucositis | Reduce incidence of mucositis. | Not significant |

(continued)

**TABLE 7.1  PRO-SELF Program Intervention** (*continued*)

| | Theoretical/ conceptual framework | Design | Sample | Measures | Results |
|---|---|---|---|---|---|
| Dodd et al. (1998–2001) | Physiology/ pathophysiology, pharmacology, self-care, Adult Learning Theory | RCT, 2-group design (pilot); self-care intervention targeted radiation therapy-induced mucositis | $N = 30$ head and neck cancer patients | Reduce incidence of mucositis. | Not significant |
| Dodd et al. (1999–2004) | Physiology/ pathophysiology, exercise training, self-care | RCT, 3-group design; individualized home-based exercise prescription | $N = 65$ with mixed cancers, cancer-related fatigue | Manage chemotherapy-related fatigue. | Ongoing |
| MacPhail et al. (1999) | Physiology/ pathophysiology, pharmacology, self-care, Adult Learning Theory | RCT, 2-group design; self-care intervention targeted oral hygiene and dietary modifications, recurrence of oral candidiasis | $N = 35$ HIV positive, oral candidiasis | Increase inter-episode time for recurrences of oral candidiasis. | Data analyses ongoing |

| | Theoretical/ conceptual framework | Design | Sample | Measures | Results |
|---|---|---|---|---|---|
| Miaskowski, Dodd, Koo, Tripathy, & Paul (2001) | Physiology/ pathophysiology, pharmacology, self-care, Adult Learning Theory | RCT, 2-group design; stratified on presence or absence of family caregiver; self-care intervention with academic detailing; targeted pain relief | $N = 200$ with mixed cancers, metastatic bone pain | Reduce pain. | PRO-SELF intervention group reported significantly less pain, shorter duration of daily pain, increased consumption of analgesics |

Self-care is a critically important dimension of healthcare for patients undergoing cancer treatment to understand and achieve. Dodd et al. (1984a, 1984b, 1988a, 1988b) found that patients reported modest levels of self-care activities used to manage the side effects of treatment. However, no self-care activities were employed to prevent the side effects of cancer treatment. Patients waited until the side effects were severe and persistent before initiating self-care measures.

With evidence that intervention is necessary, treatment information and suggestions for managing the side effects of treatment were developed and tested. Patients could use targeted information to learn about their treatment and perform self-care activities (Dodd, 1987, 1988a, 1988b). The question of whether increasing self-care activities would decrease morbidity was not posed in these early studies. Larson et al. identified that patients in high-risk situations, such as those undergoing bone marrow transplants and those undergoing intensive outpatient chemotherapy protocols, wanted to engage in self-care activities and needed these activities presented in an organized and pragmatic manner (Larson, 1995; Larson, Viele, Coleman, Dibble, & Cebulski, 1993).

Changes in clinical practice that impacted self-care were documented in a descriptive, longitudinal (6-month) study of 100 oncology outpatients and their family caregivers (Dodd, Lindsey, Larson, & Musci, 1990). First, chemotherapy protocols were becoming more complex and aggressive, causing increases in treatment-related morbidity. Second, patient management of treatment-related side effects by trial and error tended to be very costly in terms of energy and time (Dodd & Dibble, 1993). Third, with the advent of the Diagnostic Related Groups and managed care, outpatient treatment became the preferred approach for providing care to oncology patients. It was evident that the development of an effective approach for teaching patients self-care strategies was urgently needed. This approach would help oncology outpatients become proficient and competent in the management of side effects of cancer and cancer treatment. Furthermore, such an approach needed to be tested in a clinical trial format to determine its effectiveness.

This chapter describes the work the PRO-SELF team has accomplished in developing, testing, and refining a self-care intervention focused on decreasing the symptoms associated with cancer (e.g., metastatic bone pain) or cancer treatment (e.g., mucositis). This work has occurred through the collaborations with multidisciplinary team members from nursing, dentistry, medicine, exercise physiology, pharmacy, biostatistics, and social sciences. First, cancer-related interventions are discussed, then HIV/AIDS and Parkinson's disease interventions are summarized, and then the evolution of the PRO-SELF Program and future research directions are addressed.

## THE PRO-SELF PROGRAM

### Development

The development of the PRO-SELF Program encompassed several steps. First, 10 experienced clinical nurse specialists participated in a consultation seminar to determine the ideal, creative, and realistic nursing intervention to decrease the symptom morbidity associated with aggressive chemotherapy treatment. These nurses indicated that patients needed information about their disease, treatment, and side effects; instruction in essential self-care skills; and ongoing supportive nursing care. This information, instruction, and support needed to be presented in a timely and consistent manner by all nurses involved in the patient's care. Although nurses in their various treatment settings wanted to provide this comprehensive care to all their patients, for a variety of reasons (e.g., lack of time, too many patients, or too many interruptions), patients occasionally did not receive essential information related to symptom control. Also, with chemotherapy shifted to the outpatient setting, almost all the patients' self-care activities related to symptom management required management in the home without direct supervision by a healthcare provider. Initially, the development of the PRO-SELF Program to manage the symptoms of cancer and cancer treatment focused on intervening with the patient. As PRO-SELF work progressed, family caregivers were incorporated into the program.

### The Content and Process Involved in the PRO-SELF Program

Orem's Theory of Self-Care Deficit in Nursing provides the theoretical foundation of the PRO-SELF Program. Orem's theory proposes that by increasing a patient's self-care agency (abilities) the probability of obtaining desired health outcomes is increased: "Self-care is the practice of activities that individuals initiate and perform on their own behalf in maintaining life, health, and well-being" (Orem, 1995, p. 104). The four key constructs of PRO-SELF Program are self-care, therapeutic self-care demand, self-care agency, and nursing. Orem defined *therapeutic self-care demand* as "a specification of the kinds and number of care measures that are known or presumed to be regulatory of an individual's human functioning and development within some time frame" (p. 187). For example, a therapeutic self-care demand is created when a patient receiving chemotherapy experiences a side effect. *Self-care agency* is defined as "the complex acquired capability to meet one's continuing requirement for care of self" (p. 212). Using the PRO-SELF Program, the patient's self-care agency is enhanced through the provision of relevant information, the enhancement of self-care skills, and the provision of support. Nursing is needed when a deficit exists between the patient's self-care agency and the existing therapeutic self-care demands.

INFORMATION (KNOWLEDGE)

To assist patients in managing the cancer treatment experience, it has been generally believed that patients need comprehensive information on the specifics of their disease and treatment, associated symptoms, and approaches to symptom management. Frequently, the latter two areas are not addressed until patients actually experience symptoms. The first test of the PRO-SELF Program (described later) was a clinical trial that focused on reducing four side effects associated with chemotherapy: nausea, vomiting, mucositis, and infection. The written materials provided to patients contained both general information about cancer and its treatment and self-care strategies that patients could use to deal with these four side effects. The written materials were supplemented with individualized treatment-related information (Dodd et al., 1992). The findings from this first clinical trial revealed nonsignificant differences between the intervention group and the control group on the designated outcomes. Patient feedback indicated that they were overwhelmed with too much information.

Subsequently, the research team members decided to focus on only one cancer treatment symptom. The development and testing (randomized clinical trials) of the PRO-SELF Program using symptom-specific self-care strategies would provide the scientific evidence for the most effective management strategies that could be used with some of the most problematic symptoms associated with cancer and its treatment.

SELF-CARE EXERCISES (SKILLS)

In addition to information, the PRO-SELF Program emphasizes the importance of helping patients become proficient in specific skills needed to manage symptoms. Patients gain confidence that they can be successful in reducing symptoms by carrying out prescribed symptom-management strategies. Three dimensions of skill enhancement are emphasized: (a) doing the skill correctly, (b) doing the skill consistently and in a timely manner, and (c) being able to evaluate whether the prescribed activity is effective. For example, in the clinical trial that focused on reducing the morbidity associated with mucositis (described later), the patients were taught, supervised, and evaluated by return demonstration on how and when to care for their mouths (Larson et al., 1998). Every attempt is made to keep the PRO-SELF Program equipment, if needed, to a minimum and to use what most patients already have on hand (e.g., toothbrush, floss, watch, and flashlight in the mucositis trial).

SUPPORTIVE, INTERACTIVE NURSING CARE (COACHING)

Supportive care provided by nurses engaged in the patient's care is an integral part of the PRO-SELF Program. Patients undergoing cancer treatment, especially chemotherapy, often receive their care in one setting at 1- to 3-week intervals for 6 to 12 months. At each of their treatment visits, they receive chemotherapy from the nurses employed in that setting. Some settings use a primary care approach; others use a more generic approach wherein a variety of nurses provide care to patients over the course of their treatment. These treatment-setting realities were taken into account in developing the PRO-SELF Program relative to designing the supportive, interactive nursing care. The PRO-SELF Program prepares intervention nurses to listen to patients' experiences, positively reinforce their self-care activities, and give encouragement during the treatment experience.

Another aspect of the supportive interaction is telephone calls between the intervention nurse and the patient. The purpose of the telephone call varies depending on the symptom of concern. For instance, in the PRO-SELF Program that focuses on preventing mucositis, patients are instructed to call the nurse when their mouth assessment indicates potential signs of mucositis (Larson et al., 1998). These telephone calls are very directed and require only a brief interaction between the patient and nurse.

A basic premise of the PRO-SELF Program is the belief that once a relationship with the nurse is established, patients are then receptive to supportive nursing care that offers encouragement and problem-solving assistance. This interaction, in turn, allows the nurse to assess patients' self-care abilities. The PRO-SELF Program is designed to provide patients the opportunity to expand their self-care abilities throughout their cancer experience.

## Testing and Refinement of the PRO-SELF Program

The initial large-scale testing of the PRO-SELF Program occurred in a large randomized clinical trial with oncology patients receiving a select group of chemotherapy drugs. This randomized clinical trial tested the effectiveness of the PRO-SELF Program in enhancing the experimental patients' self-care abilities and reducing chemotherapy morbidity. Chemotherapy-related morbidity was defined as (a) the number and extent of chemotherapy-related complications, as measured by four major side effects: nausea, vomiting, mucositis, and infection (Dodd et al., 1992); (b) the tolerance of patients to their chemotherapy protocol as measured by the number of treatment delays, reduced chemotherapy doses, and the need to change chemotherapy agents; and, (c) healthcare resources utilization as measured by the number of emergency department visits and unscheduled hospitalizations.

This initial version of the PRO-SELF Program consisted of (a) written information on managing the four side effects and individualized information cards; (b) self-care exercises (i.e., a log where patients recorded side effects and self-care activities used to manage them) and equipment (i.e., a digital thermometer to assess their temperature and a small flashlight to examine their mouths); and (c) assistive support. Assistive support consisted of the nurses at the study sites (a) coaching the patients on how to use the PRO-SELF Program while administering the patient's treatment; (b) audiotaping these interactions so the patient could replay them at home for guidance and/or clarification of various components; (c) providing a prescriptive relaxation and imagery audiotape for the patient to use at home; and (d) providing a follow-up telephone call to the patient 24 hours after treatment to find out how patients were doing and to answer any questions. The control group patients received usual care.

This first randomized clinical trial did not demonstrate a statistically significant difference between the experimental and control groups in reducing chemotherapy morbidity. However, in an analysis of the audiotaped semistructured interactions between the patients and nurses, it was clearly evident that the patients in the PRO-SELF group perceived that they benefited from participating in the intervention (Larson et al., 1998). An analysis of these data found that the majority (91%) of the patients in the experimental group indicated that the PRO-SELF Program was helpful in managing the side effects associated with chemotherapy. The printed information was seen as the most valuable portion of the intervention; patients used the materials extensively as a reference tool and workbook.

Several patients found that tracking the four symptoms allowed them to identify problems requiring follow-up. In addition, they were able to track the improvements of these symptoms. One patient stated that using the materials produced a sense of accomplishment because she could see that she was "making it through the treatment." The follow-up telephone calls from the nurses were mentioned by many patients as "something to look forward to." Over half (53%) of the experimental patients believed that because they participated in the PRO-SELF Program they had fewer problems with their chemotherapy treatments. They indicated that by participating they had a greater sense of control, had an increased knowledge and understanding of what was occurring, and felt more empowered (Larson et al., 1998).

With this first testing of the PRO-SELF Program, it became evident that it contained too much information to learn and too many self-care skills to perform for the assessment and management of the selected side effects. In addition, two of the outcome variables occurred at such a low frequency (i.e., the side effect of infection and unscheduled hospitalizations) that there was little room to show improvement ("floor effect") in this outpatient sample.

## The PRO-SELF Mouth Aware (PSMA) Program

In a subsequent randomized clinical trial, the focus of the PRO-SELF Program was on only one symptom, namely mucositis; the dose of the intervention was reduced. The PRO-SELF Mouth Aware (PSMA) Program focused on the provision of succinct information, skills training, and support on how to carry out a systematic oral assessment and hygiene protocol (Larson et al., 1998). The PSMA Program in the second randomized clinical trial focused on decreasing chemotherapy-induced mucositis morbidity. Reducing the incidence and severity of mucositis may decrease breaks or interruptions in cancer treatments and enhance patients' chances for a cure or sustained control of their disease.

### INFORMATION (KNOWLEDGE)

The didactic content and procedures found in the PSMA Program were based on the scientific literature and clinical experience of oncology nurses and dentists. Natural history studies demonstrate that mucositis occurs shortly after chemotherapy begins. This suggests that a preventive approach may be beneficial. Therefore, the PSMA Program is initiated when the patients begin chemotherapy.

The PSMA Program incorporated principles of good oral hygiene, such as a new toothbrush for each cycle of chemotherapy or monthly and consistent, regular, and thorough brushing for approximately 90 seconds to ensure that the oral cavity is clean (Epstein, Vickers, Spinelli, & Reece, 1992; Weisdorf et al., 1989). Specific PSMA Program directions were provided for nondenture wearers and denture wearers. Patients were given a list of signs and symptoms (Barker, Loftus, Cuddy, & Barder, 1991; Carl & Emrich, 1991) that needed to be reported to the nurse in their treatment setting. Nurses performed an additional assessment to determine if mucositis was present. The didactic information and self-care exercises for the PSMA Program were contained in a concise booklet that was kept and used in the place where patients did their mouth care (in most instances, the bathroom).

SELF-CARE EXERCISES (SKILLS)

The PSMA Program emphasized the importance of helping patients become proficient in the skills they needed to achieve the best symptom management. By targeting specific skills and providing only essential information, practice, and support, nurses helped patients gain the confidence they needed to carry out the prescribed symptom-management regimen. Three aspects of skill enhancement were emphasized: learning the skill, doing the skill correctly, and doing the skill consistently.

Patients were taught, supervised, and evaluated (through a return demonstration) by a nurse on how and when to care for their mouths. Using an oral assessment guide (e.g., Dibble, Shiba, MacPhail, & Dodd, 1996; Eilers, Berger, & Peterson, 1988), the nurse taught patients how to examine their mouths. First, they learned what is normal. Then they were taught the essential aspects of mouth assessment, how to do the prescribed mouth care skills, and when to notify the nurse of any changes in their mouth. The importance of informing the nurse when any mouth problems were found was emphasized in the PSMA Program materials and during the nurse-patient interactions.

To assist patients in carrying out the PSMA Program, they were instructed to have the following on hand: soft toothbrushes, a small bottle of drinking water (unused portions were to be discarded at the end of each day), a timer or watch to ensure that they brushed their teeth for 90 seconds, a flashlight to assist them to examine their mouth, and dental floss.

SUPPORTIVE, INTERACTIVE NURSING CARE

At each of their treatment visits, patients saw and received chemotherapy from nurses; as part of the PSMA Program, nurses were taught about the purpose of the intervention and the specific information and skills patients needed to more effectively manage mucositis. However, the nurse's own style of nurse–patient interaction served as the foundation for the supportive care component of the PSMA Program. Besides establishing the parameters of the PSMA Program, nurses were free to practice their usual style of interaction on other issues important to patient care. The interaction also gave nurses the opportunity to assess and expand, when needed, patients' self-care abilities.

Nurses needed to be trained in the PSMA Program protocol and needed to commit to follow it. Ideally, they were taught how to perform a mouth assessment by a dental professional. Usually, the nurses determined if the patient had mucositis. Likewise, it was the nurse who helped the patient determine when mucositis was no longer a problem and when the specified mouth care protocol could be discontinued. The importance of calling the nurse to report problems must be emphasized to help patients overcome the common concern of not wanting to bother the busy nurse.

Although the PSMA Program has three distinct dimensions, the process is interactive. This interaction begins when the patient is introduced to the PSMA Program and continues throughout the time the patient utilizes the intervention. Thus, although the three dimensions are presented separately for clarity, in clinical practice patients are taught the PSMA Program, implement it using the information to guide their self-care practices, and, when appropriate, are encouraged to interact with the nurses in the treatment setting. Each dimension is essential, but it is the interactive process among the three dimensions that ensures the success of the PSMA Program.

In a clinical trial that tested the efficacy of three different mouthwashes (with different mechanisms of action) in preventing or treating chemotherapy-induced mucositis, theories related to the pathophysiology of chemotherapy-induced mucositis and the pharmacology of the mouthwashes supplemented Orem's self-care theory. Chemotherapy-induced mucositis morbidity was defined with direct and indirect indices: Prevention-phase direct indices included the incidence of mucositis, the time to onset of mucositis, and the severity of mucositis. Treatment-phase direct indices included days to heal, mucositis-related pain, and disruptions in food and fluid intake. Indirect indices included affective state and quality of life.

No significant differences were found between the two mouthwashes in the direct indices during the prevention phase or among the three mouthwashes in the direct indices during the treatment phase of the clinical trial (Dodd, Dibble, Miaskowski, et al., 2000). An analysis of the data from the prevention phase suggested that the PSMA Program reduced the incidence of mucositis from an *a priori* estimate of 44% to less than 26% (Dodd et al., 1996). No value was added to using costly mouthwashes to either prevent or treat mucositis beyond the benefit of practicing good oral hygiene (Dodd et al., 1996). Interestingly, one of the indirect indices, affective state, was significantly different between patients who developed mucositis and those who did not (Dodd, Dibble, Miaskowski, et al., 2001).

In another clinical trial, the PSMA Program was adapted to test the efficacy of two mouthwashes in the treatment of radiation-induced mucositis for patients who had head and neck cancers (Dodd et al., in press).

COST, CONSISTENCY, AND ADMINISTRATION

The PSMA Program booklets can be produced via desktop publishing on a personal computer. The PSMA Program is both time and cost effective in that the nurse initiates and monitors the intervention when patients have their regularly scheduled appointments. The patients then use the intervention at home. The nurse spends little additional time beyond the usual nurse-patient interactions that occur during the course of care. The initial instructions take approximately 15 minutes.

## The PRO-SELF: Pain Control (PSPC) Program

PATIENTS ONLY

A third randomized clinical trial using the PRO-SELF Program, called the PRO-SELF: Pain Control (PSPC) Program, has recently been completed and focused on reducing pain in patients with bone metastasis (Miaskowski, Dodd, Koo, Tripathy, & Paul, 1996–2001).

**Information (Knowledge)**    Following the completion of the baseline data questionnaires, patients in the PRO-SELF group were taught to keep a daily pain log, a pain medication log, and a side effects checklist. The PRO-SELF intervention nurse then conducted an *academic detailing* session. Academic detailing is an approach based on a normative reeducation program that takes into account that nonintellectual factors may affect particular behaviors (Soumerai & Avorn, 1990). This approach was used successfully to change the behaviors of clinicians regarding inappropriate prescribing (Avorn & Soumerai, 1992; Gurwitz, Noonan, & Soumerai, 1992). This randomized clinical trial was the first to use the academic detailing approach with patients.

The academic detailing session involved reviewing the answers to the knowledge and attitude questions about pain management contained in the Pain Experience Scale (Ferrell, Ferrell, Rhiner, & Grant, 1991). Patients' answers were compared to the correct answers to each of the knowledge and attitude questions. The rationale for each correct answer was provided as well as specific information or instructions related to each question. The instructions were contained in the PSPC booklet provided to the patient as written information to reinforce the teaching session. In addition, the intervention nurse reviewed patients' medication schedules and made suggestions on how to more effectively manage the pain based on the prescriptions provided by the physician.

**Self-care Exercises (Skills)**   Patients were taught how to keep a daily pain diary (to record average, worst, and least pain, and the number of hours per day in pain) and how to evaluate whether their current pain medication was effective in relieving their pain. In addition, patients were given pill boxes to remind them when and how much pain medicine they should take each week.

If doses of medications or types of medications required changing, the intervention nurse coached the patient on how to speak with the healthcare provider at the site to obtain the needed changes in the treatment plan. In addition, the intervention nurse had the patient complete the side effects checklist, reviewed the checklist, and made suggestions about how to manage side effects. If side effects required prescription medications for management, the patient was coached in how to obtain these prescriptions from the healthcare provider at the site. Patients were also informed how to contact the intervention nurse for pain management questions.

**Supportive, Interactive Nursing Care (Support That Includes Coaching)**   The PRO-SELF intervention nurse engaged in the coaching function by reviewing the content of the educational materials using a telephone interview guide during the weekly phone calls. The patients had the opportunity to ask questions about pain management and discuss any problems that they had related to their pain management. At the end of the phone call, the intervention nurse scheduled the next week's phone call or home visit. At the home visit, the patients' diaries, pain medication logs, and side effects checklists from the previous week were reviewed and modifications in the treatment plan were discussed. Patients had the opportunity to ask questions and the key points in the PSPC booklet were reviewed. On weeks 2 and 4, patients received coaching by telephone, reviewing the information from the logs, diaries, and checklists.

THE PSPC PROGRAM, PATIENT AND FAMILY CAREGIVER

A family caregiver was defined as the one individual most involved in the patient's care as designated by the patient. The patient and family caregiver dyad was randomized to either the intervention group or the control group. Family caregivers in both groups were asked to complete the Caregiver Information Questionnaire, the Pain Experience Scale (Ferrell, Ferrell, Rhiner, & Grant, 1991), and the Caregiver Reaction Assessment (Given et al., 1992). The protocol was identical to the one outlined for the patient-only group, with a few additions because the patient and the family caregiver were seen together. The additions are summarized as follows: With the telephone calls, if the patient/caregiver dyad had an extension or speaker phone, both individuals were encouraged to participate in the call. If there was only one phone, the intervention nurse spoke with the patient first and then with the family caregiver. By seeing both the patient and the family caregiver together at the home visits, discussions about differences in knowledge and attitudes about pain-control behaviors between the members of the dyad were encouraged and misconceptions were clarified.

The PSPC Program was effective in significantly diminishing patient pain. The patients who received the intervention reported significant reductions in their average and worst pain scores. These patients also increased their consumption of opioid analgesics by 50 milligrams per day. The pillboxes were helpful to remind patients of the need to refill prescriptions.

## PRO-SELF: Fatigue Control

A final cancer-related randomized clinical trial using the PRO-SELF Program is ongoing and is titled PRO-SELF: Fatigue Control. This trial tests the efficacy of an individualized home-based exercise protocol for managing chemotherapy-related fatigue (Dodd et al., 1999–2004).

## Other PRO-SELF Programs

In addition to the cancer-related PRO-SELF Programs, the research team has developed similar interventions for HIV/AIDS and Parkinson's disease patients. The HIV/AIDS intervention focuses on oral candidiasis; the Parkinson's disease intervention addresses the effects of exercise on gait and balance. Both will be briefly summarized here.

### THE PRO-SELF: CANDIDIASIS (PSC) PROGRAM

This intervention focused on increasing the interepisode time for recurrences of oral candidiasis in susceptible HIV-infected persons (MacPhail et al., 1996–1999). Patients were instructed on how to minimize the presence of exogenous sugars in the mouth through diet and oral hygiene. An additional focus was to determine whether persons who were in the PSC group self-reported the recurrence of their oral candidiasis more accurately than did persons in the control group.

The PSC Program provided instructions in three areas: oral hygiene, diet, and oral self-exam. To assist participants in performing oral hygiene and self-exam, patients were supplied with written instructions for oral hygiene, a toothbrush and/or denture brush, toothpaste and/or soap for denture cleaning, floss, a plastic mouth mirror, and a penlight. For the diet instructions, patients were given eating-habit suggestions, lists of food types to avoid, and lists of alternatives.

Data analysis is ongoing, but a preliminary inspection of the data supports the hypothesis that those participants with poorer hygiene and more dietary sugar exposure had significantly shorter intervals between lesion episodes. An advancement in clinical therapeutics (the advent of protease inhibitors) in this population greatly reduced the pool of potential participants for this randomized clinical trial and also the recidivism of oral candidiasis.

### THE PRO-SELF EXERCISE FOR PARKINSON'S DISEASE (PSEPD) PROGRAM

The PRO-SELF Exercise for Parkinson's Disease (PSEPD) Program focuses on improving primarily gait and balance. The secondary aims are to examine the effects of the gait/balance training intervention on the number of falls, quality of life, functional status, and mood.

Basic information related to Parkinson's Disease is provided to participants in the PSEPD group. The booklet includes information on the principles of the PSEPD Program, when to exercise, the do's and don'ts of exercise, and helpful hints. The intervention includes a videotape with five 1-hour exercise sessions. These videotapes were filmed in a home setting with a sample patient who has Parkinson's disease. Each of the five different exercise sessions on the videotape contains identical amounts of time in each of the three phases (i.e., warm-up, exercise, and cool-down). To avoid fatigue, different muscle groups are utilized, while another muscle group is resting. The specific exercises and their sequence is varied. Variable, random practice increases retention and the possibility that normal movements will be performed outside of the exercise session, especially complex movements (Schmidt, 1988).

During each of the clinic assessments (at baseline and at 3 and 6 months) and during the home visits (at 6 and 18 weeks), the interactions of the physical therapist and participants in the PSEDP group focus on self-care information and reinforcing self-care exercises. The physical therapist exercises with the participants of the PSEPD group at each visit while viewing a videotaped exercise session to facilitate discussion, provide feedback, and resolve any problems. Weekly phone calls to participants of the PSEPD group by the same physical therapist provide additional support during the 6-month study period. The interactions during the phone calls have a focus similar to the clinic assessments and home visits.

## HOW THE STUDIES SUPPORTED OR ALTERED THE PRO-SELF PROGRAM MODEL

Patients and their families are interested in learning about their disease and treatment and want to participate in their own care. It remains highly important to provide relevant and timely information, self-care exercises and activities, and support for patients and their families to participate. These components of the PRO-SELF Program have been tested and corroborated in the studies discussed in this chapter.

The size of the dose to be tested in the randomized clinical trials has been derived from the literature and clinical experience. Clearly, earlier empiric symptom-related work has provided the foundation for this work. For example, good systematic oral hygiene has been recognized as important in the prevention and treatment of cancer chemotherapy-induced mucositis, so to designate the twice-a-day protocol during the prevention phase and the four-times-a-day protocol during the treatment phase is not a novel idea. The prospective testing of several mouthwashes with different mechanisms of action was the innovative feature of the second randomized clinical trial.

In two of the randomized clinical trials, the intervention was individualized for the study participants. In the PSPC study, the investigators worked with the analgesics the physician had prescribed for the patient. If adequate analgesia was not being obtained, then patients were coached to use a telephone script where the patient contacted the physician and reported that the analgesics were not working.

The other individualized approach is occurring with the PRO-SELF Fatigue Control study. Study participants are given exercise prescriptions based on their baseline and subsequent performances on the treadmill test. The exercise prescription changes as patients' physical conditioning changes. In contrast, the mouthwash protocols for the PSMA study are the same across all patients. The mouthwash dose does not vary by personal, disease, or treatment characteristics.

The duration of the intervention to be tested in the randomized clinical trial has been derived from the literature and clinical experience. In the early studies, the third cycle of chemotherapy (each cycle was 3 to 4 weeks in length) was a critical event in terms of peak chemotherapy-related morbidity (the most numerous and severe side effects; Dodd, Lindsey, Larson, & Musci, 1990). This observation was validated with healthcare providers and clinicians in the San Francisco Bay area. Consequently, a 4-month study period was selected for the testing of the first generation of the PRO-SELF Program (four symptoms/side effects). For the second randomized clinical trial, the patients were followed for three complete cycles of chemotherapy (patients are most likely to have developed mucositis by then, if they are going to develop this side effect). The duration of the study period is an especially important question to ask in the PRO-SELF: Fatigue Control study. The timing of the exercise intervention is one of the study's major aims, that is, the efficacy of exercising during chemotherapy or after patients have completed chemotherapy on the primary outcome of fatigue. The PSPC study was a positive trial and was 6 weeks in length. While this study was being conducted, a meta-analysis article was published that documented the need for studies requiring a behavior change to be 12 weeks in length at a minimum.

In the PRO-SELF-related investigations, the dose and duration needed to achieve an effect have varied by the symptom being targeted for intervention. In the PSPC trial, the severity of the unrelieved pain directly affected the dose of the intervention in that the pain-management regimen was modified and the patient contacted his or her physician to report inadequate analgesia. The investigators have not incorporated the psychological status of patients when designing the duration or dose of the interventions. The reinforcement frequency of the intervention to be tested in the randomized clinical trials has been derived from earlier work by the PRO-SELF research team, other investigators, and clinical experience. The reinforcement of the PRO-SELF Program content occurs in weekly person-to-person meetings at the scheduled clinic visits, at patients' homes, or by telephone calls.

## Strengths and Weaknesses of the Original Framework

The PRO-SELF Program has been tested in samples of outpatients and some of these patients were quite ill with their disease or its treatment. This is a considerable strength of the PRO-SELF series of studies in that not just the healthiest of patients have been involved in testing the interventions. Intervention must focus on more than one symptom at a time because most —if not all—patients have to manage more than one symptom. The PSPC trial was costly in terms of personnel. Other strategies will need to be tested in place of the person-to-person interactions. The effect of delivering the PRO-SELF intervention to both the patient and family caregiver and when it should be delivered remain questions for future research.

## Future Development and Refinement

The development and incorporation of the PRO-SELF Program into clinical trials has focused on the reduction of symptom morbidity associated with chronic conditions and their treatment. Further, by carefully examining which aspects of the PRO-SELF Program are effective and by refining them for subsequent trials, the program will continue to evolve as an evidence-based framework that can support the delivery of a variety of pharmacologic and nonpharmacologic strategies to reduce the symptoms associated with the disease and treatment of chronic illnesses.

To date, the PRO-SELF Program has been tested in predominately Caucasian samples, with a racial diversity of 20% of the participants as reflected in northern California and the central valley. Future testing of the

PRO-SELF Program in more diverse samples needs to occur. The PRO-SELF Program needs to be tested in ill elderly cancer patients in order to determine the duration and intensity of the dosage required. In addition to looking at dosage requirements based on age, it would be important to know who benefits most from this intervention, who adheres to the intervention protocol, who does not, and who declines participating in a study that tests the efficacy of the PRO-SELF.

To date, the PRO-SELF Program has been tested with physical symptoms (e.g., mucositis, fatigue, and pain). Future work needs to expand to include the development and testing of the PRO-SELF Program with psychological symptoms, such as depression, anxiety, sexual dysfunction, communication with family/healthcare providers, and spirituality.

Finally, adherence to the intervention protocol has been carefully documented in the series of PRO-SELF studies; it was not in need of special attention until the nonadherence of 11 patients in the PSPC study. These patients who were experiencing metastatic bone pain were resistant to increasing their opioid use despite having considerable pain (Miaskowski, Dodd, West, et al., 2001). The reasons for their nonadherence were multifactorial and complex. Future research with the PRO-SELF Program framework will need to include a deeper understanding of nonadherence and further refinement of the intervention to reach individuals who appear to not benefit from a more generic PRO-SELF Program approach.

Currently, the national Children's Oncology Group is adopting the PRO-SELF Program for use with children who are diagnosed with cancer and their families. Another group of individuals who might benefit from the development and testing of a PRO-SELF Program is cancer survivors. All the participants in the PRO-SELF series of studies have received active treatment for their disease or symptoms. The development and testing of dietary and activity protocols using the PRO-SELF framework may hold great promise for positively affecting disease-free period and survival.

## ACKNOWLEDGMENT

Supported in part by NIH, NCI R01s CA48312; CA55555, CA64734; CA83316; NR04396. Acknowledgement is given to Dr. Patricia Larson, retired professor, School of Nursing, University of California, San Francisco, for her work on the early PRO-SELF Program.

# REFERENCES

Avorn, J., Soumerai, S. B., Everitt, D. E., Ross-Degnan, D., Beers, M. H., Sherman, D., et al. (1992). A randomized trial of a program to reduce the use of psychoactive drugs in nursing homes. *New England Journal of Medicine, 327,* 168–173.

Barker, G., Loftus, L., Cuddy, P., & Barder, B. (1991). The effects of sucralfate suspension and diphenhydramine syrup plus kaolin-pectin on radiotherapy-induced mucositis. *Oral Surgery, Oral Medicine, Oral Pathology, and Endodontics, 71,* 288–298.

Carl, W., & Emrich, L. (1991). Management of oral mucositis during local radiation and systemic chemotherapy: A study of 98 patients. *Journal of Prosthetic Dentistry, 66,* 361–369.

Devine, E. C., & Westlake, S. K. (1995). The effects of psycho-educational care provided to adults with cancer: Meta-analysis of 116 studies. *Oncology Nursing Forum, 22,* 1369–1381.

Dibble, S., Shiba, G., MacPhail, L., & Dodd, M. J. (1996). MacDibbs mouth assessment: A new tool to evaluate mucositis in the radiation therapy patients. *Cancer Practice, 4,* 135–140.

Dodd, M. (1987). Efficacy of proactive information on self-care in radiation therapy patients. *Heart Lung, 16,* 538–544.

Dodd, M., Lovejoy, N., Larson, P., Stetz, K., Lewis, B., Holzemer, W., et al. (1992). Self-care intervention to decrease chemotherapy morbidity: A randomized clinical trial. NIH, NCI R01 CA48312, 1988–1992. Final Report. Paper presented at the Seventeenth Annual Congress of the Oncology Nursing Society, San Diego, CA.

Dodd, M. J. (1984a). Measuring informational intervention for chemotherapy and self-care behavior. *Research in Nursing and Health, 7,* 43–50.

Dodd, M. J. (1984b). Patterns of self-care in cancer patients receiving radiation therapy. *Oncology Nursing Forum, 10,* 23–27.

Dodd, M. J. (1988a). Efficacy of proactive information on self-care in chemotherapy patients. *Patient Education Counseling, 11,* 215–225.

Dodd, M. J. (1988b). Patterns of self-care in patients with breast cancer. *Western Journal of Nursing Research, 10,* 7–14.

Dodd, M. J., & Dibble, S. L. (1993). Predictors of self-care: A test of Orem's model. *Oncology Nursing Forum, 20,* 272–276.

Dodd, M. J., Dibble, S. L., Miaskowski, C., MacPhail, L., Greenspan, D., Paul, S., et al. (2000). Clinical trial of the effectiveness of three commonly used mouthwashes to treat chemotherapy-induced mucositis. *Oral Surgery, Oral Medicine, Oral Pathology, Oral Radiology, and Endodontics, 90,* 39–47.

Dodd, M. J., S. Dibble, C. Miaskowski, S. Paul, L. MacPhail, D. Greenspan, et al. (2001). A comparison of the affective state and quality of life on chemotherapy patients who do and do not develop chemotherapy-induced oral mucositis. *Journal of Pain and Symptom Management, 21,* 498–505.

Dodd, M. J., P. Larson, S. L. Dibble, C. Miaskowski, D. Greenspan, L. MacPhail, et al. (1996). Randomized clinical trial of chlorhexidine versus placebo for prevention of oral mucositis in patients receiving chemotherapy. *Oncology Nursing Forum, 23,* 921–927.

Dodd, M. J., Lindsey, A. M., Larson, P., & Musci, E. (1990). Coping and self-care of cancer families: Nurse prospectus. 1986–1990. NIH NINR NR01441, 1986–1990. (Final report).

Dodd, M. J., Miaskowski, C., Greenspan, D., MacPhail, L., Shih, A., Shiba, G., et al. (in press). Radiation-induced mucositis: A randomized clinical trial of micronized sucralfate versus salt and soda mouthwashes. *Cancer Investigation.*

Dodd, M. J., Painter, P., Miaskowski, C., Paul, S., Facione, N., Tripathy, D., et al. (1999–2004). Exercise: An intervention for fatigue in cancer patients. NIH NCI, RO1 CA 83316.

Eilers, J., Berger, A. M., & Peterson, M. C. (1988). Development, testing and application of the oral assessment guide. *Oncology Nursing Forum, 15,* 325–330.

Epstein, J. B., Vickars, L., Spinelli, J., & Reece, D. (1992). Efficacy of chlorhexidine and nystatin rinses in prevention of oral complications in leukemia and bone marrow transplant. *Oral Surgery, Oral Medicine, Oral Pathology, Oral Radiology, and Endodontics, 73,* 682–689.

Fawzy, F. I., Fawzy, N. W., Arndt, L. A., & Pasnau, R. O. (1995). Critical review of psychosocial interventions in cancer care. *Archives of General Psychiatry, 52,* 100–113.

Ferrell, B. R., Ferrell, B. A., Rhiner, M., & Grant, M. (1991). Family factors influencing cancer pain management. *Postgraduate Journal of Medicine, 67,* 564–569.

Given, C. W., Given, B., Stommel, M., Collins, C., King, S., & Franklin, S. (1992). The caregiver reaction assessment (CRA) for caregivers to persons with chronic physical and mental impairments. *Research in Nursing and Health, 15,* 271–283.

Griffiths, M., & Leek, C. (1995). Patient education needs. Opinions of oncology nurses and their patients. *Oncology Nursing Forum, 22,* 139–144.

Gurwitz, J. H., Noonan, J. P., & Soumerai, S. B. (1992). Reducing the use of H2-receptor antagonists in the long-term-care setting. *Journal of the American Geriatrics Society, 40,* 359–364.

Larson, P. (1995). Perception of needs of hospitalized patients undergoing bone marrow transplant. *Cancer Practice, 17,* 173–179.

Larson, P., Miaskowski, C., MacPhail, L., Dodd, M. J., Greenspan, D., Dibble, S. L., et al. (1998). The PRO-SELF Mouth Aware Program: An effective approach for reducing chemotherapy mucositis. *Cancer Nursing, 21,* 263–268.

Larson, P. J., Viele, C. S., Coleman, S., Dibble, S. L., & Cebulski, C. (1993). Comparison of perceived symptoms of patients undergoing bone marrow transplant and the nurses caring for them. *Oncology Nursing Forum, 20,* 81–87.

MacPhail, L., Dodd, M. J., Hilton, J., Greenspan, D., Srouss, H., & Cheikh, B. (1999). Self-care intervention to prevent oral candidiasis. NIH NINR, R01 NR 043966, 1996–1999.

Meyer, T. J., & Mark, M. M. (1995). Effects of psychosocial interventions with adult cancer patients: A meta-analysis of randomized experiments. *Health Psychology, 14,* 101–108.

Miaskowski, C., Dodd, M. J., Koo, P., Tripathy, D., & Paul, S. (2001). Self-care intervention to control cancer pain. Funded by NIH, NCI R01 CA 64734, 1996–2001.

Miaskowski, C., Dodd, M. J., West, C., Paul, S., Tripathy, D., Koo, P., et al. (2001). Lack of adherence with the analgesic regimen: A significant barrier to effective cancer pain management. *Journal of Clinical Oncology, 119,* 4275–4279.

Orem, D. (1995). *Nursing: Concepts of practice* (5th ed.). St. Louis, MO: Mosby Year Book, Inc.

Schmidt, R. A. (1988). *Motor control and learning: A behaviour analysis.* Champaign, IL: Human Kinetics Publishers.

Smith, M. C., Holcombe, J. K., & Stullenbarger, E. (1994). A meta-analysis of intervention effectiveness for symptom management in oncology nursing research. *Oncology Nursing Forum, 21,* 1201–1210.

Soumerai, S. B., & Avorn, J. (1990). Principles of educational outreach ("academic detailing") to improve clinical decision-making. *Journal of the American Medical Association, 263,* 549–556.

Spiegel, D. (1995). Essentials of psychotherapeutic intervention for cancer patients. *Supportive Care in Cancer, 3,* 252–256.

Weisdorf, D. J., Bostrum, B., Raether, D., Mattingly, M., Walker, P., Pihlstrom, B., et al. (1989). Oropharyngeal mucositis complicating bone marrow transplantation: Prognostic factors and the effect of chlorhexidine mouthrinse. *Bone Marrow Transplantation, 4,* 89–95.

# 8

## Cancer-Related Fatigue

## Victoria Mock

Fatigue is the most common and debilitating symptom of cytotoxic chemotherapy, radiation therapy, or biological response modifiers, affecting 70% to 100% of cancer patients (Jacobsen et al., 1999; Longman, Braden, & Mishel, 1996; Robinson & Posner, 1992; Sitzia & Huggins, 1998). In patients with metastatic disease, the prevalence exceeds 75% and even cancer survivors report fatigue as a disruptive symptom months or years after treatment ends (Broeckel, Jacobsen, Horton, Balducci, & Lyman, 1998). Patients are often reluctant to report fatigue to care providers, fearing that modifications may be made to their cancer treatment program that may affect survival. Other patients feel that fatigue is a symptom they should be able to manage themselves. Care providers frequently do not screen for cancer-related fatigue (CRF) because they are uncertain about how to treat it. Consequently, CRF is all too often underdiagnosed and undermanaged. This chapter describes the clinical problem of fatigue in individuals diagnosed with cancer and it critiques the evidence base for common fatigue interventions.

Studies reviewed in the chapter were selected from MEDLINE® and CINAHL® searches of research published between 1985 and 2001. Articles were retrieved under the linked key terms of *cancer and fatigue*; *cancer, fatigue, and exercise*; and *cancer, fatigue, and coping*. Research studies were selected for inclusion if they were published in referenced, English language journals and reported the testing of an intervention in a sample of individuals with cancer with fatigue as a specific outcome.

This chapter begins with a brief description of the fatigue experience in cancer patients, followed by a review of the conceptual models related to CRF. The focus of the chapter is a critique of the studies testing interventions to mitigate CRF, including exercise, energy conservation, rest, and sleep, as well as stress/coping interventions such as educational preparation, stress reduction, and attention-restoring therapy. The chapter concludes with a summary of the state of the knowledge; gaps in knowledge and areas for future research are also identified.

## THE FATIGUE EXPERIENCE

CRF has been defined by the National Comprehensive Cancer Network (NCCN) Fatigue Practice Guidelines as "an unusual, persistent, subjective sense of tiredness related to cancer or cancer treatment that interferes with usual functioning" (Mock et al., 2000, p. 152). CRF is more severe, disruptive, and distressing than the fatigue experienced by healthy individuals (Andrykowski, Curran, & Lightner, 1998; Stone, Richards, & Hardy, 1998) and also less likely to be relieved by rest and sleep (Glaus, Crow, & Hammond, 1996).

In a qualitative study of CRF (Glaus et al., 1996), individuals described fatigue as having three major characteristics: physical sensations (59% of responses), such as decreased physical performance and weakness; cognitive performance (24% of responses), such as lack of concentration and decreased problem-solving ability; and affective sensations (21% of responses), such as sadness and decreased motivation. Fatigue and other side effects of treatment contribute to a reduced level of physical activity that leads to deconditioning and decreases in functional status as treatment progresses (Nail & Jones, 1995). As cancer patients are less able to engage in valued roles and activities, quality of life is affected (Ferrell, Grant, Dean, Funk, & Ly, 1996). The prevalence and incidence of CRF by cancer site or by treatment modality have not been widely investigated. One retrospective study using mailed surveys to breast cancer survivors found fatigue levels to be highest in women who received combination cancer therapies and lowest in those who received radiation alone (Woo, Dibble, Piper, Keating, & Weiss, 1998).

Central and peripheral mechanisms have been proposed to explain the cause of CRF; they can be classified into four general categories:

- Alterations in biochemistry such as the accumulation of toxic by-products of cellular damage and destruction resulting from cancer therapies;
- Changes in the production and balance of hormones, such as those involved in the stress response;
- The depletion of essential substances such as hemoglobin (resulting in anemia) or nutrients lost to hypermetabolism from tumor growth or to anorexia, diarrhea, and vomiting; and
- Deconditioning related to a prolonged reduction in one's activity level with resulting activity intolerance. (Jacobs & Piper, 1996)

The most accurate conceptualization of CRF may be multifactorial and multidimensional with biological, psychological, social, and environmental factors influencing the onset, intensity, duration, distress, and behavioral expression of the fatigue experience.

Although the specific causes of CRF remain unclear, correlates of the symptom provide guidance for interventions. Fatigue is inversely correlated with activity level and the ability to perform physical activities. Sedentary breast cancer patients with diminished exercise tolerance reported higher levels of fatigue than more active, physically fit patients (Mock, Dow et al., 1997; Mock et al., 2001, 2002). This is complicated by the common recommendations that fatigued patients get additional rest and decrease activity. A consistent decrease in the level of daily activities eventually leads to a lower tolerance for normal activity and high levels of fatigue (Berger & Farr, 1999).

CRF is also consistently correlated with anxiety, depression, and emotional stress (Irvine, Vincent, Graydon, Bubela, & Thompson, 1994). It is unclear whether fatigue results from prolonged emotional stress (characterized by anxiety, depression, and difficulty sleeping) or if high levels of fatigue cause emotional distress. Both mechanisms seem probable. Research with breast cancer patients receiving adjuvant chemotherapy or radiation therapy has indicated that the most common symptoms experienced were fatigue, difficulty sleeping, anxiety, and depression (Longman et al., 1996; Mock et al., 1994; Mock et al., 2001; Mock, Dow, et al., 1997).

Fatigue has also been positively correlated with high levels of other unmanaged symptoms, especially pain (Blesch et al., 1991). In a survey of 455 Japanese cancer patients, female gender, higher education, full-time employment status, living alone, low performance status, and depression were significantly correlated with high levels of fatigue (Akechi, Kugaya, Okamura, Yamawaki, & Uchitomi, 1999). The cancer site and duration of the disease were not associated with fatigue. Irvine et al. (1994) investigated the correlates of fatigue in 54 patients receiving radiation therapy and 47 patients receiving chemotherapy. Symptom distress and mood disturbance were the strongest correlates of fatigue. Decreases in both functional status and white blood counts were related to increases in fatigue. Fatigue levels were similar in the two types of cancer treatment. Fatigue was not related to age, employment status, or hemoglobin level. In some studies, fatigue was not found to be related to the stage of disease or the type of chemotherapy regimen (Greene, Nail, Fieler, Dudgeon, & Jones, 1994). However, in other studies, fatigue was associated with the type of cancer and chemotherapy regimen (Berger & Walker, 2001; Richardson, Ream, & Wilson-Barnett, 1998).

## CONCEPTUAL MODELS

Common intervention models for CRF can be classified into two basic categories: energy balance models and stress/coping models. The energy balance models underlie exercise, sleep enhancement, and energy conservation interventions. The stress/coping models include educational preparation and stress-reduction interventions. In the absence of tested pathophysiologic theories of CRF, behavioral-practice-oriented theories have been developed to explain and predict the fatigue experience. A review by Ream and Richardson (1999) found five frequently cited theories of CRF to be relatively unsophisticated and limited in their predictive capacity. None of these models were used in the intervention studies reported in this chapter, although it seems likely that the exercise studies of MacVicar et al. (1986, 1989) were supported by assumptions that in time became part of the subsequent Winningham Psychobiological-Entropy Model (Winningham, 1996).

As an example of an energy balance model, the Psychobiological-Entropy Model is relatively well developed and is accompanied by 10 propositional statements (Winningham, 1996; see Figure 8.1). The model defines fatigue as an energy deficit caused by illness, treatment, related symptoms, environmental influences, and inactivity. The secondary fatigue that arises from inactivity leads to a cycle of downward mobility resulting in disability. In this model, interventions are suggested to manage factors that contribute to primary fatigue as well as interventions to prevent

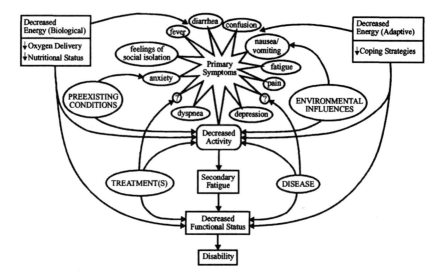

**FIGURE 8.1    The Psychobiological-Entropy Model of Functioning©**

secondary fatigue by a balance of rest and physical activity. Other energy balance models include Ryden's (1977) Conceptual Framework of Energy Expenditure and the Energy Analysis Model of Irvine et al. (1994).

An example of a stress/coping model is Aistars' (1987) Organizing Framework, in which prolonged stress is proposed as the main cause of fatigue in cancer patients. Building on Selye's Theory of Stress, the Aistars theory describes the stress of cancer diagnosis and treatment as depleting body reserves, with fatigue as the outward manifestation. The model proposes interventions directed toward stress management, good nutrition, and conservation of energy. Although a strong correlation exists between emotional distress and CRF, the mediating mechanism between them has not yet been elucidated.

The most frequently cited fatigue model is the Piper Integrated Fatigue Model (Piper, Lindsey, & Dodd, 1987; see Figure 8.2). This model, developed from a synthesis of the fatigue literature, is a comprehensive framework that identifies multiple potential biological and psychosocial factors that influence the manifestations of fatigue in cancer patients. No

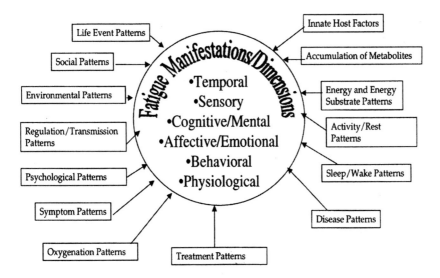

Life Event Patterns

Social Patterns

Environmental Patterns

Regulation/Transmission Patterns

Psychological Patterns

Symptom Patterns

Oxygenation Patterns

Treatment Patterns

Innate Host Factors

Accumulation of Metabolites

Energy and Energy Substrate Patterns

Activity/Rest Patterns

Sleep/Wake Patterns

Disease Patterns

Fatigue Manifestations/Dimensions

•Temporal
•Sensory
•Cognitive/Mental
•Affective/Emotional
•Behavioral
•Physiological

**FIGURE 8.2    Integrated Fatigue Model (IFM)©**

propositional statements have been identified for the model to explicate the relationships among the variables. Although the model represents well the complexity of factors in CRF and has been used extensively in descriptive and correlational studies, it needs additional development to be useful in testing interventions for fatigue.

In summary, the conceptual models for CRF are in the early stages of development and testing. Several of the models have demonstrated the potential for explaining CRF, but all need further work before being considered substantive theory.

## INTERVENTIONS FOR CANCER-RELATED FATIGUE

The most effective approach to symptom management is to identify the cause of the disturbing symptom and correct it. In the published NCCN Fatigue Practice Guidelines, the NCCN panel of experts identified five factors frequently associated with CRF and recommended that, if present, they be assessed and treated as a first step in managing the symptom. The five factors are pain, emotional distress, anemia, sleep disturbance, and thyroid disorders. Other contributors to fatigue in cancer patients—such as fluid and electrolyte imbalances, underlying cardiorespiratory disorders, and malnutrition—can be medically treated. However, in many cancer patients, no cause for CRF can be readily identified and the approach to management is a more generalized one. Despite the recognition of CRF as a significant problem over the last decade, little is understood about the underlying mechanisms of CRF and few evidence-based interventions are available to manage this distressing symptom (Ream & Richardson, 1999).

Although CRF has been identified as a major research priority for many years (Mooney, Ferrell, Nail, Benedict, & Haberman, 1991) and the symptom has been the topic of much descriptive work, few interventions have been tested to mitigate CRF. The interventions can be categorized as exercise, psychosocial treatments, preparatory education, and attention-restoring techniques for cognitive fatigue. Research on those interventions has not consistently described the theory being tested, and the relationship of these interventions to the emerging body of fatigue theory is often unclear (Ream & Richardson, 1999).

## Exercise Interventions

In the management of CRF, exercise is the intervention with the most supporting evidence of effectiveness. To date, eight reports (conducted by four research teams) have been published on studies testing the effects of exercise on fatigue during active cancer treatment and three additional reports have been done with cancer survivors as subjects (see Tables 8.1 and 8.2).

### EXERCISE DURING CANCER TREATMENT

MacVicar and Winningham conducted a series of laboratory-controlled experiments using stationary bicycles to measure the effects of an exercise intervention with women receiving adjuvant chemotherapy for breast cancer (MacVicar & Winningham, 1986; MacVicar, Winningham, & Nickel, 1989; Winningham & MacVicar, 1988; Winningham, MacVicar, Bondoc, Anderson, & Minton, 1989). Only one of their studies reported fatigue as an outcome (MacVicar & Winningham, 1986). In this study, mood disturbance and fatigue measured by the Profile of Mood States (POMS) were compared in six exercising patients, six exercising healthy women, and four patient controls.

**TABLE 8.1  Effects of Exercise on Fatigue of Cancer Patients in Treatment**

| | Theoretical/ conceptual framework* | Design | Sample | Measures** | Results |
|---|---|---|---|---|---|
| Dimeo et al. (1999) | None reported | Experimental, 2-group design; bed cycle ergometer at 50% maximum heart rate | N = 59 mixed hematologic malignancies and solid tumors; PBSCT | F = POMS, SCL-90 | Decreased fatigue and psychological distress in exercisers; no exercise outcomes reported |
| MacVicar & Winningham (1986) | None reported | Quasi-experimental, 3-group design; laboratory cycle ergometer 3 times per week for 10 weeks at 60% to 85% maximum heart rate | N = 10 breast cancer patients; CT | F = POMS EX = SLET | Increased functional capacity; decreased mood disturbance and fatigue in exercising patients and exercising nonpatients; increased mood disturbance in patient controls |

(continued)

**TABLE 8.1  Effects of Exercise on Fatigue of Cancer Patients in Treatment** (*continued*)

| | Theoretical/ conceptual framework* | Design | Sample | Measures** | Results |
|---|---|---|---|---|---|
| Mock et al. (1994) | None reported | Experimental, 2-group design; home-based walking 4 to 5 times per week for 30 minutes, plus support group | N = 14 breast cancer patients (stages I and II); CT | F = VAS EX = 12-Minute Walk Test | Increased walking ability in exercisers; decreased psychosocial distress compared to controls; less fatigue in exercisers; effects of exercise alone cannot be determined; fatigue was one item on VAS; exercise was self-reported; small sample size |
| Mock, Cameron, Tompkins, Lin, & Stewart (1997) | None reported | Experimental, 2-group design; home-based walking 4 to 5 times per week for 30 minutes; self-report | N = 46 breast cancer patients (stages I and II); RT | F = VAS and PFS EX = 12-Minute Walk Test | Increased walking ability in exercisers; decreased fatigue and other symptoms compared to controls |
| Mock et al. (2001) | None reported | Experimental, 2-group design; home-based walking 4 to 5 times per week for 30 minutes; self-report | N = 50 breast cancer patients (stages I–III); CT/RT | F = PFS EX = 12-Minute Walk Test | Increased walking ability in exercisers; decreased fatigue and other symptoms compared to controls |

| | Theoretical/ conceptual framework* | Design | Sample | Measures** | Results |
|---|---|---|---|---|---|
| Mock et al. (2002) | None reported | RCT, 2-group design; home-based walking 4 to 5 times per week for 30 minutes; self-report | $N$ = 111 breast cancer patients (stages 0–III); CT/RT | F = PFS EX = 12-Minute Walk Test | Increased walking ability in exercisers; decreased fatigue and other symptoms compared to controls; 72% adherence in EX group |
| Schwartz (1999, 2000) | None reported | Pre-experimental, 1-group design; home-based walking or patient choice of exercise 3 times per week | $N$ = 27 breast cancer patients (stages I–III); CT | F = Schwartz Cancer Fatigue Scale; VAS EX = 12-Minute Walk Test | Increased pre- to post-test walking ability; increased quality of life and less fatigue in active exercisers versus non-compliers; 60% of subjects adhered to program |

*(continued)*

**TABLE 8.1  Effects of Exercise on Fatigue of Cancer Patients in Treatment** (*continued*)

| | Theoretical/ conceptual framework* | Design | Sample | Measures** | Results |
|---|---|---|---|---|---|
| Schwartz, Mori, Gao, Nail, & King (2001) | None reported | Pre-experimental, 1-group design; home-based walking or patient choices of exercise for 8 weeks at 3 to 4 times per week for 15 to 30 minutes | $N = 61$ breast cancer patients (stage II); CT | F = VAS EX = 12-Minute Walk Test | Increased pre- to post-test walking ability; decreased fatigue in active exercisers; 61% of subjects adhered to program |

*Note: No theoretical models included in the studies are summarized here, except the theory eventually developed; models are discussed in chapter text.

**Note:

SLET = Symptom Limited Exercise Test (O$_2$ uptake)

POMS = Profile of Mood States; VAS = Visual Analogue Scale

PFS = Piper Fatigue Scale

EX = Exercise

**TABLE 8.2  Effects of Exercise on Fatigue in Cancer Survivors**

| | Theoretical/ conceptual framework* | Design | Sample | Measures** | Results |
|---|---|---|---|---|---|
| Dimeo, Rumberger, & Keul (1998) | None reported | Pre-experimental; treadmill walking at 80% of maximum heart rate | N = 5 mixed cancer survivors; post-PBSCT | EX = SLET | Increased functional capacity and distance walked for exercisers; decreased fatigue by anecdote; no fatigue measures |
| Dimeo, Tilmann et al. (1997) | None reported | Quasi-experimental; treadmill walking at 80% of maximum heart rate | N = 16 mixed hematologic malignancies and solid tumors; post-PBSCT | EX = SLET | Increased functional capacity in exercisers; less fatigue in exercisers by anecdote; no fatigue measures |
| Schwartz (1998a) | None reported | Survey retrospective; running, walking, cycling, other | N = 219 mixed cancer survivors/ exercisers; CT/RT/surgery | Questionnaire | Decreased exercise during treatment; decreased fatigue by rest and exercise |

*Note: No theoretical models included in the studies are summarized here, except the theory eventually developed; models are discussed in chapter text.

**Note:

| | |
|---|---|
| EX = Exercise | CT = Chemotherapy |
| SLET = Symptom Limited Exercise | Test RT = Radiation Therapy |

Exercisers rode stationary bicycles 3 times a week for 10 weeks at 60% to 85% of their maximum heart rate. In this quasi-experimental pre-test/ post-test design, results indicated significantly lower fatigue and mood disturbance for both groups of exercising subjects compared to the patient controls, as well as improved functional capacity for the exercisers. However, the sample size was small and the breast cancer subjects were not randomly assigned to groups. This early study was important because it indicated that cancer patients could exercise safely during active treatment and that beneficial outcomes could result. This team then conducted a larger randomized controlled trial (MacVicar et al., 1989) demonstrating important increases in functional capacity (40%) and decreased nausea (Winningham & MacVicar, 1988) in the experimental group, but fatigue was not reported in this larger study (see Table 8.3). Although no theoretical framework was named in the MacVicar and Winningham research reports, the authors describe disuse syndrome and decreases in functional capacity as affecting functional and psychological status. Winningham (1996) subsequently incorporated these concepts into the Winningham Psychobiological-Entropy Model.

Four studies employing experimental designs have been conducted by Mock et al., testing the effects of a home-based walking exercise intervention on fatigue in breast cancer patients receiving active treatment. In the first study (Mock et al., 1994), 14 women receiving adjuvant chemotherapy for breast cancer were randomly assigned to the experimental intervention or to usual care. The intervention had two components: a progressive home-based walking exercise program (30 minutes, 4 to 5 times per week) and a support group led by an Oncology Clinical Nurse Specialist. The intervention lasted from pre-test before chemotherapy treatment began to the end of treatment (4 to 6 months). All subjects in the exercise group were able to walk at least 90 minutes per week (a 30-minute session per day for 3 days a week). Study results revealed significantly higher physical functioning and psychosocial adjustment in the exercise group and higher symptom distress in the usual-care group, especially fatigue, anxiety, and difficulty sleeping. The 12-Minute Walk Test, psychosocial adjustment by the Psychosocial Adjustment to Illness Scale (PAIS), and symptoms by visual analogue scales measured physical functioning (exercise tolerance). Because the intervention in this study included both exercise and support, benefits could not be clearly attributed to one component versus the other.

In the second study by Mock, Dow, et al. (1997), the home-based walking program was tested in 46 women receiving radiation therapy following

**TABLE 8.3  Effects of Exercise on Nonfatigue Outcomes in Cancer Patients**

| | Theoretical/ conceptual framework* | Design | Sample | Measures** | Results |
|---|---|---|---|---|---|
| Dimeo, Tilmann et al. (1997) | None reported | Experimental; bed cycle ergometer at 50% of maximum heart rate | N = 68 mixed hematologic malignancies and solid tumors; PBSCT | EX = SLET, complications LOS | Increased functional capacity; decreased complications of transplant; decreased LOS in exercisers versus controls; no fatigue or psychosocial outcomes |
| MacVicar, Winningham, & Nickel (1989) | None reported | Experimental laboratory cycle ergometer 3 times per week for 10 weeks at 60% to 85% of maximum heart rate | N = 45 breast cancer patients; CT | EX = SLET | Increased functional capacity in exercisers; no psychosocial or fatigue outcomes |
| Segar et al. (1998) | None reported | Experimental, cross-over; aerobic exercise 4 times per week for 10 weeks at 60% of maximum heart rate | N = 24 breast cancer survivors | Beck Depression; Stait Anxiety | Decreased anxiety and depression in exercisers; subjects deleted if less than 89% adherence (20%) |

*(continued)*

**TABLE 8.3** Effects of Exercise on Nonfatigue Outcomes in Cancer Patients *(continued)*

| | Theoretical/ conceptual framework* | Design | Sample | Measures** | Results |
|---|---|---|---|---|---|
| Winningham & MacVicar (1988) | None reported | Experimental; laboratory cycle ergometer 3 times per week for 10 weeks at 60% to 85% of maximum heart rate | N = 42 breast cancer patients; CT | EX = SLET Nausea = SCL_90 | Decreased nausea; fatigue not a reported outcome; single nausea item |
| Winningham et al. (1989) | None reported | Experimental; laboratory cycle ergometer 3 times per week for 10 weeks at 60% to 85% of the maximum heart rate | N = 24 breast cancer patients; CT | EX = SLET weight, body fat | Decreased body fat in exercisers; increased body fat in controls; no information on diet; some subjects on Prednisone; no fatigue outcome |

*Note: No theoretical models included in studies are summarized here, except the theory eventually developed; models are discussed in chapter text.
**Note:

EX = Exercise    SLET = Symptom Limited Exercise Test    CT = Chemotherapy conservative surgery for breast cancer. Subjects randomized to exercise were given an individualized exercise prescription and assigned to walk 4 to 5 days per week at 60% to 80% of their maximum heart rate for progressive intervals up to 30 minutes per day. Both the visual analogue scale and the Piper Fatigue Scale (PFS) were used to measure fatigue. Study results demonstrated increased physical functioning on the 12-Minute Walk Test as well as significantly lower levels of fatigue, difficulty sleeping, and emotional distress for subjects who walked at least 90 minutes weekly (30 minutes 3 times a week) for the 6 weeks of radiation therapy. Fatigue was correlated with anxiety ($r = .60$), depression ($r = .61$), and difficulty sleeping ($r = .54$) at a significant level of $p < .001$ for all. There was an inverse relationship between the amount of exercise and difficulty sleeping ($r = -.42$, $p = .008$).

The most recent studies reported by Mock et al. (2001, 2002) were multi-institutional clinical trials conducted by a team of oncology nurse researchers interested in fatigue and other symptoms. A pilot study in 2001 tested the home-based walking program with 50 breast cancer patients (receiving chemotherapy or radiation therapy) at five cancer centers. Results included physical functioning measured by the 12-Minute Walk Test, mood disturbance measured by the POMS, fatigue measured by the PFS, and quality of life measured by the Medical Outcome Study Short Form-36. The pilot project to develop the methods for a subsequent randomized, controlled clinical trial was complicated by a diffusion-of-treatment effect related to the adherence of subjects to the group assignment. Fifty percent of the subjects assigned to usual care walked during treatment at levels as high as the exercise group. Furthermore, 30% of subjects assigned to exercise did not meet the minimum levels for that group. Data were analyzed and indicated significant differences between the groups in the study results of physical functioning, fatigue, mood, difficulty sleeping, and quality of life.

The subsequent randomized, controlled clinical trial by Mock et al. (2002) enrolled 111 sedentary women receiving chemo or radiation therapy for breast cancer. Subjects were randomly assigned to the home-based walking exercise program (*Every Step Counts®*; Mock, Cameron, Tompkins, Lin, & Stewart, 1997) or to usual care during the course of their treatment at five cancer centers. Similar outcomes and instruments to those of the pilot project were used in this study. Seventy-two percent of the subjects assigned to exercise adhered to the exercise intervention. Mean walk time was 120 minutes weekly (30 minutes daily for 4 days per week). Crossovers were also a challenge in this study, as 30% of the subjects assigned to usual care walked more than 60 minutes per week, an increase from their baseline sedentary level. A data-analysis approach was used in consideration of the adherence issue. Results indicated a significant difference between groups on the PFS scores. Emotional distress and difficulty sleeping were significantly lower in exercising subjects.

An adaptation theoretical framework was used in each of the four Mock et al. studies: the Roy Adaptation Model (Roy & Andrews, 1991) for the two early studies and the Levine Conservation Model (Fawcett, 1995) for recent studies. The proposition being tested was that successful adaptation in physiologic and psychosocial modes would result in less symptom distress and higher levels of physical functioning and quality of life. The exercise intervention was hypothesized to facilitate adaptation to the cancer diagnosis and treatment. The four studies offer support for the hypothesis, but the mediating mechanisms underlying the effects of exercise on fatigue remain unclear.

Schwartz has published several research reports of a home-based exercise intervention with breast cancer patients receiving adjuvant chemotherapy. The first publication (Schwartz, 2000) reported results in 27 subjects in a single group pre-test/post-test design. The exercise intervention was an 8-week, low-intensity aerobic program; 60% of women adopted the exercise program, as demonstrated by increased distance on the 12-Minute Walk Test at post-test. Women who adhered exercised an average of 140 minutes weekly (35 minutes 4 days a week). Caltrac® accelerometers worn during exercise periods measured the exercise intensity. Fatigue was reported in a daily log using visual analogue scales. Exercise adherers were compared to those who did not adhere, revealing significantly higher functional ability in the exercising subjects. Patterns of fatigue varied over the chemotherapy cycle, with more increases in average fatigue and worst fatigue in the nonexercisers. However, the comparison of fatigue levels of adherers to nonadherers raises questions of selection bias.

Although no theoretical framework is described in the Schwartz (2000) study, exercise is suggested as retarding functional declines, weakness, and fatigue in diseases associated with inactivity. A separate publication of the same study (Schwartz, 1999) reporting the quality of life outcomes of the research, as measured by the Quality of Life Index, indicated that fatigue is the mediating variable through which exercise affects quality of life. In a strong inverse relationship, fatigue accounted for 71% of the variance in quality of life.

Schwartz, Mori, Gao, Nail, and King (2001) tested a home-based, low-to-moderate-intensity exercise program in 61 breast cancer patients over two cycles of chemotherapy. In a one-group, pre-test/post-test design, all the women were instructed to exercise using an aerobic activity of their choice for 15 to 30 minutes 3 to 4 days a week. Sixty-one percent of the subjects adopted the exercise program and showed improvements in functional ability as measured by the 12-Minute Walk Test. Study results revealed that the intensity of subjects' fatigue as measured daily on visual analogue scales declined as the duration of the exercise increased. Women who exercised experienced less severe fatigue than nonexercisers. Exercisers also experienced a significant carry-over effect of exercise on fatigue, but the effect lasted only one day. In general, fatigue declined as calorie expenditure increased. However, reported levels of current fatigue increased in subjects who exercised over 60 minutes per session. No specific framework was described for this study.

Methylphenidate, a psychostimulant, is being tested with exercise to help manage fatigue. In a preliminary study by Schwartz, Masood, Thompson, and Chahal (2001), 12 newly diagnosed melanoma patients beginning high-dose interferon were instructed to exercise 4 days per week and take methylphenidate daily. Although all 12 subjects adhered to exercise, only 67% adhered to the medication due to side effects. Energy levels were reported as higher in those who took methylphenidate than those who did not. The potential role of methylphenidate to manage fatigue needs further investigation.

Dimeo, Stieglitz, Novelli-Fischer, Fetscher, and Keul (1999) conducted the only reported exercise study of fatigue results during hospitalization for peripheral blood stem cell transplantation. Using a sample of 59 subjects with mixed hematologic malignancies and solid tumors, patients in the training group stationary biked 30 minutes daily with a bed ergometer at an intensity of 50% of cardiac reserve. The POMS (short form) and the Symptom Check List (SCL-90-R) measured the psychological results. Fatigue was assessed on a subscale of both instruments. Psychologic variables were measured at baseline and on the day of discharge. The exercising group experienced decreases in psychological distress and a nonsignificant increase in fatigue scores. Although no theoretical model was described for the study, the exercise intervention is discussed as treatment for an impairment of physical performance related to deconditioning during a prolonged treatment and hospitalization.

EXERCISE FOLLOWING CANCER TREATMENT

A few studies have explored exercise to decrease fatigue in cancer survivors who have completed treatment. Dimeo, Tilmann, et al. (1997) evaluated aerobic exercise in the rehabilitation of 32 patients following high-dose chemotherapy and autologous peripheral blood stem cell transplantation. The patients trained in a progressive program, walking on treadmills 5 days a week for 6 weeks. In this quasi-experimental design, maximum performance improvements were significantly higher for the exercise group than for a group of 16 nonexercising control-group subjects. Personal interviews were used to assess patients' feelings of fatigue and experiences of limitations in daily activities. At post-test, no patient in the training group, but four patients in the control group (25%), reported feeling fatigued by daily activities. This study would have been strengthened by a formal fatigue measure.

Dimeo, Rumberger, and Keul (1998) investigated the effects of an aerobic exercise program on fatigue and the physical performance of five cancer survivors suffering from severe fatigue. Using a one-group pre-test/post-test design, the investigators implemented a progressive program of treadmill walking tailored to the fitness level of each subject, guided by training heart rates and periodic checks of serum lactate concentration. Maximal performance, training speed, and training distance all improved significantly from pre-test to post-test for the group. Subjective reports as well as the resumption of daily activities indicated a reduced fatigue level for subjects. However, no standardized measure of fatigue was used in the study.

Schwartz (1998a) conducted a cross-sectional mailed survey of 219 cancer survivors to examine the physical activity patterns of individuals who identified themselves as athletes. This survey would assess patient exercise behavior and fatigue levels during cancer treatment. The majority of respondents reported decreasing their activity level during treatment, but they used exercise to decrease CRF.

A variety of studies have been conducted to investigate nonfatigue outcomes of exercise in cancer patients. The results of many of these studies have indicated support for theories related to CRF, such as improved functional capacity (Dimeo, Rumberger, & Keul, 1998; Dimeo, Tilmann, et al., 1997; MacVicar et al., 1989; Segal et al., 2001), decreased anxiety and depression (Segar et al., 1998), and increased quality of life (Young-McCaughan & Sexton, 1991). Furthermore, the cumulative volume of studies on exercise in cancer patients in treatment as well as survivors indicates that this health-promoting activity has many positive benefits for cancer patients and few notable risks.

## SUMMARY OF EXERCISE EFFICACY IN CANCER-RELATED FATIGUE

Although the 11 studies reviewed here have been limited in number and sample sizes, the designs have all been a form of experimental design and the results have been unequivocal. All the investigations have demonstrated significantly lower levels of fatigue in subjects who exercised when compared to controls. In addition, emotional distress and sleep disturbance results were significantly lower in those who exercised.

## TYPES AND DURATIONS OF EXERCISE

The forms of exercise reported in the studies described previously were varied, but all were considered aerobic. Some exercise programs were supervised in a laboratory or clinical setting (Dimeo et al., 1999; MacVicar & Winningham, 1986), while a greater number were unsupervised home-based programs. Studies have indicated that subjects do better in the more convenient home-based settings (Segal et al., 2001). Although the home-based exercise program lacks the control of a supervised exercise program, it is more cost-effective and is easily promoted to women. The dose of exercise was also varied but stayed in a range known to achieve a training effect: 60% to 85% of the maximum heart rate in sessions of about 30 minutes 3 to 4 days a week.

In the 2001 research report by Schwartz et al., a dose–response outcome was described with fatigue levels inversely related to three increasing levels of exercise observed in the subjects. The length of the exercise programs in the 11 studies ranged from 6 weeks for patients in radiation therapy to 4 to 6 months for chemotherapy and during the often lengthy hospitalization for peripheral blood stem cell transplantation. This suggests that a wide range of doses of exercise is effective and no minimum effective dose has been established in this population. Schwartz et al. did find that women who exercised more than 60 minutes a session were most likely to report *increased* levels of fatigue, suggesting a maximum effective dose, at least within the context of an 8-week training program. No serious adverse events have been reported in any of the studies, although this may reflect the convention of not including this information in research reports. Most studies used criteria to exclude high-risk patients.

Aerobic exercise interventions have a powerful effect on CRF. Significant differences have been seen between experimental and control groups even with small sample sizes of 6 to 10 subjects per group in laboratory studies and 22 to 24 subjects per group in home-based exercise studies. Fatigue levels were 40% to 50% lower in exercising subjects.

POPULATIONS STUDIED

The populations studied have been limited to female breast cancer patients with the exception of Dimeo's work with both male and female patients undergoing peripheral blood stem cell transplantation. Mean ages of the breast cancer samples have ranged from 44 to 53 years. The sample characteristics in studies that collected these data have reflected a high educational level (greater than 12 years in every case) and a limited ethnic diversity, with primarily Caucasian subjects. Breast cancer stages of 0 to III have been included and several types of cancer treatments have been represented, with the notable exception of biological response modifier therapy, in which fatigue is a dose-limiting toxicity. In studies of breast cancer patients receiving chemotherapy, the protocols have primarily been cyclophosphamide and doxorubicin, or cyclophosphamide, methotrexate, and 5-fluorouracil.

In studies with control groups, the intensity of chemotherapy regimens was evaluated and controlled. No studies reported the prevalence of anemia or whether subjects were receiving colony-stimulating factor medications, although this information would be helpful in interpreting results related to fatigue. Therefore, the study results have limited generalizability to individuals with other cancer diagnoses, older individuals or children, and minorities.

ADHERENCE OBSERVED

Adherence to exercise is a challenge for healthy individuals, with a reported drop-out rate of about 50% (Dishman, 1998), and is surely more difficult for cancer patients undergoing active cancer treatment. Adherence rates averaged 60% in the Schwartz studies where adherence was defined as pre-test to post-test improvement on the 12-Minute Walk Test, averaged 70% to 80% in the Mock et al. studies by self-report on diaries of minutes walked, and were not clearly reported by Dimeo or MacVicar. In the supervised laboratory and clinical sites, subjects either adhered by catching up on missed sessions or dropped out of the study. In the home-based exercise studies, subjects were retained even though they exercised at a level less than that defined as adherence in the study.

Adherence to exercise was determined in the studies either by direct observation in clinical sites or by logs kept by the subjects who walked at home. Adherence is correlated with prior exercise history, body mass index, and the subjects' educational level (Courneya & Friedenreich, 1999; Mock, Dow et al., 1997; Pickett et al., 2002; Sallis, Hovell, & Hofstetter, 1992).

Several of the home-based exercise studies report prior exercise history and one study (Mock et al., 2002) enrolled only sedentary individuals to decrease the amount of spontaneous exercise in the control group. In the randomized studies, intention to treat was the approach to data analysis when adherence was 70% or greater (Dimeo et al., 1999; MacVicar & Winningham, 1986; Mock et al., 1994; Mock, Dow, et al., 1997). However, in the studies where crossovers were common, both intention to treat and a compliance/dose–response approach to analysis were used (Mock et al., 2001; Mock et al., 2002).

MEASURES

The effects of exercise on functional capacity or exercise performance were measured at pre-test and post-test by cycle ergometer (Dimeo et al., 1999; MacVicar & Winningham, 1986), treadmill test (Dimeo et al., 1998; Dimeo, Tilman, et al., 1997), or the 12-Minute Walk Test (Mock et al., 1994, 2001, 2002; Mock, Dow, et al., 1997; Schwartz, 1999, 2000, 2001). The 12-Minute Walk is a submaximal test of functional capacity in which subjects walk briskly under controlled conditions for 12 minutes, and the distance walked is the subject's score (Steele, 1996). Only two (Schwartz, 2000, 2001) of the home-based unsupervised exercise studies used an objective measure to quantify the subjects' activity during exercise sessions. The other studies relied upon subjects' self-reported exercise data on diaries or questionnaires, obviously a more subjective and potentially less valid measure.

Fatigue was measured by visual analogue scales (Mock et al., 1994; Mock, Dow, et al., 1997; Schwartz, 1999, 2001), by the POMS fatigue subscale (Dimeo et al., 1999; MacVicar and Winningham, 1986; Mock et al., 2001), by the PFS (Mock et al., 2001, 2002; Mock, Dow, et al., 1997), by the Schwartz Cancer Fatigue Scale (Schwartz, 1998b), or by anecdote during interviews (Dimeo et al., 1997, 1998).

The fatigue instruments are all self-reports and all are considered to be valid and reliable, having been used previously in cancer populations. Although the single-item visual analogue scale measures only the magnitude of the symptom, the 22-item, more comprehensive PFS (Piper, 1998) yields a total score plus four dimensions of fatigue: behavioral/severity, sensory, cognitive/mood, and affective. The POMS fatigue subscale sums the number and severity of fatigue-like symptoms currently experienced by the subject. The Schwartz Cancer Fatigue Scale is a newly developed six-item scale that has received limited use in research to date (Schwartz, 1998b).

The measures were collected at pre-test or baseline before the exercise program began and at post-test at the end of the exercise program. In four of the studies, the program was designed to extend through the cancer treatment, so the pre-test was also before cancer treatment was begun and post-test measures were collected just before cancer treatment ended, or, in one case, 30 days later (Mock et al., 1994). In the Schwartz studies (2000, 2001), patients were followed over two cycles of chemotherapy. The time of post-test in the peripheral blood stem cell transplantation patients was just before discharge from the hospital, creating a variable length to the exercise program. Few studies have followed subjects past the post-test period to see whether subjects continue to exercise and what happens to fatigue levels if they do or do not.

## Energy Conservation Interventions

Energy conservation, along with additional rest, may be the most frequent CRF treatment recommendation by care providers as well as the most frequent self-care activity of fatigued patients (Richardson & Ream, 1997). The underlying assumption is that energy can be stored in the body so that additional amounts will be available when needed or that rest is restorative and will diminish CRF as it does fatigue in healthy individuals. Although studies are in progress, currently no evidence is available for testing this theory in cancer patients. The conservation of energy is a common approach to care for patients with cardiac or respiratory disease when exertion beyond tolerance accrues an oxygen deficit with resultant high levels of fatigue. No evidence exists that a similar oxygen deficit is present in CRF, with the exception of moderate to severe anemia in some cancer patients. Furthermore, decreasing activity to "save" energy contributes to deconditioning and decreased activity tolerance. However, using limited energy to perform highly valued activities, instead of mundane tasks that can be delegated, may increase personal satisfaction and quality of life.

## Sleep and Rest Interventions

Clinical recommendations for additional rest and sleep have been common advice by care providers to patients who report CRF. Sleep disturbance is frequently reported as a distressing symptom by cancer patients (Longman, Braden, & Mishel, 1996; Mock et al., 2001; Mock, Dow, et al., 1997; Owen, Parker, & McGuire, 1999). Although universal human experience indicates that sleep deprivation results in fatigue, the relationship between sleep disturbance and fatigue in cancer patients has been inadequately explored (Lee, 2001).

Berger studied the relationships among activity, sleep, and fatigue in breast cancer patients receiving chemotherapy (Berger, 1998; Berger & Farr, 1999; Berger & Higginbotham, 2000; Berger & Walker, 2001). Frequent night awakenings affected 50% of the sample and were accompanied by lower levels of daytime activity, more daytime napping, and high levels of fatigue (Berger & Farr, 1999). The strongest association with fatigue was the number of night awakenings. The use of continuous-activity measurement by actigraphy has been a strength of these studies.

Cancer patients who try additional rest and sleep to manage CRF do not report it to be particularly effective (Graydon, Bubela, Irvine, & Vincent, 1995). However, these results may be related to poor quality of nocturnal sleep or other factors. Studies testing sleep interventions to decrease CRF are just beginning.

## Stress and Coping Interventions

### EDUCATIONAL PREPARATION

An extensive body of research has documented the beneficial effects of providing patients with preparatory knowledge about their disease and treatment, including sensory information. Some of these studies have included cancer patients receiving radiation therapy (Johnson, Nail, Lauver, King, & Keys, 1988). The assumption of preparatory information and education is that patients who receive valid information about what to anticipate develop accurate expectations and are less likely to experience the stress that accompanies unforeseen problems. Patients can prepare for side effects and learn management and coping strategies. In the case of CRF, patients will interpret the symptom as an expected side effect of treatment rather than an indication that their cancer treatment is not working or that their disease is progressing—interpretations that increase anxiety and depression. However, the limited research on education and preparatory information for cancer patients has not focused specifically on fatigue as an outcome, but has demonstrated decreased disruption in usual activities and more positive emotional outcomes (Johnson, 1999).

### STRESS REDUCTION

Psychosocial interventions aimed at stress reduction and improved coping have also been used to manage fatigue. In research evaluating support groups for individuals with cancer, the experimental group demonstrated less depression and fatigue, as well as greater vigor than the control group on the POMS (Fawzy et al., 1990).

A comprehensive coping strategy program (CCSP) was tested in a randomized controlled clinical trial (Gaston-Johansson et al., 2000) to reduce pain, fatigue, nausea, and psychological distress in 110 breast cancer patients undergoing autologous bone marrow transplantation (ABMT). The subjects were well educated, primarily married, Caucasian women with high incomes. The CCSP included components of preparatory information, cognitive restructuring, and relaxation with guided imagery. The preparatory information, delivered by a clinical social worker and accompanied by printed material, covered symptom management, the use of positive coping self-statements, and the importance of avoiding distorted thinking. Participants were taught muscle relaxation accompanied by guided imagery and were given an audiotape to use in practicing the relaxation daily from baseline until 7 days after transplant.

The CCSP was found to significantly reduce fatigue combined with nausea 7 days post-ABMT, but no significant differences took place in the two groups in fatigue alone. Both fatigue and nausea were measured with visual analogue scales. The effect size of the CCSP on fatigue outcomes in this study was .35, a small effect, and the study was powered for medium effect. A larger sample size might have revealed more differences between groups.

Cimprich (1992, 1993, 2001) has described a model of cognitive or attentional fatigue in cancer patients. The theory proposes that, based on principles from the field of cognitive neuropsychology, attentional fatigue follows intense mental effort and is manifested as a decreased capacity to direct attention to perform activities such as problem solving or planning. According to the theory, the act of concentrating involves a global neural inhibitory mechanism that blocks competing stimuli during purposeful activity. This capacity to block distractions, defined as *directed attention*, is essential to purposeful cognitive functioning. During stressful situations, such as those that occur during the increased demands of life-threatening illness and treatment, directed attention may become impaired with a resulting loss of concentration.

In a descriptive, comparative study, 95 older women with newly diagnosed breast cancer were tested before surgery and were followed for 3 months postsurgery. Compared to women of similar age without breast cancer, the women with breast cancer scored significantly lower on measures of their capacity for direct attention before surgery, with a gradual improvement in scores by 3 months. At 3 months, the breast cancer group still reported significantly higher scores than the control group on fatigue and loss of concentration as measured by the McCorkle and Young (1978) Symptom Distress Scale.

Cimprich (1993) developed and tested an attention-restoring intervention in post-surgical breast cancer patients with a controlled experimental design. The intervention involved restorative experiences with the natural environment, such as gardening, watching birds or wildlife, and caring for pets, with the specific choice of activities selected by the subjects in a tailored fashion. Subjects performed the selected activities for 20 to 30 minutes at least three times a week. Subjects in the experimental group demonstrated enhanced attentional capacity on a variety of neurocognitive tests and returned to work earlier than the control group.

The research in this field is preliminary and needs further development. However, because individuals with CRF have described a cognitive component, the relationship between physical feelings of fatigue and attentional fatigue deserves exploration. Studying the effects of an exercise program on cognitive functioning or of a restorative intervention on physical tiredness might reveal more about the relationship of physical and psychological aspects of CRF.

In summary, the nonexercise interventions have been less well tested than exercise interventions but have considerable potential as additional therapies for CRF.

## SUMMARY AND RECOMMENDATIONS FOR FUTURE RESEARCH

Much progress has occurred in the research on CRF since an initial appraisal in 1991 (Irvine, Vincent, Graydon, Bubela, & Thompson) and a state-of-the-science report in 1994 (Winningham et al.). Most of this work has been descriptive or correlational, but a growing body of reports has focused on testing interventions. In the absence of effective medications to treat CRF, behavioral interventions to manage the symptom have predominated, with exercise as the most widely tested intervention.

Although theories to explain CRF have been described, most research studies have not tested these theories in a manner that clearly contributes to theory development. The populations studied have primarily been breast cancer patients and samples have been limited in regard to ethnicity, socioeconomic status, age, and gender. Little research has focused on fatigue management in palliative care.

Small sample sizes, a lack of control groups, and other forms of methodologic rigor have limited research designs. A need exists to report and control variations in the type and intensity of chemotherapy or other cancer treatments that are concurrent with fatigue interventions. In addition, subject characteristics—such as age, educational level, comorbid conditions, and the stage of disease—that may affect adherence to interventions or the measurement of efficacy should be controlled in research designs. Addressing these issues could lead to more effective interventions tailored to patient characteristics and to disease and treatment factors.

A growing variety of fatigue instruments are available for use in research, but current evidence comparing these in differing research situations is insufficient to guide investigators in their selection. Evidence suggests that tailoring interventions to individuals' needs and situations is helpful and sometimes essential for effectiveness. However, evidence-based guidelines for performing this tailoring are not yet available for most interventions. Based on these and other identified gaps in the current knowledge of interventions for CRF, the following recommendations are suggested for future research in the field. First, additional investigations are necessary at all levels, especially at the intervention-testing level. Current fatigue theories must be tested, along with the development of new theories. These theories should then be put into practice; all research should be guided by theory.

Studies must make use of more rigorous research designs with larger sample sizes and larger control groups, with healthy controls and attentional controls as appropriate. Further, research must rely upon a greater standardization of interventions to facilitate replication and increase internal validity. Studies must further investigate correlations of fatigue to provide directions for future interventions. Psychometric research must be conducted using both existing and new fatigue instruments; comparisons of instruments should be undertaken. More objective instruments and outcomes should be relied upon to increase validity and reliability. An example of this would be the use of instruments such as actigraphy to measure the dose of exercise in home-based programs.

More diverse populations and samples of cancer patients should be targeted, especially in regard to ethnicity, cultural health beliefs and practices, socioeconomic status, age, and type of cancer. Research should explore fatigue in recurrent disease and in palliative care. Interventions should be tested across the types of cancer treatments, including chemotherapy, radiation therapy, biotherapy, hormonal therapy, and surgery.

Researchers should focus on elucidating the mediating mechanisms for every intervention to facilitate our understanding of CRF. Further, research must more comprehensively report study results in regard to refusals, withdrawals, adherence rates, and adverse events. Also, exercise and other interventions should be tailored, within standardized guidelines, to increase efficacy, adherence, and patient acceptability. The secondary outcomes of fatigue interventions—such as survival, quality of life, and immune function—should be studied. Researchers should determine the effectiveness of clinical practice guidelines for managing fatigue. Interventions to improve sleep quality as a treatment for fatigue should be tested along with stress-reducing interventions to manage fatigue. Finally, studies should compare exercise and psychosocial interventions in a factorial design.

Although much work is yet to be done, it is reassuring that several large-scale clinical studies of CRF are currently under way, investigating interventions such as the conservation of energy and sleep facilitation, as well as exercise with prostate and colorectal cancer patients during treatment and post-cancer treatment. The management of CRF will be more effective when a variety of evidence-based interventions are available to prevent and treat this distressing symptom.

## REFERENCES

Aistars, J. (1987). Fatigue in the cancer patient: A conceptual approach to a clinical problem. *Oncology Nursing Forum, 14*(6), 25–30.

Akechi, T., Kugaya, A., Okamura, H., Yamawaki, S., & Uchitomi, Y. (1999). Fatigue and its associated factors in ambulatory cancer patients: A preliminary study. *Journal of Pain and Symptom Management, 17*, 42–48.

Andrykowski, M. A., Curran, S. L., & Lightner, R. (1998). Off-treatment fatigue in breast cancer survivors: A controlled comparison. *Journal of Behavior Medicine, 21*, 1–18.

Berger, A. M. (1998). Patterns of fatigue and activity and rest during adjuvant breast cancer chemotherapy. *Oncology Nursing Forum, 25*, 51–62.

Berger, A. M., & Farr, L. (1999). The influence of daytime inactivity and nighttime restlessness on cancer-related fatigue. *Oncology Nursing, 26*, 1663–1671.

Berger, A. M., & Higginbotham, P. (2000). Correlates of fatigue during and following adjuvant breast cancer chemotherapy: A pilot study. *Oncology Nursing Forum, 27*, 1443–1448.

Berger, A. M., & Walker, S. N. (2001). An explanatory model of fatigue in women receiving adjuvant breast cancer chemotherapy. *Nursing Research, 50*, 42–52.

Blesch, K., Paice, J., Wickham, R., Harte, N., Schnoor, T., Purl, S., et al. (1991). Correlates of fatigue in people with breast or lung cancer. *Oncology Nursing Forum, 18*, 81–87.

Broeckel, J. A., Jacobsen, P. B., Horton, J., Balducci, L., & Lyman, G. H. (1998). Characteristics and correlates of fatigue after adjuvant chemotherapy for breast cancer. *Journal of Clinical Oncology, 16*, 1689–1696.

Cimprich, B. (1992). Attentional fatigue following breast cancer surgery. *Research in Nursing & Health, 15*, 199–207.

Cimprich, B. (1993). Developing an intervention to restore attention in cancer patients. *Cancer Nursing, 16*, 83–92.

Cimprich, B. (2001). Attention and symptom distress in women with and without breast cancer. *Nursing Research, 50*, 86–94.

Courneya, K. S., & Friedenreich, C. M. (1999). Physical exercise and quality of life following cancer diagnosis: A literature review. *Annals of Behavioral Medicine, 21*, 171–179.

Dimeo, F., Fetscher, S., Lange, W., Mertelsmann, R., & Keul, J. (1997). Effects of aerobic exercise on the physical performance and incidence of treatment-related complications after high-dose chemotherapy. *Blood, 90*, 3390–3394.

Dimeo, F. C., Rumberger, B. G., & Keul, J. (1998). Aerobic exercise as therapy for cancer fatigue. *Medicine and Science in Sports and Exercise, 30*, 475–478.

Dimeo, F. C., Stieglitz, R. D., Novelli-Fischer, U., Fetscher, S., & Keul, J. (1999). Effects of physical activity on the fatigue and psychologic status of cancer patients during chemotherapy. *Cancer, 85*, 2273–2277.

Dimeo, F. C., Tilmann, M. H. M., Bertz, H., Kanz, L., Mertelsmann, R., & Keul, J. (1997). Aerobic exercise in the rehabilitation of cancer patients after high dose chemotherapy and autologous peripheral stem cell transplantation. *Cancer, 79*, 1717–1722.

Dishman, R. K. (Ed.). (1998). Overview to *Exercise adherence* (pp. 1–9). Champaign, IL: Human Kinetics.

Fawcett, J. (1995). Levine's Conservation Model. In J. Fawcett & M. Fithian (Eds.), *Analysis and evaluation of conceptual models of nursing* (3rd ed., pp. 165–215.) Philadelphia: F.A. Davis.

Fawzy, F. I., Cousins, N., Fawzy, N. W., Kemeny, M., Elashoff, R., & Morton, D. (1990). A structured psychiatric intervention for cancer patients: I. Changes over time in methods of coping and affective disturbance. *Archives of General Psychiatry, 47*, 720–725.

Ferrell, B. R., Grant, M., Dean, G. E., Funk, B., & Ly, J. (1996). "Bone tired": The experience of fatigue and its impact on quality of life. *Oncology Nursing Forum, 23*, 1539–1547.

Gaston-Johansson, F., Fall-Dickson, J. M., Nanda, J., Ohly, K. V., Stillman, S., Krumm, S., et al. (2000). The effectiveness of the comprehensive coping strategy program on clinical outcomes in breast cancer autologous bone marrow transplantation. *Cancer Nursing, 23*, 277–285.

Glaus, A., Crow, R., & Hammond, S. (1996). A qualitative study to explore the concept of fatigue/tiredness in cancer patients and in healthy individuals. *Supportive Care in Cancer, 4*, 82–86.

Graydon, J. E., Bubela, N., Irvine, D., & Vincent, L. (1995). Fatigue-reducing strategies used by patients receiving treatment for cancer. *Cancer Nursing, 18*, 23–28.

Greene, D., Nail, L. M., Fieler, V. K., Dudgeon, D., & Jones, L. S. (1994). A comparison of patient-reported side effects among three chemotherapy regimens for breast cancer. *Cancer Practice, 2*, 57–62.

Irvine, D., Vincent, L., Bubela, N., Thompson, L., & Graydon, J. (1991). A critical appraisal of the research literature investigating fatigue in the individual with cancer. *Cancer Nursing, 14*, 188–199.

Irvine, D., Vincent, L., Graydon, J. E., Bubela, N., & Thompson, L. (1994). The prevalence and correlates of fatigue in patients receiving treatment with chemotherapy and radiotherapy: A comparison with the fatigue experience by healthy individuals. *Cancer Nursing, 17*, 367–378.

Jacobs, L. A., & Piper, B. F. (1996). The phenomenon of fatigue and the cancer patient. In R. McCorkle, M. Grant, M. Frank-Stromborg, & S. Baird (Eds.), *Cancer nursing: A comprehensive textbook* (2nd ed., pp. 1193–1206). Philadelphia: W.B. Saunders Company.

Jacobsen, P. B., Hann, D. M., Azzarello, L. M., Horton, J., Balducci, L., & Lyman, G. H. (1999). Fatigue in women receiving adjuvant chemotherapy for breast cancer: Characteristics, course, and correlates. *Journal of Pain and Symptom Management, 18*, 233–242.

Johnson, J. (1999). Self-regulation theory and coping with physical illness. *Research in Nursing & Health, 22*, 435–438.

Johnson, J., Nail, L., Lauver, D., King, K., & Keys, H. (1988). Reducing the negative impact of radiation therapy. *Cancer, 61*, 46–51.

Lee, K. A. (2001). Sleep and fatigue. *Annual Review of Nursing Research, 19*, 249–273.

Longman, A. L., Braden, C. J., & Mishel, M. H. 1996. Side effects burden in women with breast cancer. *Cancer Practice, 4*, 274–280.

MacVicar, M. G., & Winningham, M. L. (1986). Promoting the functional capacity of cancer patients. *Cancer Bulletin, 38*, 235–239.

MacVicar, M. G., Winningham, M. L., & Nickel, J. L. (1989). Effects of aerobic interval training on cancer patients' functional capacity. *Nursing Research, 38*, 348–351.

McCorkle, R., & Young, K. (1978). Development of a symptom distress scale. *Cancer Nursing, 1*, 373–378.

Mock, V., Atkinson, A., Barsevick, A., Cella, D., Cimprich, B., Cleeland, C., et al. (2000). National Comprehensive Cancer Network Oncology Practice Guidelines for Cancer-Related Fatigue. *Oncology, 14*, 151–161.

Mock, V., Burke, M. B., Sheehan, P. K., Creaton, E., Winningham, M., McKinney-Tedder, S., et al. (1994). A nursing rehabilitation program for women with breast cancer receiving adjuvant chemotherapy. *Oncology Nursing Forum, 21*, 899–908.

Mock, V., Cameron, L. A., Tompkins, C., Lin, E., & Stewart, K. (1997). *Every Step Counts: A walking exercise program for persons living with cancer.* Baltimore: Johns Hopkins University.

Mock, V., Davidson, N., Ropka, M. E., Pickett, M., Poniatowski, B., Stewart, K. J., et al. (2002). Exercise manages fatigue during breast cancer treatment: A randomized controlled trial.

Mock, V., Dow, K. H., Meares, C., Grimm, P., Dienemann, J., Haisfield-Wolfe, M. E., et al. (1997). Effects of exercise on fatigue, physical functioning, and emotional distress during radiation therapy for breast cancer. *Oncology Nursing Forum, 24,* 991–1000.

Mock, V., Pickett, M., Ropka, M., Lin, E., Stewart, K., Rhodes, V., et al. (2001). Fatigue and quality of life outcomes of exercise during cancer treatment. *Cancer Practice, 9,* 119–127.

Mooney, K. H., Ferrell, B. R., Nail, L. M., Benedict, S. C., & Haberman, M. R. (1991). Oncology Nursing Society Research Priorities Survey. *Oncology Nursing Forum, 18,* 1381–1388.

Nail, L. M., & Jones, L. S. (1995() Fatigue as a side effect of cancer treatment: Impact on quality of life. *Quality of Life, 4,* 8–13.

Owen, D. C., Parker, K. P., & McGuire, D. B. (1999). Comparison of subjective sleep quality in patients with cancer and healthy subjects. *Oncology Nursing Forum, 26,* 1649–1651.

Pickett, M., Mock, V., Ropka, M. E., Cameron, L., Coleman, M., & Podewils, L. (in press). Adherence to moderate intensity exercise during breast cancer treatment. *Cancer Practice.*

Piper, B. F., Dibble, S., Dodd, M. J., Weiss, M. C., Slaughter, R., & Paul, S. (1998). Revised Piper Fatigue Scale: Psychometric evaluation in women with breast cancer. *Oncology Nursing Forum, 25,* 677–684.

Piper, B., Lindsey, A., & Dodd, M. (1987). Fatigue mechanisms in cancer patients: Developing a nursing theory. *Oncology Nursing Forum, 14*(6), 17–23.

Ream, E., & Richardson, A. (1999). From theory to practice: Designing interventions to reduce fatigue in patients with cancer. *Oncology Nursing Forum, 26,* 1295–1303.

Richardson, A., & Ream, E. (1997). Self-care behaviours initiated by chemotherapy patients in response to fatigue. *International Journal of Nursing Studies, 34,* 35–43.

Richardson, A., Ream, E., & Wilson-Barnett, J. (1998). Fatigue in patients receiving chemotherapy: Patterns of change. *Cancer Nursing, 21,* 17–30.

Robinson, K. D., & Posner, J. D. (1992). Patterns of self-care needs and interventions related to biologic response modifier therapy: Fatigue as a model. *Seminar in Oncology Nursing, 8*(Suppl. 4), 17–22.

Roy, C., & Andrews, H. A. (1991). *The Roy Adaptation Model. The definitive statement.* Norwalk, CT: Appleton and Lange.

Ryden, M. (1977). Energy: A crucial consideration in the nursing process. *Nursing Forum, 16,* 71–82.

Sallis, J. F., Hovell, M. F., & Hofstetter, C. R. (1992). Predictors of adoption and maintenance of vigorous physical activity in men and women. *Preventative Medicine, 21,* 237–251.

Schwartz, A. L. (1998a). Patterns of exercise and fatigue in physically active cancer survivors. *Oncology Nursing Forum, 25*, 485–491.

Schwartz, A. L. (1998b). Reliability and validity of the Schwartz Cancer Fatigue Scale. *Oncology Nursing Forum, 25*, 711–717.

Schwartz, A. L. (1999). Fatigue mediates the effect of exercise on quality of life. *Quality of Life Research, 8*, 529–538.

Schwartz, A. L. (2000). Daily fatigue patterns and effect of exercise in women with breast cancer. *Cancer Practice, 8*, 16–24.

Schwartz, A. L., Masood, N., Thompson, J. A., & Chahal, A. F. (2001). Aerobic exercise and methylphenidate for fatigue of interferon in malignant melanoma. *Proceedings of 6th National Conference on Cancer Nursing Research, 77*.

Schwartz, A. L., Mori, M., Gao, R., Nail, L. M., & King, M. E. (2001). Exercise reduces daily fatigue in women with breast cancer receiving chemotherapy. *Medicine and Science in Sports and Exercise, 33*, 718–723.

Segal, R., Evans, W., Johnson, D., Smith, J., Colletta, S., Gayton, J., et al. (2001). Structured exercise improves physical functioning in women with stages I and II breast cancer: Results of a randomized controlled trial. *Journal of Clinical Oncology, 19*, 657–665.

Segar, M. L., Katch, V. L., Roth, R. S., Garcia, A. W., Portner, T. I., Glickman, S. G., et al. (1998). The effect of aerobic exercise on self-esteem and depressive and anxiety symptoms among breast cancer survivors. *Oncology Nursing Forum, 25*, 107–113.

Sitzia, J., & Huggins, L. (1998). Side effects of cyclophosphamide, methotrexate, 5-fluorouracil (CMF) chemotherapy for breast cancer. *Cancer Practice, 6*, 13–21.

Steele, B. (1996). Timed walking tests of exercise capacity in chronic cardiopulmonary illness. *Journal of Cardiopulmonary Rehabilitation, 16*, 25–33.

Stone, P., Richards, M., & Hardy, J. (1998). Fatigue in patients with cancer. *European Journal of Cancer, 34*, 1670–1676.

Winningham, M. (1996). Fatigue. In S. Groenwald, M. H. Frogge, M. Goodman, & C. H. Yarbro (Eds.), *Cancer symptom management* (pp. 42–58). Boston: Jones & Bartlett.

Winningham, M., Nail, L., Burke, M., Brophy, L., Cimprich, B., Jones, L., et al. (1994). Fatigue and the cancer experience: State of the knowledge. *Oncology Nursing Forum, 24*, 23–36.

Winningham, M. L., & MacVicar, M. G. (1988). The effects of aerobic exercise on patient reports of nausea. *Oncology Nursing Forum, 15*, 447–450.

Winningham, M. L., MacVicar, M. G., Bondoc, M., Anderson, J. I., & Minton, J. P. (1989). Effect of aerobic exercise on body weight and composition in patients with breast cancer on adjuvant chemotherapy. *Oncology Nursing Forum, 16*, 683–689.

Woo, B., Dibble, S. L., Piper, B. F., Keating, S. B., & Weiss, M. C. (1998). Differences in fatigue by treatment methods in women with breast cancer. *Oncology Nursing Forum, 25*, 915–920.

Young-McCaughan, S., & Sexton, D. L. (1991). A retrospective investigation of the relationship between aerobic exercise and quality of life in women with breast cancer. *Oncology Nursing Forum, 18*, 751–757.

# 9

## Pain Management

### Christine Miaskowski

The undertreatment of cancer pain is a significant clinical problem (Jacox, Carr, & Payne, 1994; Ward et al., 1993). Unrelieved pain has serious negative consequences (e.g., depression, fatigue, and decreases in quality of life) for both cancer patients (Burrows, Dibble, & Miaskowski, 1998; Glover, Dibble, Dodd, & Miaskowski, 1995; Miaskowski, Zimmer, Barrett, Dibble, & Wallhagen, 1997) and their family caregivers (Miaskowski, Zimmer, et al., 1997; Miaskowski, Kragness, Dibble, & Wallhagen, 1997). Much of the research on cancer pain has focused on determining the epidemiology of cancer pain (Bonica, 1985; Cleeland et al., 1994; Portenoy et al., 1992) as well as the professional, patient, and organizational barriers to effective cancer pain management (Cleeland et al., 1994; Jacox et al., 1994; Ward et al., 1993). The focus on epidemiological research was warranted to define the scope and magnitude of the problem. In addition, the identification of the major barriers to effective cancer pain management laid the foundation to design intervention studies.

In an excellent review, Allard, Maunsell, Labbe, and Dorval (2001) pointed out that the majority of intervention studies in cancer pain management have attempted to improve clinician knowledge and attitudes, while a smaller number of studies have focused on changing clinician behaviors. Of note, far fewer studies have focused on improving patient and family caregiver *knowledge and attitudes* regarding cancer pain management (see Table 9.1; Clotfelter, 1999; Ferrell, Grant, Chan, Ahn, & Ferrell, 1995; Glajchen & Moul, 1996; Walker, 1992). Even fewer studies have tested the effectiveness of interventions to change patient and family caregiver *behaviors* regarding cancer pain management (see Table 9.2; Dalton, 1987; de Wit et al., 1997; Ferrell, Ferrell, Ahn, & Tran, 1994; Miaskowski et al., 2002; Rimer et al., 1987; Ward, Donovan, Owen, Grosen, & Serlin, 2000).

The purpose of this chapter is to summarize and critique some of the studies focused on improving patient and family caregiver knowledge and attitudes, and changing their behaviors regarding cancer pain management. Computer searches of MEDLINE® (from 1962 to 2001) and CINAHL® (from 1982 to 2001) have been done to identify intervention studies aimed at increasing patient and family caregiver knowledge and changing behaviors regarding cancer pain management. The search terms used were *cancer pain management*, *intervention*, and *education*. Additional references have been located by reviewing the reference lists of the studies identified through the computer searches. Brief summaries of these two groups of studies are presented and critiqued. In addition, this research literature is synthesized in terms of the provision of recommendations for clinical practice. The chapter concludes with recommendations for future research.

## INTERVENTION STUDIES TO CHANGE KNOWLEDGE

As shown in Table 9.1, four intervention studies have focused on changing cancer patient (Clotfelter, 1999; Glajchen & Moul, 1996; Walker, 1992) or family caregiver (Ferrell et al., 1995) knowledge regarding pain management. Only one of the studies is a randomized clinical trial (Clotfelter, 1999). The other three quasi-experimental studies utilize a pre- and post-test design or only conduct a post-test following a teleconference intervention (Glajchen & Moul, 1996). All four of these studies use a targeted intervention. A *targeted* intervention, in the context of this chapter, is one in which all the study participants in the intervention group receive an identical intervention. This targeted intervention can be contrasted with a *tailored* intervention, in which study participants receive an intervention structured to meet their specific learning needs.

Walker (1992) provided patients with a leaflet that contained information on controlled-release morphine tablets and complementary methods of pain control. Patients were interviewed 1 week after the intervention to evaluate pain relief scores, satisfaction with pain relief, and knowledge scores. Ferrell et al. (1995) had family caregivers of elderly patients with cancer-related pain participate in a three-part educational program on the

**TABLE 9.1  Summary of the Intervention Studies Focused on Changing Cancer Patient Knowledge Regarding Pain Management**

| | Theoretical/ conceptual framework | Design | Sample | Measures | Results |
|---|---|---|---|---|---|
| Clotfelter (1999) | None reported | RT, experimental targeted intervention: 14-minute video; 2-week duration of study | $N = 36$ elderly breast, prostate, and lung cancer patients recruited from a private oncology practice | Pain intensity; visual analogue scale | Patients in experimental group had significantly lower pain-intensity scores (16.3) than patients in control group (29.4); both groups experienced increases in pain intensity overall in 2-week period between pre- and post-test. |
| Ferrell, Grant, Chan, Ahn, & Ferrell (1995) | Conceptual model: impact of pain on quality of life | Quasi-experimental, pre- and post-test design; targeted intervention: 3-part educational program; 7-week duration of study | $N = 50$ family caregivers of elderly breast, GU organs, bone, connective tissue, and skin cancer patients identified by patients as person most involved in care and pain management | Quality of life; knowledge regarding pain measurement; caregiver burden | 1-week postintervention, significant improvements in psychological and social well-being, and overall quality of life; improved family caregiver knowledge about pain management; no caregiver burden data reported. |

| | Theoretical/ conceptual framework | Design | Sample | Measures | Results |
|---|---|---|---|---|---|
| Glajchen & Moul (1996) | None reported | Quasi-experimental design with follow-up post-test; targeted intervention: 25-minute presentation, followed by 10-minute question and answer; no data provided on time from intervention to post-test | $N = 107$ men with advanced-stage prostate cancer recruited from the community | Decrease misconceptions about pain management | 86% knew pain from prostate cancer could be controlled; 95% knew pain did not signify recurrent disease; 93% believed they would not become addicted to the pain medication; 73% stated pain medicine should not be withheld until absolutely necessary. |

*(continued)*

**TABLE 9.1  Summary of the Intervention Studies Focused on Changing Cancer Patient Knowledge Regarding Pain Management (*continued*)**

| | Theoretical/ conceptual framework | Design | Sample | Measures | Results |
|---|---|---|---|---|---|
| Walker (1992) | None reported | Quasi-experimental, pre- and post-test design; targeted intervention: leaflet on pain control, patient pain diaries; the length of time for intervention not reported; 1-week duration of study | $N = 11$ patients discharged from a cancer hospital | Satisfaction with pain relief; pain relief scores; knowledge scores | No significant changes on satisfaction with pain relief found following the provision of pain leaflet; patients stated that the use of complementary methods increased pain relief; knowledge scores regarding pain management increased in 91% of the surviving patients ($n = 10$). |

pharmacologic and nonpharmacologic management of pain. Family caregivers were asked to complete questionnaires that evaluated knowledge regarding pain management, quality of life, and caregiver burden at 4 and 7 weeks after enrollment in the study. In the third intervention study (Glajchen & Moul, 1996), a teleconference format was used to teach men with advanced prostate cancer about cancer pain management. Men were interviewed by phone following the teleconference to determine how effective the educational program was in reducing misconceptions regarding cancer pain management. In the fourth targeted intervention study (Clotfelter, 1999), patients were randomized to receive either standard care or view a 14-minute educational video on cancer pain management. Pain intensity scores were measured 2 weeks after the intervention.

All the studies (Ferrell et al., 1995; Glajchen & Moul, 1996; Walker, 1992) except the one by Clotfelter (1999) evaluated whether patient or family caregiver knowledge of cancer pain management improved following the intervention. The authors of all three educational intervention studies reported that patient and family caregiver knowledge of cancer pain management improved following the intervention. However, details were insufficient to determine the magnitude of the change in knowledge following the various interventions. Interestingly, in the study by Clotfelter, patients who received the educational intervention had significantly lower pain intensity scores (16.3) than patients in the control group (29.4) 2 weeks after the intervention, even though both groups experienced increases in pain intensity overall in the 2-week period between the pre- and post-test. In addition, the patients in this study reported relatively low levels of pain intensity.

## INTERVENTION STUDIES TO CHANGE BEHAVIOR

As shown in Table 9.2, in the past 15 years, only six intervention studies focused on changing patient behaviors regarding cancer pain management (Dalton, 1987; de Wit et al., 1997; Ferrell et al., 1994; Miaskowski et al., 2002; Rimer et al., 1987; Ward et al., 2000). Of note, with the exception of the study by Ferrell et al. (1994), all these studies were randomized clinical trials. In addition, three of these studies incorporated both targeted and tailored aspects into the intervention protocol (de Wit et al., 1997; Miaskowski et al., 2002; Rimer et al., 1987).

The studies by Dalton (1987) and Ward et al. (2000) need to be considered pilot studies. Dalton's study recruited 30 patients randomized to

**TABLE 9.2  Summary of the Intervention Studies Focused on Changing Cancer Patient Behaviors Regarding Pain Management**

| | Theoretical/ conceptual framework | Design | Sample | Measures | Results |
|---|---|---|---|---|---|
| Dalton (1987) | Melzack and Wall's theory of pain perception; McCaffery's guidelines for non-invasive, nonpharmacologic pain-control modalities | RCT, pre- and post-test design; targeted intervention; 60-minute educational intervention, followed by a 10-minute phone call; 10-day duration of study | $N = 30$ breast, multiple myeloma, and colon cancer patients recruited from outpatient oncology clinics in a large private teaching hospital | Knowledge of pain management; patient attitude regarding ability to decrease or control pain; pain intensity; pain when performing activities of daily living | Knowledge scores of patients in intervention group increased; no differences between groups regarding patient attitude toward ability to decrease or control pain; no differences between groups on pain intensity and pain when performing activities of daily living. |

| | Theoretical/conceptual framework | Design | Sample | Measures | Results |
|---|---|---|---|---|---|
| de Wit et al. (1997) | None reported | Prospective, longitudinal RT, pre- and post-test design; targeted and tailored intervention: 30- to 60-minute educational session in hospital; two 5- to 10-minute follow-up phone calls; 8-week duration of study | N = 313 oncology patients recruited from a specialized cancer center | Pain intensity; pain knowledge; quality of life | Pain-intensity scores decreased for patients in intervention group without district nursing; patients in both intervention groups had significant increases in pain knowledge scores; Pain Education Program (PEP) had no effect on quality of life. |
| Ferrell, Ferrell, Ahn, & Tran (1994) | Conceptual model of the impact of pain on quality of life | Quasi-experimental, pre- and post-test design; targeted intervention: 3-part educational program; 7-week duration of study | N = 80 breast, prostate, colon, lung, and melanoma patients recruited from 2 institutions not described | Knowledge; pain intensity; medication use; quality of life | Significant improvements in knowledge following intervention; patients reported improvement in pain-intensity scores; amount of medication taken increased over the duration of the study; no data reported on whether quality-of-life scores changed following intervention. |

*(continued)*

**TABLE 9.2  Summary of the Intervention Studies Focused on Changing Cancer Patient Behaviors Regarding Pain Management** (*continued*)

| | Theoretical/ conceptual framework | Design | Sample | Measures | Results |
|---|---|---|---|---|---|
| Miaskowski et al. (2002) | Orem's self-care theory, academic detailing, nurse coaching | RCT; targeted and tailored intervention: 60- to 90-minute teaching session; subsequent 60-minute home visits; 30-minute follow-up phone calls; 8-week duration of study | Breast, prostate, and lung cancer outpatients recruited from 7 outpatient settings; all patients experiencing pain from bone metastasis | Pain-intensity scores; knowledge about pain management; pain medication intake | Significant decreases found in average, worst, and least pain-intensity scores for patients in PRO-SELF© group compared to standard-care group; significant increases in knowledge for patients in the PRO-SELF group compared to standard-care group; patients in PRO-SELF group increased intake of opioids by 38 mg/day compared to standard-care group who increased opioid intake by 18 mg/day. |

| | Theoretical/ conceptual framework | Design | Sample | Measures | Results |
|---|---|---|---|---|---|
| Rimer et al. (1987) | None reported | RCT with a Solomon 4-group design; targeted and tailored intervention: 15-minute counseling session and print materials; 4-week duration of study | $N = 177$ lung, colorectal, and breast cancer outpatients from a comprehensive cancer center and $n = 53$ oncology outpatients from 2 community hospitals | Self-reported pain; implementation and adherence with pain-control regimen; recognition of and experience of side effects; misconceptions about tolerance and addiction | 44% of patients in experimental group and 24% in control group reported no or mild pain; experimental group was more likely to take pain medication on correct schedule and in correct dosage; experimental group was more likely to believe that side effects of medications could be prevented; experimental group was less fearful of addiction and tolerance. |
| Ward, Donovan, Owen, Grosen, & Serlin (2000) | None reported | RCT; tailored: 10-minute session about side effect management with follow-up phone calls; 8-week duration of study | $N/F = 100\%$, $M$ age = 58; ovarian, endometrial, uterine, and cervical cancers | Barriers questionnaire; pain management index; medication side effects checklist; brief pain inventory (pain intensity and interference); FACT-G | Barrier scores decreased for all patients; no differences were found between groups regarding analgesic intake, side effects, pain-intensity scores, quality of life; pain-interference scores decreased in both groups. |

receive either standard care or a 60-minute educational intervention in the outpatient clinic. This intervention was designed to increase the knowledge and use of self-management methods and to change attitudes toward their ability to manage pain and their self-report of pain. Although knowledge regarding pain management increased in both groups of patients, no differences were found between the two groups in pain intensity, the level of interference pain caused in activities, or a measure of patient attitude regarding one's ability to decrease or control pain. In the study by Ward et al., 43 patients were randomized to either a standard-care group or an intervention group that received an individually tailored intervention. Similar to the findings by Dalton, barrier scores decreased for both groups of patients. However, no differences were found in any of the other outcome measures (i.e., pain intensity scores, the use of adequate analgesic intake, pain interference scores, side effects, and quality-of-life scores).

All three studies utilizing targeted and tailored approaches as part of the intervention (i.e., de Wit et al., 1997; Miaskowski et al., 2002; Rimer et al., 1987) provided evidence that patients in the intervention group reported significant increases in knowledge and changes in behaviors that resulted in improvements in cancer pain management. In the study by Rimer et al., an oncology nurse conducted interactive and structured counseling sessions and provided educational materials on cancer pain management. Patients were interviewed 4 weeks after enrolling in the study. A higher percentage of patients (44%) in the intervention group reported mild or no pain than patients in the control group (24%). In addition, patients in the intervention group reported that they were more likely to take their pain medication in the correct dose and on the correct schedule. However, this information was not verified by evaluating patient analgesic prescriptions or actual intake. Finally, patients in the intervention group reported less fear of addiction and tolerance.

In the study by de Wit et al. (1997), patients were first stratified based on whether they would or would not receive district nursing (i.e., home care nursing) and then randomized to either standard care or a targeted and tailored intervention called the Pain Education Program (PEP). The tailored portion of the intervention consisted of a one-on-one session with a nurse prior to discharge from the hospital. This session, which lasted 30 to 60 minutes, focused on areas that the patient and nurse identified as areas with a knowledge deficit. Patients were given an audiotape of this targeted educational session. The targeted portion of the intervention consisted of having patients record pain intensity scores (using a 0 to 10 scale) twice a day in a diary. In addition, patients were given a pain brochure that consisted of two parts. Part 1, the targeted part, contained general information aimed at all cancer patients with chronic pain and described the possible causes of pain, pain control, nonadherence, and misconceptions. Part 2, the tailored part, consisted of nine supplementary sheets of paper with specific information about different cancer treatments. Patients were given only those sheets applicable to them. Patients were phoned at home 3 and 7 days following the intervention to determine if they had any questions. Patients in both intervention groups (i.e., those with and without district nursing) reported significant increases in knowledge about cancer pain management. However, decreases in pain intensity scores were only found in patients in the intervention group without district nursing. The reason for this finding is not clear.

In the study by Miaskowski et al. (2002), patients were randomized to either standard care or the targeted and tailored pain management intervention called the PRO-SELF Pain Control Program (PSPC) (see Chapter 7 for a detailed description of the program). The intervention and coaching sessions took place in patients' homes. Participating patients and their family caregivers received an educational program tailored to their specific needs. In addition, they were coached over a period of 6 weeks to change their behaviors regarding pain management. Significant improvements in the knowledge of cancer pain management were found in intervention-group patients. In addition, intervention-group patients reported significant decreases in pain intensity scores and increased their intake of opioid analgesics by 38 milligrams (expressed in morphine equivalents) per day.

## CRITICAL CHARACTERISTICS OF INTERVENTION STUDIES IN CANCER PAIN MANAGEMENT

In the past 15 years, only 10 intervention studies have been published focusing on changing patient or family caregiver knowledge and/or behaviors regarding cancer pain management (see Tables 9.1 and 9.2). A critical question to ask at this time is: What have we learned from these studies? To attempt to answer this question, these 10 studies were examined for similarities and differences in terms of seven critical characteristics: theoretical/conceptual frameworks, participant characteristics, the instruments used to measure the study results, the length of time for the intervention, the duration of the study, the outcome measures evaluated, and whether the changes in the outcome measures were clinically significant. A change in an outcome measure was considered clinically significant if the change was greater than or equal to half the standard deviation of the baseline measure.

## Theoretical/Conceptual Frameworks

Half of the studies reported a theoretical or conceptual framework (Dalton, 1987; Ferrell et al., 1994, 1995; Miaskowski et al., 2002; Ward et al., 2000). However, none of the frameworks are similar. The frameworks range from physiologic theories of pain perception (Dalton, 1997) to self-care theory and coaching (Miaskowski et al., 2002). Perhaps one way to design more effective intervention studies is to use a more focused behavioral theory as the basis for designing an intervention to change patient behaviors regarding pain management.

## Participant Characteristics

A total of 1,028 patients were enrolled in these 10 intervention studies. This number is extremely small considering the magnitude of the cancer pain problem. In fact, epidemiologic data suggest that 50% of oncology patients receiving active treatment for their cancer and 90% of terminally ill cancer patients experience moderate to severe pain (Bonica, 1985; Cleeland et al., 1994; Jacox et al., 1994; Portenoy et al., 1992). The mean age of the patients ranged from 55.5 to 67.7 years. This age range is fairly narrow and does not reflect the age range of individuals diagnosed with cancer. Of note, only one study focused specifically on elderly patients with cancer pain (Ferrell et al., 1994). The sex distribution of most of the studies was evenly divided between men and women. Given the recent reports of sex differences in pain and analgesic responses (for a review, see Miaskowski, Gear, & Levine, 2000), researchers should evaluate for sex differences in chronic cancer pain and in the effectiveness of interventions to improve cancer pain management. Of note, the majority of the studies have recruited patients with breast, prostate, or lung cancer.

## Measures

All the studies used appropriate instruments to measure the results of interest. However, when the information is reviewed, with the exception of numeric rating scales for pain intensity, a real heterogeneity exists in the number and types of instruments used in these 10 studies. The instruments that have the most sensitivity to detect changes in pain intensity, knowledge, and quality of life as a result of interventions to improve cancer pain management remain to be determined.

## Length of the Intervention

The intervention sessions ranged in time from 14 to 90 minutes. In addition, in four of the studies (Clotfelter, 1999; Glajchen & Moul, 1996; Rimer et al., 1987; Walker, 1992), the intervention was administered as a single educational session. In the other six studies, some type of opportunity was provided to additionally reinforce the educational intervention or enable a nurse to coach the patient to change his or her behavior regarding cancer pain management. The lack of consistency in the length of time for the intervention makes it impossible to determine the optimal length of time for a cognitive-behavioral intervention to improve cancer pain management.

## Duration of the Study

As with the length of time for the intervention, the effectiveness of the intervention was measured at a minimum of 1 week and at a maximum of 8 weeks. Given the fact that cancer patients can experience chronic pain associated with cancer and/or cancer treatment for several years, the duration of all these studies is extremely short.

## Outcome Measures

The most important outcome measures for intervention studies to improve cancer pain management include an evaluation of changes in knowledge regarding cancer pain management, changes in pain intensity, a measure of medication use or adherence with the analgesic regimen, and an evaluation of changes in mood or quality of life. These types of measures will reflect key outcomes for any cognitive-behavioral intervention focused on improving cancer pain management. Only the Ferrell et al. (1994) study of elderly cancer patients included all four of these outcome measures.

## Clinically Significant Changes in the Outcome Measures

As stated previously, a change in an outcome measure was considered clinically significant if the change was greater than or equal to half the standard deviation of the baseline measure. The majority of the intervention studies did not provide the appropriate data to determine whether the changes noted in the various outcome measures were clinically significant changes. To date, the only intervention study that produced clinically significant decreases in pain intensity scores and clinically significant increases in knowledge scores regarding cancer pain management was the study conducted by Miaskowski et al. (2002). Investigators need to provide the data to determine whether the changes that occur as a result of an intervention study are clinically significant changes.

## DIRECTIONS FOR FUTURE RESEARCH

Intervention studies targeted to improve cancer pain management among patients with cancer and their families are extremely limited. Over the past 15 years, only 10 studies were conducted that attempted to test the interventions to increase patient or family caregiver knowledge or improve behaviors regarding cancer pain management. Based on this review of the literature, studies that combine targeted and tailored approaches as part of the intervention appear to be the most effective in increasing knowledge and teaching behaviors that improve cancer pain management.

Future studies in this area will need to determine the "dose response" for a behavioral intervention in cancer pain management. For example, is it more effective to teach and coach a patient on a daily basis for 2 weeks or to meet with the patient on a weekly or monthly basis to improve pain management results? In addition, what is the optimal mode of delivering a behavioral intervention for cancer pain management (e.g., one-on-one teaching, videotape, audiotape, computer-assisted instruction, or group-teaching sessions)?

Additional research needs to be done to determine whether the effects of an intervention are sustained after it is completed. No studies have stopped an intervention and continued to evaluate patients for a period of time after the cessation of the intervention. The sustainability of the intervention is a critical factor to assess, because cancer pain is a chronic pain problem that can persist for years. Ideally, any intervention that improves outcomes would provide patients with the required skills to maintain effective pain management practice.

Another question that needs to be answered is whether different types of interventions need to be designed and whether different interventions would be more effective for different types of cancer pain (e.g., acute versus chronic pain or somatic versus neuropathic pain). Recently, Woolf et al. (Mannion & Woolf, 2000; Woolf & Decosterd, 1999; Woolf & Max, 2001) suggested that newer approaches to pain management should be based on underlying pain mechanisms. This concept of mechanistically based pain treatments needs to be considered when cognitive-behavioral interventions are designed to improve cancer pain management.

Another area for future research is the impact of other types of acute (e.g., a toothache or fractured limb) and chronic pain (e.g., arthritis) for the patient already experiencing cancer-related pain. As the population ages and is likely to have more chronic pain in addition to cancer pain, it becomes critical to understand the interaction effects among multiple pain problems, how these interaction effects influence patient results, and whether different types of interventions need to be used to effectively manage pain in patients with single or multiple types of pain problems.

An additional topic for future research is to determine how to more accurately assess a clinically significant reduction in pain following a behavioral intervention. Although changes in pain intensity scores are used in both pharmacologic and nonpharmacologic studies of cancer pain management, these scores may not reflect clinically significant effects. Better outcome measures may prove to be changes in functional status, changes in satisfaction with pain relief, changes in the amount of pain relief, or increased analgesic consumption without increased side effects.

Myriad questions need to be answered regarding the most effective interventions to improve cancer pain management. All the future intervention studies need to focus on changing patient and family caregiver behaviors to produce clinically significant results.

## ACKNOWLEDGMENT

This work was supported in part by a grant (R01 CA 64734) from the National Cancer Institute. Additional support for the author's program of research was provided through unrestricted grants from Janssen Pharmaceutica and Purdue Pharma LP.

## REFERENCES

Allard, P., Maunsell, E., Labbe, J., & Dorval, M. (2001). Educational interventions to improve cancer pain control: A systematic review. *Journal of Palliative Medicine, 4*, 191–203.

Bonica, J. J. (1985). Treatment of cancer pain: Current status and future needs. In H. L. Fields, R. Dubner, & F. Cervero (Eds.), *Proceedings of the Fourth World Congress on Pain: Advances in pain research and Therapy* (pp. 589–616). New York: Raven Press.

Burrows, M., Dibble, S. L., & Miaskowski, C. (1998). Differences in outcomes among patients experiencing different types of cancer-related pain. *Oncology Nursing Forum, 25*, 735–741.

Cleeland, C. S., Gonin, R., Hatfield, A. K., Edmonson, J. H., Blum, R. H., Stewart, J. A., et al. (1994). Pain and its treatment in outpatients with metastatic cancer. *New England Journal of Medicine, 330*, 592–596.

Clotfelter, C. E. (1999). The effect of an educational intervention on decreasing cancer pain intensity in elderly people with cancer. *Oncology Nursing Forum, 26*, 27–33.

Dalton, J. (1987). Education for pain management: A pilot study. *Patient Education and Counseling, 9*, 155–165.

de Wit, R., van Dam, F., Zandbelt, L., van Buuren, A., van der Heijden, K., Leenhouts, G., et al. (1997). A pain education program for chronic cancer pain patients: Follow-up results from a randomized clinical trial. *Pain, 73*, 55–69.

Ferrell, B. R., Ferrell, B. A., Ahn, C., & Tran, K. (1994). Pain management for elderly patients with cancer at home. *Cancer, 74*, 2139–2146.

Ferrell, B. R., Grant, M., Chan, J., Ahn, C., & Ferrell, B. A. (1995). The impact of cancer pain education on family caregivers of elderly patients. *Oncology Nursing Forum, 22*, 1211–1218.

Glajchen, M., & Moul, J. W. (1996). Teleconferencing as a method of educating men about managing advanced prostate cancer and pain. *Journal of Psychosocial Oncology, 14*, 73–87.

Glover, J., Dibble, S. L., Dodd, M. J., & Miaskowski, C. (1995). Mood states of oncology outpatients does pain make a difference? *Journal of Pain and Symptom Management, 10*, 120–128.

Jacox, A., Carr, D., & Payne, R. (Eds.). (1994). *Management of cancer pain. Clinical practice guideline no. 9* (AHCPR Publication No. 94–0592). Rockville, MD: Agency for Health Care Policy and Research, U.S. Department of Health and Human Services, Public Health Service.

Mannion, R. J., & Woolf, C. J. (2000). Pain mechanisms and management: A central perspective. *Clinical Journal of Pain, 16*(Suppl. 3), 144–156.

Miaskowski, C., Kragness, L., Dibble, S., & Wallhagen, M. (1997). Differences in mood states, health status, and caregiver strain between family caregivers of oncology outpatients with and without cancer-related pain. *Journal of Pain and Symptom Management, 13*, 138–147.

Miaskowski, C., Zimmer, E. F., Barrett, K. M., Dibble, S. L., & Wallhagen, M. (1997). Differences in patients' and family caregivers' perceptions of the pain experience influence patient and caregiver outcomes. *Pain, 72*, 217–226.

Miaskowski, C., Gear, R. W., & Levine, J. D. (2000). Sex-related differences in analgesic responses. In R. B. Fillingim (Ed.), *Sex, gender, and pain: Progress in pain research and management* (Vol. 17, pp. 209–230). Seattle, WA: IASP Press.

Miaskowski, C., Dodd, M., West, C. M., Paul, S., Schumacher, K., Tripathy, P., et al. (2002). A randomized clinical trial of the effectiveness of the PRO-SELF Pain Control Program in improving cancer pain management. Manuscript submitted for publication.

Portenoy, R. K., Miransky, J., Thaler, H. T., Horung, J., Bianchi, C., Cibas-Knog, I., et al. (1992). Pain in ambulatory patients with lung and colon cancer. Prevalence, characteristics, and effect. *Cancer, 70,* 1616–1624.

Rimer, B., Levy, M. H., Keintz, M. K., Lox, L., Engstrom, P. F., & MacElwee, N. (1987). Enhancing cancer pain control regimens through patient education. *Patient Education and Counseling, 10,* 267–277.

Walker, J. R. (1992). A study to develop and assess the value of a leaflet on pain control for patients taking MST in the community. *Palliative Medicine, 6,* 65–73.

Ward, S., Donovan, H. S., Owen, B., Grosen, E., & Serlin, R. (2000). An individualized intervention to overcome patient-related barriers to pain management in women with gynecological cancers. *Research in Nursing and Health, 23,* 393–405.

Ward, S. E., Goldberg, N., Miller-McCauley, V., Mueller, C., Nolan, A., Pawlik-Planek, D., et al. (1993). Patient-related barriers to management of cancer pain. *Pain, 52,* 319–324.

Woolf, C. J., & Decosterd, I. (1999). Implications of recent advances in the understanding of pain pathophysiology for the assessment of pain in patients. *Pain, 6*(Suppl.), 141–147.

Woolf, C. J., & Max, M. B. (2001). Mechanism-based pain diagnosis: Issues for analgesic drug development. *Anesthesiology, 95,* 241–249.

# 10

## Complementary and Alternative Therapy Interventions Used by Cancer Patients

## Gwen Wyatt

C omplementary and alternative medicine (CAM) is rapidly expanding and becoming a more complex arena. Multiple questions emerge around even the simplest of considerations and even address what to call this area of care. Is CAM complementary, alternative, integrative, holistic, traditional, unconventional, natural, or something else entirely? Beyond naming and identification questions are the questions of which practices fit this new field of care, which do not, and which modalities are in transition between this new field and conventional medicine. Another key question is, what are the necessary standards that a modality must measure up to in order to enter mainstream medicine? Finally, who is using these therapies, and for treatment of what symptoms or conditions?

The purpose of this chapter will be to outline the state of the science for evidence-based CAM therapies. The chapter begins with the current nomenclature and categories. The next section addresses the body of survey work on the prevalence of CAM therapies. Finally, five areas of CAM therapies will be assessed for their evidence base; each of the five areas includes a table with study components, a section on clinical results, and a section addressing directions for future research.

A computerized database search was first conducted, including MED-LINE® and CINAHL® from 1990 to the present. Key search words were included as well as phrases such as *cancer therapies, complementary therapies, alternative therapies*, and *cancer and CAM therapies*. Review articles and meta-analysis articles were assessed. The Cochrane Report was reviewed (Ezzo, Berman, Vickers, & Linde, 2000). Therapies that had two or more data-based publications were considered for inclusion. Once a study was selected for inclusion, citations within that publication were reviewed for additional research on the specific therapy.

Clearly, controversy surrounds each possible label for CAM. For some, *alternative* means in place of conventional medicine. *Unconventional* has a negative connotation and produces a fear response for some. Many *natural* therapies and medicines are not healthy or safe, such as tobacco (Drew & Myers, 1997). *Traditional* is often confused with conventional medicine, but in fact can mean the practices indigenous to a particular culture or population. *Complementary* most often refers to the use of modalities in conjunction with conventional medical care. For clarity, the National Center for Complementary and Alternative Medicine (NCCAM) definition will be used here: "[CAM] practices are best described as those not presently considered an integral part of conventional medicine" (NCCAM, 2000). Although we can propose terminology, it is important to remember that it is the individual who determines whether a therapy is complementary or alternative. That is, it is the patient who chooses whether to seek conventional medical care in addition to going to the herbal supplement store or the massage therapist.

## QUALIFICATIONS FOR MAINSTREAM MEDICINE

Despite the burgeoning interest in the utilization of CAM therapies, their efficacy and safety in the research literature has not received any overwhelming support (Vickers et al., 1997). However, at our current state of the science, a number of therapies are moving from CAM to mainstream, such as acupuncture (Ernst and White, 1998), St. John's wort (Linde et al., 1996), and chiropractics (Kaptchuk & Eisenberg, 1998). A variety of requirements constitute conventional medical practice (Gatchel & Maddrey, 1998; Vickers et al., 1997). Methods need to be subjected to randomized clinical trials that can be replicated, providers need to have specific credentials, such as licensure or certification (Geddes & Henry, 1997), and therapies need to demonstrate a consistent impact on health outcomes

(Jonas, 1998). The list of CAM practices changes over time as new therapies are proven to be safe, effective, and accepted as mainstream healthcare practices (NCCAM, 2000). Although various therapies have received numerous categorizations, the most widely relied upon is the NCCAM system.

## NATIONAL CENTER FOR COMPLEMENTARY AND ALTERNATIVE MEDICINE CATEGORIES

The categories for CAM therapies have been defined by NCCAM and correspond with how CAM therapies are typically found in the literature and on the Internet. The NCCAM categories have evolved in an effort to represent areas of interest in the most accurate and inclusive manner. The current five categories are mind–body interventions, biologically based therapies, manipulative and body-based methods, energy therapies, and alternative medical systems. Descriptions of the categories as well as examples of specific therapies within each category are as follows:

- *Mind–body intervention therapies* employ a variety of techniques to facilitate the mind's capacity to affect the body and various symptoms. Typical examples are meditation and guided imagery.
- *Manipulative and body-based methods* focus on the manipulation and/or movement of the body. Example therapies include chiropractic therapy, osteopathic manipulation, and reflexology.
- *Biologically based therapies* include practices, interventions, and products that often overlap with conventional therapies, including special diets. This category also encompasses less conventional therapies such as shark cartilage, bee pollen, and herbs.
- *Energy therapies* focus either on fields believed to originate from within the body (biofields) or those from external sources (electromagnetic fields). Examples of biofield work are Therapeutic Touch and Reiki, both of which are practices of body-energy alignment. Electromagnetic fields include the unconventional use of magnetic fields or alternating current fields.
- *Alternative medical systems* include complete systems of theory and practice that have evolved independently of, and often prior to, the conventional biomedical approach, such as Eastern Ayurveda medicine or homeopathic medicine (NCCAM, 2000).

## Prevalence of Complimentary and Alternative Therapies

The work of Eisenberg et al. (1993) was clearly the introduction of CAM into mainstream science. In 1993, the *New England Journal of Medicine* published the feature article entitled "Unconventional Medicine in the United States: Prevalence, Costs, and Patterns of Use." This national survey revealed that 33.8% of Americans were using at least one CAM therapy per year, at an average cost per visit of $27.60. The highest use was in the 25 to 49 age group, those who had relatively more education, and those with higher incomes than nonusers. In addition, 72% of the people using CAM therapies were not informing their primary health provider. An estimated 425 million visits for CAM therapies were reported to be made annually by participants. This number exceeded the number of annual visits to all U.S. primary care providers during this same time period (i.e., 388 million).

Following this published survey, the single most significant event occurred in the CAM movement: the National Institutes of Health (NIH) established an Office for the Study of Unconventional Medical Practices in 1993. The creation of this office charted a legitimate scientific course for the field and provided confirmation that such research has merit. This office authorized practitioners and scientists to demonstrate whether CAM therapies actually have the potential to change the clinical course and outcome of illness using the tools of rigorous science (Guzzetta, 1996). In 1998, this office was elevated to a center and renamed the National Center for Complementary and Alternative Medicine. NCCAM now funds centers of research at major institutions and provides funding to individual investigators.

Between 1990 and 2000, a variety of new refereed journals on CAM therapies appeared and began publishing in this rapidly growing field (see Table 10.1). Well-established professional journals are now also open to publishing evidence-based work on CAM. The creation of new journals and the openness of established journals to disseminate CAM-related work is are additional markers of mainstream acceptance (Cassileth, 1999b).

Many surveys have followed the initial assessment of the use of CAM therapies. In 1998, Eisenberg et al. conducted a follow-up survey to the 1993 report that assessed the use of the same 18 therapies, that is, relaxation techniques, herbal medicine, massage, chiropractic, spiritual healing, megavitamins, self-help groups, imagery, commercial diets, folk remedies, lifestyle diets, energy healing, homeopathy, hypnosis, biofeedback, acupuncture, and prayer. The definition of CAM therapies used in both surveys was "interventions neither taught widely in medical schools nor generally available in

**TABLE 10.1    Sample of Refereed Periodicals Devoted to CAM Therapies**

| Journal Name* | Publisher | Frequency of Publication |
|---|---|---|
| *Alternative Medicine Review* | Thorne Research, Inc. | Bimonthly |
| *Alternative Therapies in Health and Medicine* | InnoVision Communications | Bimonthly |
| *Complementary and Alternative Medicine at the NIH/National Institutes of Health* | Office of Alternative Medicine, Department of Health and Human Services, Public Health Service, NIH | Quarterly |
| *Complementary Health Practice Review* | Springer Publishing Company | Three times per year |
| *Focus on Alternative and Complementary Therapies* | Pharmaceutical Press, Inc. | Quarterly |
| *Integrative Medicine* | Elsevier Science, Inc. | Quarterly |
| *International Journal of Integrative Medicine* | Impakt Communications, Inc. | Bimonthly |
| *Journal of Alternative and Complementary Medicine: Research on Paradigm, Practice, and Policy* | Mary Ann Liebert, Inc. | Quarterly |
| *Scientific Review of Alternative Medicine* | Prometheus Books, Inc. | Semiannually |

*Note: A complete list of the 43 titles may be obtained from *Ulrich's International Periodicals Directory* (39th ed.), New Providence, NJ: R. R. Bowler.

U.S. hospitals" (Eisenberg et al., 1993, p. 246; Eisenberg et al., 1998, p. 1569; Kessler et al., 2001, p. 263). The percentage of Americans using CAM therapies rose from 33.8% in 1990 to 42.1% in 1997, and the estimated out-of-pocket expenditures rose from $13.7 billion in 1990 to $27 billion in 1997. Further, Wyatt, Friedman, Given, Given, and Beckrow (1999) reported that among 700 older, mixed-diagnosis cancer patients, 33% were independent of prescriptions from the health system but using some form of CAM. In another cancer-specific study, Wyatt, Given, Given, and Beckrow (2001) assessed 240 women with early stage breast cancer and found that 55% used CAM therapies during their cancer treatment. Finally, based on 26 surveys of cancer patients from 13 countries (including five patients from the U.S.), the average prevalence of CAM across all studies was 31% (Ernst & Cassileth, 1998).

Although surveys report consumer interest in access to CAM therapies, it is critical to acknowledge the state of the science. Even though consumer interest is peaked, evidence-based applications are running far behind. The broadest area of research to date is in the survey work on the prevalence of these therapies. Next in frequency are the data-based studies utilizing a pretest/post-test design without control groups. Finally, the randomized clinical trials have only, in the last 7 to 10 years, begun the huge task of testing for safety and efficacy.

## Rationale for Patient Use

Individuals, especially cancer patients, are becoming more interested in how CAM therapies can augment the treatment received from the conventional healthcare system (Jonas, 1998). Paltiel et al. (2001) pointed out that, further, cancer patients are a highly vulnerable population, often looking for a cure or relief of symptoms from nearly any source and often at whatever price is requested.

Some predictors of CAM use in the general population include a higher educational level, poorer health status, a holistic orientation toward health, a transformational experience that altered the individual's worldview, a classification in a cultural group committed to environmentalism and/or feminism, an interest in spirituality and personal growth, and having the following health problems: anxiety, back problems, chronic pain, or urinary tract problems (Astin, 1998). Richardson, Sanders, Palmer, Greisinger, and Singletary (2000) found that predictors for CAM use were younger persons, females, persons who had surgery as part of their cancer treatment, persons undergoing chemotherapy, and indigent persons. The best predictors for CAM use among cancer patients tend to be their demographics: female, better educated, of higher socioeconomic status, and younger than those who do not use CAM (Casselilth, 1999b).

## Interventions and Their Evidence Base

Using the five NCCAM categories as a framework, practices being employed by cancer patients where an evidence base supports the therapy or practice will be discussed. As with all CAM therapies, the knowledge base is only emerging. In terms of cancer care, multiple therapies are currently under investigation, and those will be highlighted. At least one example from each of the five NCCAM categories is included. The selection was based on the history of the therapy with cancer patients, the potential promise as a new therapy with cancer patients, and the uniqueness of the therapy with cancer patients. For instance, in the mind–body categories, imagery research with a cancer population began over 30 years ago and has expanded since that time. Also in this category is a new area of investigation showing promise with cancer patients: music. Therefore, both imagery and music are included. Further, in the manipulative and body-based therapies, reflexology was selected due to its potential unique contribution to cancer patients.

In reviewing the five NCCAM categories, the discussion will begin with a definition of the practice or therapy, and then describe the mechanism of action (whenever information is available), current research (with an emphasis on randomized clinical trials), the impact on clinical results, and, finally, directions for future research.

## NCCAM Category 1: Mind—Body Interventions

NCCAM Category 1 therapies engage mental activity to influence the body. Guided imagery and music will be the examples discussed here; each of these therapies has been used with cancer patients (see Tables 10.2A and 10.2B for study summaries).

### Guided Imagery: Definition

Guided imagery has been recognized for its potential to provide supportive care to cancer patients since the early work of Simonton, Matthews-Simonton, and Sparks (1980). Guided imagery is based on the premise that health-promoting images can help the mind interpret a health crisis in a calmer manner and will elicit fewer physiological stress responses (Gruber et al., 1993). When a person feels less stress, the body functions in a more balanced and stable manner, which may help decrease symptoms (Horowitz & Breitbart, 1993).

### Guided Imagery: Mechanism of Action

Several assumptions have been put forth as to the mechanism of action for guided imagery. Sloman (1995) suggested that imagery practice for people with cancer increases one's sense of control, reduces feelings of helplessness and hopelessness, provides a calming diversion, and breaks the pain–anxiety tension cycle. Stephens (1993) provided the explanation that imagery works by reframing cognitive pathways associated with symptoms. Dossey, Keegan, Guzzetta, and Kolkmeier (1995) proposed that the right hemisphere of the brain translates messages such as feelings, attitudes, and beliefs so they can be understood by the autonomic nervous system. Once translated, a link between the conscious processing of information and a physiologic change is bridged. The mechanism of action for guided imagery appears to be a variety of factors, all of which involve the elicited relaxation response (Benson, Beary, & Carol, 1974).

Guided Imagery: Current Research

Current research has found guided imagery to have a positive effect on cancer patients' pain experiences. Favorable outcomes have been found for patients undergoing chemotherapy and radiation, and it supports a variety of areas such as pain, nausea, emotional well-being, quality of life, spiritual well-being, immune system changes, and functional status.

Guided Imagery and Chemotherapy

Walker et al. (1999) studied 96 women with advanced breast cancer. They found that the experimental group who received the combination of relaxation and guided imagery scored significantly better on quality of life ($p < .03$) and emotional health ($p < .02$) than the standard-care group (control group). Burish, Carey, Krozely, and Grego (1987) and Burish, Snyder, and Jenkins (1991) conducted a variety of studies assessing the usefulness of guided imagery in combination with various cognitive therapies. Burish and Jenkins (1992) found a significant decrease in nausea ($p < .05$) and anxiety ($p < .05$) during chemotherapy, and physiological arousal after chemotherapy ($p < .05$). Troesch, Rodehaver, Delaney, and Yanes (1993) reported significant ($p < .001$) improvement in nausea and vomiting among 28 patients receiving Cisplatin infusions when compared to a standard-care group. Given, Wyatt, Given, and Kozachik (2001) studied 100 cancer patients undergoing chemotherapy and found that guided imagery either alone or in combination with reflexology showed, using a paired t-test from pre- to post-test, a significant reduction in scores of depression ($p < .05$) and anxiety ($p < .003$). It also showed a significant enhancement of mean scores for spirituality ($p < .03$) and quality of life ($p < .001$).

## GUIDED IMAGERY AND RADIATION

Kolcaba and Fox (1999) investigated 53 women undergoing radiation therapy for early stage breast cancer. The Radiation Comfort Questionnaire was administered before radiation treatment began, during the course of radiation treatments, and after the completion of treatments. The experimental group receiving guided imagery delivered via audiotape demonstrated a significant impact on improved comfort ($p < .05$) over the control group (conventional care). Richardson et al. (1997) found that among 47 women with breast cancer who were undergoing radiation and/or chemotherapy, those who had guided imagery training demonstrated an improved but nonsignificant change in coping skills ($p < .07$), vigor ($p < .08$), and functional status ($p < .07$).

## GUIDED IMAGERY AND THE IMMUNE SYSTEM

Gruber et al. (1993) utilized a 24-week training session for 13 women with stage I breast cancer. The sessions included training in guided imagery, relaxation, and biofeedback. Pre- and post-intervention immune system markers were compared. Significant effects were found in natural killer cell activity ($p < .017$), mixed lymphocyte responsiveness ($p < .001$), concanavalin A responsiveness ($p < .001$), and the number of peripheral blood lymphocytes ($p < .01$).

## GUIDED IMAGERY AND PAIN

Syrjala, Donaldson, Davis, Kippes, and Carr (1995) utilized a four-group design with 94 bone marrow transplant patients. They found a significant ($p < .009$) decrease in oral mucositis pain for two of the intervention groups: a group using imagery plus relaxation and a group receiving a package of cognitive-behavioral coping skills that included imagery and relaxation. However, the cognitive-behavioral coping skills group did not have significantly better outcomes than the imagery plus relaxation alone group. An Australian study conducted by Sloman (1995) investigated 67 intermediate and advanced stage cancer patients, predominately men with a mean age of 64 years. This three-group design compared an intervention that included nurse-delivered imagery plus relaxation against an audiotaped version of the intervention and a no-treatment control group. Both the audiotaped and nurse-delivered groups had comparable, significant ($p < .03$) improvements in four parameters of pain: sensation, intensity, severity, and nonopioid analgesia intake. Baider, Uziely, and DeNour (1994) intervened with guided imagery and muscle relaxation, and of the 86 cancer patients who completed the 6-session program, they found improvements in psychological distress measures ($p < .02$), which were sustained over time (up to 6 months).

## GUIDED IMAGERY: AN IMPACT ON CLINICAL OUTCOMES

Based on the literature reviewed, guided imagery can be useful in reducing cancer pain, chemotherapy-related nausea and vomiting, anxiety and depression, and in enhancing biological markers, spirituality, and functional status. This is a therapy with little potential for adverse reactions, and therefore it fits into a low-risk class of therapies. On the other hand, guided imagery has not been successful in reducing tumor progression or increasing survival time (Doan, 1998; Jacobson, Workman, & Kronenberg, 2000).

## GUIDED IMAGERY: FUTURE DIRECTIONS

The majority of studies have tested guided imagery in combination with other therapies. Future research needs to focus on assessing guided imagery independently, utilizing standardized outcome measures for comparison, using samples adequate to attain sufficient statistical power, and employing longitudinal designs that will track the outcomes, hence the benefits, over time.

## MUSIC THERAPY: DEFINITION

Music therapy is the intentional use of music or sound to induce health and healing (Woodham & Peters, 1997). Munro and Mount (1978) defined music therapy as the controlled use of music and its influence on the human being to aid in physiological, psychological, and emotional integration during treatment of an illness or disability.

## MUSIC THERAPY: MECHANISM OF ACTION

Many theories exist as to why music may be therapeutic. The entrainment process is one possible theory that involves two objects vibrating at similar frequencies to cause a mutual resonance (Moranto, 1993). Music may entrain physiological functions such as heart rate, pulse, or breathing. Entrainment is based on both the tempo and the mood of the music (Bonny, 1986). Guzzetta (1995) suggested a second theory that the pitch and rhythm of music has an impact on psychophysiologic responses due to their direct effect on the limbic system. Further, musical vibrations in harmony with a

**TABLE 10.2A Evidence-based CAM Therapies for Cancer Patients: Mind–body Interventions—Guided Imagery**

| | Theoretical/ conceptual framework | Design | Sample | Measures | Results |
|---|---|---|---|---|---|
| Baider, Uziely, & DeNour (1994) | None reported | Nonrandomized, 3-group design; 1 time per week for 90 minutes over 6 weeks | $N = 86$ mixed diagnosis participants | Multiple Locus of Control, Impact of Events Scale (IES), Brief Symptom Inventory (BSI) | Decreased psychological distress; decreased avoidance of disease |
| Burish, Carey, Krozely, & Greco (1987) | None reported | RCT, 2-group design; 1 to 3 sessions 30 to 45 minutes before first CT session for a total of 5 during CT sessions | $N = 24$ mixed diagnosis participants receiving CT | Multiple Affect Adjective Checklist (MAAC), Post-CT Rating Scales, Home Record Form (HRF) | Decreased nausea, anxiety, vomiting, blood pressure, pulse rates, dysphoria |
| Burish & Jenkins (1992) | None reported | RCT, 6-group design; 45 minutes per CT session for a total of 5 sessions; practice daily at home with audiotape | $N = 81$ mixed diagnosis participants receiving IV outpatient CT | MAAC, Post-CT rating scales, nurse rating scales | Decreased nausea and anxiety during CT; decreased physiologic arousal after CT |

| | Theoretical/conceptual framework | Design | Sample | Measures | Results |
|---|---|---|---|---|---|
| Burish, Snyder, & Jenkins (1991) | None reported | RCT, 4-group design; 45 minutes per CT session for a total of 5 sessions | $N = 60$ mixed diagnosis participants receiving CT | MAAC, Post-CT Rating Scales, HRF, Sickness Impact Profile (SIP), Family Rating Scale, Knowledge Questionnaire | Decreased negative affect, vomiting |
| Given, Wyatt, Given, & Kozachik (2001) | Wyatt Quality of Life | Nonrandomized, pre- and post-test, 1-group design; 20 minutes per day for 8 weeks | $N = 100$ mixed diagnosis participants receiving CT | CES-D, Spielberger State Trait Anxiety Inventory (STAI), Cella Quality of Life, Spirituality Subscale of Long-term Quality of Life Scale (LTQL) | Increased spirituality, quality of life; decreased depression, anxiety |

*(continued)*

**TABLE 10.2A  Evidence-based CAM Therapies for Cancer Patients: Mind–body Interventions—Guided Imagery** *(continued)*

| | Theoretical/ conceptual framework | Design | Sample | Measures | Results |
|---|---|---|---|---|---|
| Gruber et al. (1993) | None reported | RCT, two-group design; one session per week, practice twice daily with audiotape for 9 weeks | N = 13 breast cancer patients | Minnesota Multi-phasic Personality Inventory (MMPI), Millon Behavioral Health Inventory (MBHI), Sarason Social Support Scale, Rotter Locus of Control, Affects Balance Scale (ABS), Greer Mental Adjustment to Cancer Scale (MAC) | Increased natural killer cells, mixed lymphocytes, concanavalin A, peripheral blood lymphocytes |
| Jacobson, Workman, & Kronenberg (2000) | None reported | Meta-analysis of articles from 1980 to 1997 | N = 51 studies; all studies included at least some breast cancer patients | | Most had positive trends, but none showed that CAM therapy altered disease progression for breast cancer |

| | Theoretical/ conceptual framework | Design | Sample | Measures | Results |
|---|---|---|---|---|---|
| Kolcaba & Fox (1999) | Kolcaba's Comfort Theory | RCT, 2-group design; 20 minutes per day throughout RT and 3 weeks post-treatment | $N = 53$ breast cancer patients (stage I or II) beginning RT | State Anxiety Inventory (SAI), Radiation Therapy Comfort Questionnaire (RTCQ) | Increased comfort |
| Richardson et al. (1997) | None reported | RCT, 3-group design; one 60-minute session per week; practice 2 times per day for 20 minutes with audiotape over 6 weeks | $N = 47$ breast cancer patients (excluding stage IV) | Functional Assessment of Cancer Treatment-Breast (FACT-B), POMS-brief, Ways of Coping with Cancer (WOC-CA), Duke-UNC Functional Social Support Questionnaire (DUFSS), Duke-UNC Health Profile (DUHP) | Decreased stress |
| Sloman (1995) | None reported | RCT, 3-group design; two 30-minute sessions per week; practice twice daily and any time experiencing pain over 2 weeks | $N = 67$ intermediate to advanced stage, mixed diagnosis participants | Short Form McGill Pain Questionnaire (SF-MPA) | Decreased pain sensation, pain intensity, pain severity, nonopioid PRN analgesia |

*(continued)*

305

**TABLE 10.2A  Evidence-based CAM Therapies for Cancer Patients: Mind–body Interventions—Guided Imagery** *(continued)*

| | Theoretical/ conceptual framework | Design | Sample | Measures | Results |
|---|---|---|---|---|---|
| Syrjala, Donaldson, Davis, Kippes, & Carr (1995) | None reported | RCT, 4-group design; two 90-minute initial training sessions; 30-minute booster sessions 2 times per week over 5 weeks during treatment | *N* = 94 bone marrow transplant participants | Oral pain VAS, Nausea VAS, Symptom Checklist-90-revised (SC-90-R), Post-treatment Evaluation | Decreased treatment-related pain |
| Troesch, Rodehaver, Delaney, & Yanes (1993) | Orem's Self-care Theory | RCT, 2-group design; 20-minute tape used prior to CT, next morning, following evening over 3 CT cycles | *N* = 28 mixed diagnosis participants receiving CT | Rhodes Index of Nausea and Vomiting Form 2 (INV-2), Chemotherapy Experience Scale (CES), Subject Demographics and Emetic Response Tool (DERT) | Described overall CT experience more positively; no difference in nausea or vomiting |

| Theoretical/<br>conceptual<br>framework | Design | Sample | Measures | Results |
|---|---|---|---|---|
| Walker et al. (1999) | | | | |
| None reported | RCT, 2-group design; 5 training sessions during 18 weeks of CT, practice daily at home with audiotape | $N = 96$ breast cancer patients receiving CT | L-scale of Exsenck Personality Questionnaire-revised (EPQ), Courtawd Emotional Control Scale (CEC), Rotterdan Symptom Checklist (RSC), Global Self-reported Quality of Life (GQOL), Mood Rating Scale (MRS), Structured Clinical Interview for Diagnosis DSM-III (SCID), Hospital Anxiety and Depression Scale (HADS) | Increased quality of life, relaxation; decreased psychological symptoms |

patient's personal vibration pattern may produce healing by restoring normal functions. Beck (1991) stated that music is effective for pain management via distraction, enhancing a patient's sense of control, improving mood, and facilitating the release of endorphins. Although the various theories are preliminary, the mechanism of action may involve entrainment, the limbic system, distraction, or a combination of these factors.

## MUSIC THERAPY: CURRENT RESEARCH

Music therapy has been available and used professionally since the founding of the National Association for Music Therapy in 1950 and has been part of healthcare since Aristotle reported flute music to be healing in the fourth century B.C. (Krebs, 1999). However, scientific research has only begun to be documented for cancer patients; two studies addressed supportive care, but were not specific to cancer patients (Gallager, Huston, Nelson, Walsh, & Steele, 2001; Heiser, Chiles, Fudge, & Gray, 1997).

A variety of small studies have been conducted with cancer patients. In 1991, Beck investigated a convenience sample of 15 cancer outpatients using a crossover design, with patients as their own controls. While participants were receiving music therapy, they demonstrated a significant ($p <$ .02) decrease in the need for analgesics as compared to when they were not utilizing music therapy. Another study involved 39 patients undergoing high-dose chemotherapy for bone marrow transplants. Patients were randomly assigned either to a conventional antiemetic care group or a conventional care plus music therapy intervention group. Patients in the intervention group experienced significantly ($p <$ .02) less nausea and vomiting than the control group (Ezzone, Baker, Rosselet, & Terepka, 1998).

Boldt (1996) assessed the benefits of 10 music sessions versus 2 or 3 music sessions among six bone marrow transplant patients. Nonstatistical benefits were noted with both lengths of time; however, the patients who attended 10 sessions showed improvements in not only comfort and relaxation, but also endurance. Sabo and Michael (1996) utilized a convenience sample receiving chemotherapy for the first time. The experimental group received taped music and a message from their physician; participants in the control group received customary care alone. A significant difference was found between pre- and postintervention scores on state anxiety scores for the experimental group ($p <$ .001), while no change took place over time for the control group.

Standley (1992) investigated 15 adult chemotherapy patients using a 4-group design: (a) music during chemotherapy treatments 1 through 4, (b) music during chemotherapy treatments 2 through 5, and (c) two nonmusic control groups. The music treatment groups began listening to tapes while waiting for the nurse to prepare and administer the chemotherapy agents; the control groups did not listen to music. Data were collected when they entered the chemotherapy room, prior to chemotherapy infusion, 15 minutes after beginning infusion, and at the conclusion of the treatment. Both intervention groups had less nausea, less vomiting, a longer time before the onset of nausea, faster passing of "chemo time," less anxiety, and less tension.

Burns (2001) intervened with eight mixed-diagnosis volunteers who had cancer history but were not currently in treatment. Using a random assignment into two groups, the intervention group received 10 weekly sessions of music with guided imagery, and the controls received standard care. The intervention group showed nonsignificant but higher scores on both mood and quality of life than controls at post-test measures.

### MUSIC THERAPY: IMPACT ON CLINICAL OUTCOMES

The few studies available demonstrate promise for this CAM therapy in the treatment of cancer-related symptoms, specifically pain, nausea, vomiting, and anxiety. There seem to be few, if any, precautions necessary with music therapy. It can be considered a low-risk, easy-to-use, and potentially moderate benefit intervention.

### MUSIC THERAPY: FUTURE DIRECTIONS

Larger studies with more standardization are needed. Design poses a challenge because music is an individualized experience. The musical choice needs to be incorporated along with patient mood, emotional state, physical health status, and cultural or religious choices (Gerdner & Buckwalter, 1999). These unique personal features make music therapy a difficult form of CAM to test in all but the most carefully controlled studies. Music interventions could be strengthened by a careful description of the dosage (frequency and duration) of the therapy. Music therapy is relatively inexpensive and a volunteer or family member can help implement the therapy.

## NCCAM Category 2: Manipulative and Body-based Methods

NCCAM Category 2 therapies are focused on manipulation and/or movement of the body. Reflexology will be the example used in this section.

**TABLE 10.2B Evidence-based CAM Therapies for Cancer Patients: Mind-body Interventions—Music Therapy**

| | Theoretical/ conceptual framework | Design | Sample | Measures | Results |
|---|---|---|---|---|---|
| Beck (1991) | Investigator-developed model based on psychological and physiological pain | Randomized crossover design; 45-minute cassette twice daily for 3 days | $N = 15$ mixed diagnosis participants | Abbreviated version of McGill Pain Questionnaire (MPQ), Present Pain Intensity Scale (PPI), Pain VAS, Mood VAS | Decreased pain |
| Boldt (1996) | None reported | Nonrandomized 2-group design; 10 sessions for group 1; 2 to 3 sessions for group 2 | $N = 6$ bone marrow transplant participants | End-of-study questionnaire including pain, nausea, comfort, and relaxation | Increased (nonsignificant) relaxation, comfort, and endurance |
| Burns (2001) | None reported | Randomized, pre- and post-test, 2-group design; 90 to 180 minutes per week for 10 weeks | $N = 8$ mixed diagnosis participants | POMS, Quality of Life-cancer (QOL-CA) | Increased (nonsignificant) mood and quality of life |

| | Theoretical/ conceptual framework | Design | Sample | Measures | Results |
|---|---|---|---|---|---|
| Ezzone, Baker, Rosselet, & Terepka (1998) | Etiology of nausea and vomiting | Randomized 2-group design; 45-minute cassette 3 times (6, 9, and 12 hours after each CT infusion) | $N = 6$ bone marrow transplant participants | Nausea Thermometer VAS, Feel Bad Scale | Decreased nausea and vomiting |
| Sabo & Michael (1996) | Neuman's Systems Model | Two-group design; during CT sessions 1 through 4 | $N = 97$ participants, adults receiving first CT | Spielberger State Anxiety Inventory (SSAI), Cancer Chemotherapy and Side Effects Inventory | Decreased state anxiety |
| Smith, Casey, Johnson, Gwede, & Riggin (2001) | None reported | Randomized two-group design; during five weeks of RT | $N = 42$ participants, men receiving RT for abdominal or pelvic malignancies | State Trait Anxiety Inventory (STAI) | Decreased (nonsignificant) state anxiety |

*(continued)*

**TABLE 10.2B  Evidence-based CAM Therapies for Cancer Patients: Mind–body Interventions—Music Therapy** (*continued*)

| | Theoretical/ conceptual framework | Design | Sample | Measures | Results |
|---|---|---|---|---|---|
| Standley (1992) | None reported | Randomized four-group design; during CT sessions 1 through 4 or CT sessions 2 through 5 | $N = 15$ mixed diagnosis participants receiving CT | Post-test Questionnaire | Increased (non-significant) time before onset of nausea, passing of "chemo time," decreased (non-significant) nausea, anxiety, and tension |

REFLEXOLOGY: DEFINITION

Reflexology is a specialized foot massage based on the premise that the foot has reflexes that mirror the rest of the body. One speculation is that the nerve endings in the feet connect with different areas of the body, and the direct pressure on a specific area of the foot stimulates the corresponding area of the body (Byers, 1996). (See Table 10.3 for study summaries.)

REFLEXOLOGY: MECHANISM OF ACTION

Multiple mechanisms of action have been put forth for reflexology. One possible explanation is that this type of massage may alter baroreceptor reflex sensitivity to produce the reported benefits (Frankel, 1997). Stephenson, Weinrich, and Tavakoli (2000) summarized other possible theories on the mechanism of action as put forth by Dossey et al. (1995). One theory suggests that lactic acid is deposited in microcrystals in the feet, and reflexology crushes the crystals and allows for the free flow of energy. The theory of proprioceptive nervous receptors states that a connection exists between the areas of the feet and the body organs, and that reflexing the feet affects the organs. This process, in turn, produces a relaxing effect by relieving tension and stress. The relaxation response then affects the autonomic nervous system, which finally affects the endocrine, immune, and neuropeptide systems. The last theory is a psychological explanation that reflexology is simply a method of showing care and concern for patients. The relaxation response and the psychological explanation of caring appear to be the primary mechanisms of action associated with improvements in health status.

REFLEXOLOGY: CURRENT RESEARCH

Two intervention studies involving cancer patients were found in the literature. Stephenson, Weinrich, and Tavakoli (2000) conducted a study with 23 hospitalized lung and breast cancer patients. The majority of the sample was female, Caucasian, and over 65 years of age. Following a 30-minute reflexology treatment, a significant ($p < .02$) reduction took place in state anxiety for both lung and breast cancer patients. For breast cancer patients, a significant ($p < .05$) decrease in pain also occurred. Hodgson (2000) conducted a 40-minute reflexology treatment on 12 palliative care cancer patients on days 1, 3, and 5 of their hospitalization. Despite a small sample size, significant changes were found in quality of life ($p < .004$) and ease of breathing ($p < .03$) when compared to the placebo reflexology group.

**TABLE 10.3  Evidence-based CAM Therapies for Cancer Patients: Manipulative and Body-based Reflexology Methods**

| | Theoretical/ conceptual framework | Design | Sample | Measures | Results |
|---|---|---|---|---|---|
| Given, Wyatt, Given, & Kozachik (2001) | Wyatt Quality of Life | Nonrandomized pre- and post-test, 1-group design; 20 minutes per week for 8 weeks | $N = 100$ mixed diagnosis participants during CT | CES-D, Spielberger State Trait Anxiety Inventory (STAI), Cella Quality of Life, Spirituality Subscale of Long-term Quality of Life Scale (LTQL) | Increased spirituality and quality of life; decreased anxiety, depression, and severity of symptoms |
| Hodgson (2000) | None reported | RCT, 2-group design; 40 minutes during days 1, 3, 5 of hospitalization | $N = 12$ mixed diagnosis participants in palliative care | Variation of Holmes and Dickerson VAS | Increased quality of life and ease of breathing |
| Stephenson, Weinrich, & Tavakoli (2000) | None reported | RCT, 2-group design; 1 time for 30 minutes | $N = 23$ participants with breast and lung cancer | Short-Form McGill Pain Questionnaire (SF-MPQ), Anxiety VAS | Decreased anxiety and pain (breast cancer patients only |

314

Given et al. (2001) recently completed a study in which reflexology, along with guided imagery, was a major component with a mixed-diagnosis sample of 100 cancer patients undergoing chemotherapy. The majority of participants were female (70%), the largest percentage had breast cancer (49%), and were age 51 to 60 (43%). Patients who engaged in a weekly (8 sessions) reflexology program with their family caregiver, using either reflexology alone or in combination with imagery, demonstrated a significant improvement in mean scores from pre- to post-test for anxiety ($p < .01$), depression ($p < .02$), spirituality ($p < .04$), severity of symptoms ($p < .01$), and quality of life ($p < .04$).

REFLEXOLOGY: IMPACT ON CLINICAL OUTCOMES

From the research available, it appears that reflexology may be efficacious for a reduction of anxiety, depression, symptom severity, and pain, as well as improvements in spirituality and quality of life.

REFLEXOLOGY: FUTURE DIRECTIONS

The impact of reflexology on psychosocial parameters—such as anxiety, depression, spirituality, and quality of life—is worthy of further testing, as well as the impact on physical symptom relief. The use of standardized interventions (including dosage) and instruments is critical to provide a basis for future comparison work. A large-scale randomized clinical trial with longitudinal measures would contribute to an enhanced understanding of this noninvasive and popular therapy (Byers, 1996; Risberg, Lund, Wist, Kaasa, & Wilsgaard, 1998; Risberg, Lund, & Wist, 1995; Risberg, Lund, Wist, Dahl et al., 1995). Challenges to controlled studies are the numerous implementation variables, such as who performs the therapy (family versus therapist). To date, reflexology remains in the low-risk class of therapies.

# NCCAM Category 3: Biologically Based Therapies

NCCAM Category 3 therapies often include products or practices that overlap with conventional therapies. Herbal therapy is the exemplar that will be used for this section (see Table 10.4 for study summaries).

HERBAL THERAPY: DEFINITION

Herbal therapy is referred to as herbalism or botanical medicine and involves the use of herbs for their therapeutic value. An herb is a plant or

**TABLE 10.4  Evidence-based CAM Therapies for Cancer Patients: Biologically Based Herbal Therapies**

| | Theoretical/ conceptual framework | Design | Sample | Measures | Results |
|---|---|---|---|---|---|
| DiPaola et al. (1998) | None reported | Nonrandomized 1-group design and a minimum of four 320 mg PC-SPES capsules per day (estrogenic herbal combination) for 2 weeks | $N = 8$ advanced prostate cancer patients | Standardized questionnaire | Decreased serum testosterone and PSA |
| Sun et al. (1999) | None reported | Nonrandomized 3-group design and 30G of freeze-dried powder per day (of selected vegetables known to contain anti-tumor components), followed for 24 months or until death | $N = 11$ stage III and IV nonsmall cell lung cancer patients | Clinical observations and verbal reports only | Increased weight maintenance and survival of patients |

plant extract containing a variety of chemical substances that act upon the body (Kastner & Burroughs, 1996).

## HERBAL THERAPY: MECHANISM OF ACTION

Herbal products create the greatest dilemma in oncology (Decker & Schulmeister, 2000). Most herbal products are readily available at health supplement stores; however, they do not have the scientific evidence of the efficacy or toxicity to which the healthcare industry is accustomed (Paulsen, 1998). Currently, advice is based on judgment rather than science (Eisenberg, 1997), and this has the potential for legal liability (Wyandt & Williamson, 1999). An underlying assumption exists that the mechanism of action is a biochemical interaction similar to pharmaceuticals.

## HERBAL THERAPY: CURRENT RESEARCH

Some herbs have shown success in symptom management, but not specifically with cancer patients. A meta-analysis was conducted on St. John's wort (*Hypericum perforatum*), including 23 randomized trials ($N = 1757$ outpatients) with mild to moderate depressive disorders. St. John's wort was found to be significantly ($p < .05$) more effective than a placebo (Linde et al., 1996). Shelton et al. (2001) investigated 200 adults with major depression and found that St. John's wort was not effective for major depression. It is important to make the distinction between the significant results reported in the meta-analysis that consisted of patients with mild to moderate depression (Linde et al., 1996) versus the Shelton et al. (2001) study showing nonsignificant results among patients with major depression.

A meta-analysis reported that kava (*Piper methysticum*) was effective in reducing anxiety (Pittler & Ernst, 2000), and ginger (*Zingiber officinalis*) has demonstrated effectiveness with chemotherapy-induced nausea in a meta-analysis of randomized clinical trials (Ernst & Pittler, 2000). Valerian (*Valeriana officinalis*) has also shown promise in a meta-analysis of clinical trials for the treatment of insomnia (Stevinson & Ernst, 2000). Although each of these herbs may contribute to symptom management, they have not been tested specifically with cancer patients.

Studies specific to cancer patients include two herbal combinations. A combination of eight traditional Chinese herbs, referred to as PC-SPES, has shown a significant ($p < .05$) reduction in prostate-specific antigen levels and decreased serum testosterone concentrations among men with advanced prostate cancer. This study was conducted with a small sample of eight men, all experiencing side effects after taking the herbal combination. All eight men experienced breast tenderness and loss of libido, and one suffered a venous thrombosis. The investigators caution that although PC-SPES has potent estrogenic activity that may benefit men with prostate cancer, it is still an unregulated mixture of herbs that can confound standard therapies (DiPaola et al., 1998).

Another combination of 16 Chinese vegetables has shown a significant ($p < .01$) effect on quality and quantity of life among 11 patients with non-small cell lung cancer. Compared to the control group, the intervention group survived approximately 15 months versus 4 months for the control group. Further, no clinical signs of toxicity were found during the 24-month study period. In addition to extended survival time, the treatment was associated with improved weight maintenance and higher Karnofsky performance status (Sun et al., 1999).

HERBAL THERAPY: IMPACT ON CLINICAL OUTCOMES

Herbal therapies currently showing the most hope in cancer care come from the Far Eastern Chinese medicine system. It appears that combinations of herbs, rather than a single herb, may have necessary antitumor effects.

HERBAL THERAPY: FUTURE DIRECTIONS

Many areas need further investigation, including drug–herb interactions; standardized potency, purity, and dosage of herbal preparations; and scientific clinical trials (Tatro, 1999). Concerns abound related to biologically based therapies such as herbs. Cancer patients undergoing treatment must be cautioned to inform their conventional providers of all use of herbal remedies (Eisenberg, 1997). Undesirable chemotherapy–herbal interactions may occur because the herbs contain various chemicals that have not been tested for safety (Cassileth, 1999b; Jonas, 1996).

Several over-the-counter herbs have anticoagulation properties that can cause excessive bleeding during surgery (Ang-Lee, Moss, & Yuan, 2001). Other herbs can cause photosensitivity, leading to skin reactions during radiation therapy (Drew & Myers, 1997; Gordon, Rosenthal, Hart, Sirota, & Baker, 1995). Other biologically based cancer therapy investigations have been suspended, such as the Gerson treatment that used liquefied raw calf liver injections (Green, 1992) due to a number of patients developing sepsis. Communication between the health provider and the cancer patient is essential, because each CAM therapy must be evaluated for its interaction effect with conventional treatment, its safety, and its efficacy (Cassileth, 1999a; Montbriand, 1995). Until scientifically sound data can support the use of herbs, their use should be advised with extreme caution.

## NCCAM Category 4: Energy Therapies

NCCAM Category 4 therapies focus on fields that originate from within the body (biofields) or from external sources (electromagnetic fields). The exemplar for this section is therapeutic touch (see Table 10.5 for study summaries).

THERAPEUTIC TOUCH: DEFINITION

This therapy is based on the framework established by nursing theorist Martha Rogers in "The Science of Unitary Human Beings" (Rogers, 1990). Therapeutic touch is the rebalancing of the patient's energy field (Wyatt, 1989). The practitioner works in the patient's energy field, which extends 3 to 5 inches beyond the physical surface of the body. The practitioner uses his or her hands to make gentle strokes from head to toe within the energy field. The goal is to attain a greater uniformity of balance throughout the patient's field, which is believed to promote health.

THERAPEUTIC TOUCH: MECHANISM OF ACTION

The basic assumption is that human beings are energy fields in mutual and simultaneous interaction with the environmental field surrounding the body, and that energy can be moved intentionally from one person to another (Krieger, 1993). Therefore, according to Meehan (1993), therapeutic touch is a change that occurs in the human–environment energy field patterning as the practitioner assumes a meditative state of awareness, recognizes his or her own unitary nature and integrity with the environmental field, and focuses his or her intent to help the patient.

Weber (1989) has put forth a second theory, a general energy field framework. This theory proposes a fundamental, unitary, universal flow of energy within which all matter, consciousness, and events are grounded and interconnected. Support for this view is found in the basic organization of the universe through quantum field theory, where "quanta" can manifest as either particles of matter or an interacting field (Bohm, 1973).

**TABLE 10.5   Evidence-based CAM Therapies for Cancer Patients: Therapeutic Touch**

| | Theoretical/ conceptual framework | Design | Sample | Measures | Results |
|---|---|---|---|---|---|
| Giasson & Bouchard (1998) | Martha Roger's Science of Unitary Human Beings Model | RCT, 2-group design; 3 treatments for 15 to 20 minutes per day for 4 days | $N = 20$ mixed diagnosis participants for terminal cases | Well-being VAS, based on Edmonton Symptom Assessment Scale | Increased well-being |
| Sodergren (1993) | None reported | RCT, three-group design; over three CT cycles | $N = 80$ mixed diagnosis participants receiving CT | Self-report data on positive and negative effects, disruption in usual activity, symptom distress, and symptom severity | Decreased symptom distress severity before and after CT |

THERAPEUTIC TOUCH: CURRENT RESEARCH

The majority of research has not been conducted with cancer patients, but has focused on symptom management. The three most investigated areas have been anxiety (Gagne & Toye, 1994; Simington & Laing, 1993; Turner, Clark, Gauthier, & Williams, 1998), stress response (Olson et al., 1997; Olson, Sneed, Bonadonna, Ratliff, & Dias, 1992), and pain (Gordon, Merenstein, D'Amico, & Hudgens, 1998; Meehan, 1993; Peck, 1997; Turner et al., 1998). Supportive care via therapeutic touch in these areas (anxiety, stress, and pain) may also enhance the quality of life for cancer patients.

Sodergren (1993) investigated 80 cancer patients experiencing anticipatory nausea and vomiting during the course of chemotherapy. Participants were randomly assigned to one of four groups: a therapeutic touch group, an information group, a progressive relaxation group, and a no-treatment control group. Interventions were implemented prior to chemotherapy. When compared to the control group, the therapeutic touch group demonstrated a decrease in symptom severity ($p < .001$) before chemotherapy and reduced symptom distress before ($p < .001$) and after ($p < .01$) chemotherapy.

Giasson and Bouchard (1998) studied 20 terminally ill cancer patients in palliative care. Participants were randomly assigned to the therapeutic touch group or the control group (who were given a structured rest period). Three treatments were administered to each group over a 4-day period of time. Each treatment lasted 15 to 20 minutes and was given at the same time of day, and 1 hour following a regularly prescribed analgesic. The intervention group showed a significant ($p < .002$) increase in their sense of well-being from pre- to post-test, whereas the control group showed a decrease in well-being. The well-being scale used was a visual analogue scale that measured pain, nausea, depression, anxiety, shortness of breath, activity, appetite, relaxation, and inner peace.

THERAPEUTIC TOUCH: IMPACT ON CLINICAL OUTCOMES

Among cancer patients, initial work has been done with symptom improvement during and after chemotherapy, and improved well-being for terminally ill cancer patients. Therapeutic touch has never been reported to have caused harm to anyone; therefore, it falls into the low-risk class of interventions.

THERAPEUTIC TOUCH: FUTURE DIRECTIONS

Clearly, therapeutic touch research is still in its beginning stages of development, but it offers encouragement in the area of symptom management. Many methodological variations have been reported in the research. Future studies to test the efficacy of therapeutic touch will benefit from consistency across studies, a standardized protocol, and population-specific trials. Perhaps the most compelling area of investigation would be the empirical validation of the energy interaction central to this therapy (Egan, 1998).

## NCCAM Category 5: Alternative Medical Systems

Beginning with the conventional biomedical model (allopathic medicine), treatment in these systems focuses on the physical body, with specific interest in the structure of tissues and movement, and the transformation of chemicals within cells. Currently, osteopathic medicine is practiced in a manner similar to conventional allopathic medicine while maintaining its origins in manipulation therapy. The classic osteopathic and chiropractic modes emphasize connections and communications between bones, nerves, and muscles and the rest of the physical body.

Other systems move further from the conventional model, such as homeopathy, which views the physical body as having three significant layers and the body/person as having three distinct aspects (Vithoulkas, 1980). Shamanism engages nonmaterial and normally invisible realms (Ingerman, 1991). The Ayurveda system is based on the classification of people into one of three body types, with specific remedies for disease- and health-promoting regimens for each (Casselith, 1999b). The exemplar of an alternative medical system is traditional Oriental medicine, which consists of a group of techniques and methods, including acupuncture, Oriental massage, and qi gong (NCCAM, 2001). For this category, acupuncture will be explored (see Table 10.6 for study summaries).

**Acupuncture: Definition**   The practice of acupuncture originated in China over 5,000 years ago. It is based on the belief that deficiencies or excesses of energy (chi) in the body are manifested as illnesses. To correct the imbalance, needles are inserted into subcutaneous or muscular tissue at specific points along energy channels (Calliet, 1994).

**TABLE 10.6  Evidence-based CAM Therapies for Cancer Patients: Alternative Medical Systems Acupuncture**

| | Theoretical/ conceptual framework | Design | Sample | Measures | Results |
|---|---|---|---|---|---|
| Filshie, Penn, Ashley, & Davis (1996) | None reported | Nonrandomized, pre- and post-test, 1-group design; 1 treatment of 6 key acupuncture points for 10 minutes | *N* = 20 participants experiencing cancer-related breathlessness | Dyspnea VAS, Hospital Anxiety and Depression Scale (HAD), Borg Scale, Pain VAS, Anxiety VAS, Relaxation VAS | Increased relaxation; decreased breathlessness and anxiety (90 minutes after treatment) |
| He, Friedrich, Ertan, Muller, & Schmidt (1999) | Traditional Chinese Medicine (TCM) | Nonrandomized two-group design; six key acupuncture points, plus individualized points; third, fifth, and seventh postoperative days | *N* = 80 participants, breast cancer (with axillary node dissection) | Pain VAS | Increased pain relief, arm movement (fourteenth post-op day) |
| Xu, Liu, Li, & Xu 1995) | Traditional Chinese Medicine (TCM) | Nonrandomized, post-test, 1-group design; 2 key acupuncture points 15 minutes daily for 2 weeks | *N* = 92 participants, abdominal cancer (liver, gastric, colon) | Verbal reports only | Increased (nonsignificant) pain relief for nearly all mild to moderate pain; 72 percent of participants experiencing severe pain reported some relief (controlled pain for 1 month) |

## ACUPUNCTURE: MECHANISM OF ACTION

Twelve main energy channels (meridians) are believed to exist throughout the body that impact specific internal organs. Along these meridians are over 461 acupuncture points. Depending on the person's illness, specific points are stimulated through the use of needles. The result is a draining of excess energy or the restoring of deficiencies (Kastner & Burroughs, 1996).

## ACUPUNCTURE: CURRENT RESEARCH

The use of acupuncture for cancer pain relief is a relatively new area of investigation, and the best studies to date are international. German investigators He, Friedrich, Ertan, Muller, and Schmidt (1999) reported effective relief of pain ($p < .001$) and improved arm movement ($p < .001$) after axillary lymphadenectomy for 48 breast cancer patients (14 days after surgery) when compared to 32 comparable control patients who did not receive acupuncture. This was a nonrandomized study with unequal groups. Xu, Liu, Li, and Xu (1995) reported on 92 metastatic cancer patients with abdominal cancer pain who were treated for 2 weeks with acupuncture. Nearly all patients (99%) with mild to moderate pain and 72% of those with severe pain were controlled for one month. This study used only a post-test measure and did not employ a control group. Filshie, Penn, Ashley, and Davis (1996) investigated breathlessness directly related to malignancy. Using a pre-test/post-test design with 20 inpatients, significant improvements were found in breathlessness ($p < .005$), relaxation ($p < .005$), and anxiety ($p < .001$) 90 minutes after one 10-minute treatment of acupuncture.

## ACUPUNCTURE: IMPACT ON CLINICAL OUTCOMES

The main area of focus thus far has been on pain management, breathlessness, relaxation, and anxiety for cancer patients.

## ACUPUNCTURE: FUTURE DIRECTIONS

Clearly, acupuncture has a unique set of variables; the scientific process will need to be applied more stringently in future work. Randomized designs and pre- and post-testing are needed to distinguish within- and between-group differences.

## SUMMARY

As the consumer demand for CAM therapies continues to rise, science must move ahead with research in this area. Specifically, we need to know more about the symptoms for which each therapy is effective, we must identify appropriate and sensitive outcome measures, we need to determine the most effective delivery method for each type of intervention, and we need to discern the optimum dose and duration of each therapy.

In terms of the five categories established by the NCCAM, the category of mind–body interventions is the lowest risk and could be engaged in with self-monitored feedback on efficacy. Biologically based therapies are often seen as the highest risk because they involve the ingestion or injection of unregulated substances. Manipulative and body-based methods are generally lower risk and could be initiated at a moderate level to test their impact. Energy therapies are currently the least understood; for the most part, they involve fields not always measurable or clearly defined. Finally, alternative medical systems will need much work to disentangle which elements are effective, which are benign, and which do not contribute to the desired health outcome. CAM is an exciting frontier in healthcare, but there is still more to learn. Although the extensive survey work on who uses CAM therapies is well documented, we still need to assess the nonusers and explore why they do not choose to employ these therapies. Further randomized clinical trials will help establish the efficacy-by-therapy parameters based on demographics, such as gender, age, cancer site, and stage. As we become more informed about these therapies, health providers will need to sort out which CAM therapies have an evidence base and exercise caution with those that still involve anecdotal outcomes and remain unproven.

## REFERENCES

Ang-Lee, M. K., Moss, J., & Yuan, C. S. (2001). Herbal medicines and perioperative care. *Journal of the American Medical Association, 286,* 208–216.

Astin, J. A. (1998). Why patients use alternative medicine. *Journal of the American Medical Association, 279,* 1548–1553.

Baider, L., Uziely, B., & DeNour, A. K. (1994). Progressive muscle relaxation and guided imagery in cancer patients. *General Hospital Psychiatry, 16,* 340–347.

Beck, S. (1991). The therapeutic use of music for cancer-related pain. *Oncology Nursing Forum, 18,* 1327–1337.

Benson, H., Beary, J., & Carol, M. (1974). The relaxation response. *Psychiatry, 37,* 37–46.

Boldt, S. (1996). The effects of music therapy on motivation, psychological well-being, physical comfort, and exercise endurance of bone marrow transplant patients. *Journal of Music Therapy, 33*, 164–188.

Bonny, H. (1986). Music and healing. *Music Therapy, 6*, 3–12.

Burish, T., Carey, M., Krozely, M., & Greco, F. (1987). Conditioned side effects induced by cancer chemotherapy: Prevention through behavioral treatment. *Journal of Consulting and Clinical Psychology, 55*, 42–48.

Burish, T. G., & Jenkins, R. A. (1992). Effectiveness of biofeedback and relaxation training in reducing the side effects of cancer chemotherapy. *Health Psychology, 11*, 17–23.

Burish, T. G., Snyder, S. L., & Jenkins, R. A. (1991). Preparing patients for cancer chemotherapy: effect of coping preparation and relaxation interventions. *Journal of Consulting and Clinical Psychology, 59*, 518–525.

Burns, D. (2001). The effect of the bonny method of guided imagery and music on the mood and life quality of cancer patients. *Journal of Music Therapy, 38*, 51–65.

Byers, D. C. (1996.) *Better health with foot reflexology: The original Ingham Method.* St. Petersburg, FL: Ingham Publishing, Inc.

Calliet, R. (1994). *Pain: Mechanisms and management.* Philadelphia: F.A. Davis Company.

Cassileth, B. R. (1998). Overview of alternative/complementary medicine. *Cancer Practice, 6*, 243–245.

Cassileth, B. R. (1999a). Complementary therapies: Overview and state of the art. *Cancer Nursing, 22*, 85–90.

Cassileth, B. R. (1999b). Evaluating complementary and alternative therapies for cancer patients. *CA—Cancer Journal for Clinicians, 49*, 362–75.

Decker, G. M., & Schulmeister, L. (2000). Reporting adverse events associated with herbal products. *Clinical Journal of Oncology Nursing, 4*, 137–138.

DiPaola, R. S., Zhang, H., Lambert, G. H., Meeker, R., Licitra, E., Rafi, M. M., et al. (1998). Clinical and biologic activity of an estrogenic herbal combination (PC-SPES) in prostate cancer. *New England Journal of Medicine, 339*, 785–791.

Doan, B. D. (1998). Alternative and complementary therapies. In J. C. Holland, W. Breitbart, R. McCorkle, M. Loscalzo, P. B. Jacobsen, M. S. Lederberg, et al. (Eds.), *Psycho-oncology* (pp. 817–827). Oxford: Oxford University Press.

Dossey, B. M., Keegan, L., Guzzetta, C. E., & Kolkmeier, L. G. (1995). *Holistic nursing: A handbook for practice* (2nd ed.). Gaithersburg, MD: Aspen.

Drew, A. K., & Myers, S. P. (1997). Safety issues in herbal medicine: Implications for the health professions. *Medical Journal of Australia, 166*, 538–541.

Druss, B. G., & Rosenheck, R. A. (1999). Association between use of unconventional therapies and conventional medical services. *Journal of the American Medical Association, 282*, 651–656.

Eisenberg, D. M. (1997). Advising patients who seek alternative medical therapies. *Annals of Internal Medicine, 127*, 61–69.

Eisenberg, D., Davis, R., Ettner, S., Appel, S., Rompay, M., & Kessler, R. (1998). Trends in alternative medicine uses in the United States, 1990–1997. *Journal of the American Medical Association, 280*, 1569–1575.

Eisenberg, D., Kessler, R., Foster, C., Norlock, F., Calkins, D., & Deldanco, T. (1993). Unconventional medicine in the United States. *The New England Journal of Medicine, 328*, 246–252.

Egan, E. C. (1998). Therapeutic touch. In M. Snyder & R. Lindquist (Eds.), *Complementary/alternative therapies in nursing* (3rd ed., pp. 49–62). New York: Springer Publishing.

Ernst, E., & Cassileth, B. R. (1998). The prevalence of complementary/alternative medicine in cancer: A systematic review. *Cancer, 83*, 777–782.

Ernst, E., & Pittler, M. H. (2000). Efficacy of ginger for nausea and vomiting: A systematic review of randomized clinical trials. *British Journal of Anesthesiology, 84*, 367–371.

Ernst, E., & White, A. R. (1998). Acupuncture for back pain: A meta-analysis of randomized controlled trials. *Archives of Internal Medicine, 158*, 2235–2241.

Ezzo, J., Berman, B. B., Vickers, A., & Linde, K. (2000). Complementary medicine and the Cochrane Collaboration in P. B. Fontanarosa (Ed.), *JAMA and archives journals alternative medicine: An objective assessment* (pp. 584–587). Chicago: American Medical Association.

Ezzone, S., Baker, C., Rosselet, R., & Terepka, E. (1998). Music as an adjunct to antiemetic therapy. *Oncology Nursing Forum, 25*, 1551–1556.

Filshie, J., Penn, K., Ashley, S., & Davis, C. (1996). Acupuncture for the relief of cancer-related breathlessness. *Palliative Medicine, 10*, 145–150.

Frankel, B. S. M. (1997). The effect of reflexology on baroreceptor reflex sensitivity, blood pressure and sinus arrhythmia. *Complementary Therapies in Medicine, 5*, 80–84.

Gagne, D., & Toye, R. C. (1994). The effects of therapeutic touch and relaxation therapy in reducing anxiety. *Archives of Psychiatric Nursing, 7*, 184.

Gallagher, L. M., Huston, M. J., Nelson, K. A., Walsh, D., & Steele, A. L. (2001). Music therapy in palliative medicine. *Supportive Care in Cancer, 9*, 156–161.

Gatchel, R. J., & Maddrey, A. M. (1998). Clinical outcome research in complementary and alternative medicine: An overview of experimental design and analysis. *Alternative Therapies in Health and Medicine, 4*(5), 36–42.

Geddes, N., & Henry, J. K. (1997). Nursing and alternative medicine. Legal and practice issues. *Journal of Holistic Nursing, 15*, 271–281.

Gerdner, L. A., & Buckwalter, K. C. (1999). Music therapy. In G. M. Bulechek & J. C. McCloskey (Eds.), *Nursing interventions: Effective nursing treatments* (3rd ed., pp. 451–468). Philadelphia: WB Saunders.

Giasson, M., & Bouchard, L. (1998). Effect of therapeutic touch on the well-being of persons with cancer. *Journal of Holistic Nursing, 16*, 383–398.

Given, C. W., Wyatt, G. K., Given, B. A., & Kozachik, S. L. (2001). Acceptance and use of complementary therapy by cancer patients and family members: Final project report to the Walther Cancer Institute. East Lansing, MI: Michigan State University.

Gordon, A., Merenstein, J. H., D'Amico, F., & Hudgens, D. (1998). The effects of therapeutic touch on patients with osteoarthritis of the knee. *The Journal of Family Practice, 47*, 271–277.

Gordon, D. W., Rosenthal, G., Hart, J. Sirota, R., & Baker, A. L. (1995). Chaparral ingestion: The broadening spectrum of liver injury caused by herbal medications. *Journal of the American Medical Association, 273,* 489–490.

Green, S. (1992). A critique of the rationale for cancer treatment with coffee enemas and diet. *Journal of the American Medical Association, 268,* 3224–3227.

Gruber, B., Hersh, S., Hall, N., Waletzky, L., Kunz, J., & Carpenter, J., et al. (1993). Immunological responses of breast cancer patients to behavioral interventions. *Biofeedback and self regulation, 18,* 1–22.

Guzzetta, C. E. (1996). Alternative therapies: What's the fuss? *Nurse Investigator, 3*(2), 1–2.

Guzzetta, C. (1995). Music therapy: Hearing the melody of the soul. In B. Dossey, L. Keegan, C. Guzzetta, & L. Kolkmeier (Eds.), *Holistic nursing* (pp. 670–698). Gaithersburg, MD: Aspen.

He, J. P., Friedrich, M., Ertan, A. K., Muller, K., & Schmidt, W. (1999). Pain-relief and movement improvement by acupuncture after ablation and axillary lymphadenectomy in patients with mammary cancer. *Clinical and Experimental Obstetrics and Gynecology, 26,* 81–84.

Heiser, R. M, Chiles, K., Fudge, M., & Gray, S. E. (1997). The use of music during the immediate postoperative recovery period. *AORN Journal, 65,* 777–778, 781–785.

Hodgson, H. (2000). Does reflexology impact on cancer patients' quality of life? *Nursing Standard, 14*(31), 33–38, 43.

Horowitz, S., & Breitbart, W. (1993). Relaxation and imagery for symptom control in cancer patients. In W. Breitbart & J. Holland (Eds.), *Psychiatric aspects of symptom management in cancer patients* (pp. 147–172). Washington, DC: American Psychiatric Press, Inc.

Ingerman, S. (1991). *Soul retrieval: Mending the fragmented self.* San Francisco: HarperCollins.

Jacobson, J. S., Workman, S. B., & Kronenberg, F. (2000). Research on complementary/alternative medicine for patients with breast cancer: A review of the biomedical literature. *Journal of Clinical Oncology, 18,* 668–683.

Jonas, W. B. (1998). Alternative medicine—Learning from the past, examining the present, advancing to the future. *Journal of the American Medical Association, 280,* 1616–1618.

Jonas, W. B. (1996). Safety in complementary medicine. In E. Ernst (Ed.), *Complementary medicine: An objective appraisal* (pp. 126–149). Oxford: Butterworth-Heinemann.

Kaptchuk, T. J., & Eisenberg, D. M. (1998). Chiropractic: Origins, controversies, and contributions. *Archives of Internal Medicine, 158,* 2215–2224.

Kastner, M. & Burroughs, H. (1996). *Alternative healing: The complete A–Z guide to more than 150 alternative therapies.* New York: Henry Holt and Company.

Kessler, R. C., Davis, R. B., Foster, D. F., Van Rompay, M. I., Walters, E. E., Wilkey, S. A., et al. (2001). Long-term trends in the use of complementary and alternative medical therapies in the United States. *Annals of Internal Medicine, 135,* 262–268.

Kolcaba, K., & Fox, C. (1999). The effects of guided imagery on comfort of women with early stage breast cancer undergoing radiation therapy. *Oncology Nursing Forum, 26,* 67–72.

Krebs, L. U. (1999). Mind-body interventions. In G. M. Decker (Ed.), *An introduction to complementary and alternative therapies* (pp. 2–27). Pittsburgh, PA: Oncology Nursing Press, Inc.

Krieger, D. (1993). *Accepting your power to heal: The personal practice of therapeutic touch.* Santa Fe: Bear.

Linde, K., Ramirez, G., Mulrow, C. D., Pauls, A., Weidenhammer, W., & Melchart, D. (1996). St. John's Wort for depression—An overview and meta-analysis of randomized clinical trials. *British Medical Journal, 313,* 253–258.

Meehan, T. C. (1993). Therapeutic touch and postoperative pain: A Rogerian research study. *Nursing Science Quarterly, 6,* 69–77.

Micozzi, M. S. (1996). Characteristics of complementary and alternative medicine. In M. Micozzi (Ed.), *Fundamentals of complementary and alternative medicine* (pp. 3–8). New York: Churchill Livingstone.

Montbriand, M. J. (1995). Decision tree model describing alternate health care choices made by oncology patients. *Cancer Nursing, 18,* 104–117.

Moranto, C. (1993). Application of music in medicine. In M. Heal & T. Wogram (Eds.), *Music therapy in health and education* (pp. 153–174). London: Kingsley.

Munro, S., & Mount, B. (1978). Music therapy in palliative care. *Canadian Medical Association Journal, 119,* 1029–1034.

NCCAM. (2000, September 25). Expanding horizons of healthcare. *Five year strategic plan, 2001–2005.* 1–49.

NCCAM. (2001). Major domains for complementary and alternative medicine. NCCAM information for consumers and practitioners. Retrieved September 10, 2001, from http://nccam.nih.gov/fcp/classify.

Olsen, M., Sneed, N., Bonadonna, R., Ratliff, J., & Dias, J. (1992). Therapeutic touch and post-hurricane Hugo stress. *Journal of Holistic Nursing, 10,* 120.

Olsen, M., Sneed, N., Lavia, M., Virella, G., Bonadonna, R., & Michel, Y. (1997). Stress-induced immunosuppression and therapeutic touch. *Alternative Therapies in Health and Medicine, 3,* 68–74.

Paltiel, O., Avitzour, M., Peretz, T., Cherny, N., Kaduri, L., Pfeffer, R. M., et al. (2001). Determinants of the use of complementary therapies by patients with cancer. *Journal of Clinical Oncology, 19,* 2439–2448.

Paulsen, S. M. (1998). Use of herbal products and dietary supplements by oncology patients—Informed decisions? *Highlights in Oncology Practice, 15,* 94–106.

Peck, S. D. E. (1997). The effectiveness of therapeutic touch for decreasing pain in elders with degenerative arthritis. *Journal of Holistic Nursing, 15,* 176.

Pittler, M. H. & Ernst, E. (2000). Efficacy of kava extract for treating anxiety: Systematic review and meta-analysis. *Journal of Clinical Psychopharmacology, 20,* 84–89.

Richardson, M., Sanders, T., Palmer, J., Greisinger, A., & Singletary, E. (2000). Complementary/alternative medicine use in a comprehensive cancer center and the implications for oncology. *Journal of Clinical Oncology, 18,* 2505–2514.

Richardson, M. A., Post-White, J., Grimm, E. A., Moye, L. A., Singletary, S. E., & Justice, B. (1997). Coping, life attitudes, and immune responses to imagery and group support after breast cancer treatment. *Alternative Therapies, 3*, 62–70.

Risberg, T., Lund, E., & Wist, E. (1995). Use of non-proven therapies: Differences in attitudes between Norwegian patients with non-malignant disease and patients suffering from cancer. *Acta Oncologica, 34*, 893–898.

Risberg, T., Lund, E., Wist, E., Dahl, O., Sundstrom, S., Andersen, O., et al. (1995). The use of non-proven therapy among patients treated in Norwegian oncological departments: A cross-sectional national multicentre study. *European Journal of Cancer, 31A*, 1785–1789.

Risberg, T., Lund, E., Wist, E., Kaasa, S., & Wilsgaard, T. (1998). Cancer patients use of unproven therapy: A 5-year follow-up study. *Journal of Clinical Oncology, 16*, 6–12.

Rogers, M. E. (1990). Nursing: Science of unitary, irreducible, human beings: Update 1990. In E. A. M. Barrett (Ed.), *Vision of Rogers' science-based nursing* (pp. 5–11). New York: National League for Nursing.

Sabo, C. E., & Michael, S. R. (1996). The influence of personal message with music on anxiety and side effects associated with chemotherapy. *Cancer Nursing, 19*, 283–289.

Shelton, R. C., Keller, M. B., Gelenberg, A., Dunner, D. L., Hirschfeld, R., Thase, M. E., et al. (2001). Effectiveness of St. John's Wort in major depression. A randomized clinical trial. *Journal of the American Medical Association, 285*, 1978–1986.

Simington, J. A., & Laing, G. P. (1993). Effects of therapeutic touch on anxiety in the institutionalized elderly. *Clinical Nursing Research, 2*, 438.

Simonton, O. C., Matthews-Simonton, S., & Sparks, T. F. (1980). Psychological intervention in the treatment of cancer. *Psychosomatics, 21*, 226–227, 231–233.

Sloman, R. 1995. Relaxation and the relief of cancer pain. *Nursing Clinics of North America, 4*, 697–709.

Smith, M., Casey, L., Johnson, D., Gwede, C., & Riggin, O. Z. (2001). Music as a therapeutic intervention for anxiety in patients receiving radiation therapy. *Oncology Nursing Forum, 28*, 855–862.

Sodergren, K. A. (1993). The effect of absorption and social closeness on responses to educational and relaxation therapies in patients with anticipatory nausea and vomiting during cancer chemotherapy. Unpublished doctoral dissertation, University of Minnesota.

Standley, J. M. (1992). Clinical applications of music and chemotherapy: The effects on nausea and emesis. *Music Therapy Perspectives, 10*, 27–35.

Stephens, R. (1993). Imagery: A strategic intervention to empower clients: Part I—Review of research literature. *Clinical Nurse Specialist, 7*, 170–174.

Stephenson, N., Weinrich, S., & Tavakoli, A. (2000). The effects of foot reflexology on anxiety and pain in patients with breast and lung cancer. *Oncology Nursing Forum, 27*, 67–72.

Stevinson, C., & Ernst, E. (2000). Valerian for insomnia: A systematic review of randomized clinical trials. *Sleep Medicine, 1*, 91–99.

Sun, A. S., Ostadal, O., Ryznar, V., Dulik, I., Dusek, J., Vaclavik, A., et al. (1999). Phase I/II study of stage III and IV non-small cell lung cancer patients taking a specific dietary supplement. *Nutrition and Cancer, 34*, 62–69.

Syrjala, K. L., Donaldson, G. W., Davis, M. W., Kippes, M. E., & Carr, J. E. (1995). Relaxation and imagery and cognitive-behavioral training reduce pain during cancer treatment: A controlled clinical trial. *Pain, 63*, 489–498.

Tatro, D. S. (1999). *Drug interactions with herbal products. Facts and comparisons: The review of natural products.* St. Louis: Wolters Kluwer.

Troesch, L. M., Rodehaver, C. B., Delaney, E. A., & Yanes, B. (1993). The influence of guided imagery on chemotherapy-related nausea and vomiting. *Oncology Nursing Forum, 20*, 1179–1185.

Turner, J., Clark, A., Gauthier, D., & Williams, M. (1998). The effect of therapeutic touch on pain and anxiety in burn patients. *Journal of Advanced Nursing, 28*, 10–20.

Vickers, A., Cassileth, B., Ernst, E., Fisher, P., Goldman, P., Jonas, W., et al. (1997). How should we research unconventional therapies? A panel report from the Conference on Complementary and Alternative Medicine Research Methodology, National Institutes of Health. *International Journal of Technology Assessment in Health Care, 13*, 111–121.

Vithoulkas, G. (1980). *The science of homeopathy.* New York: Grove Press.

Walker, L., Walker, M., Ogston, K., Heys, S., Ah-See, A., Miller, I., et al. (1999). Psychological, clinical and pathological effects of relaxation training and guided imagery during primary chemotherapy. *British Journal of Cancer, 80*, 262–268.

Weber, R. (1989). A philosophical perspective on touch. In K. E. Barnard & T. B. Brazelton, (Eds.), *Touch: The foundation of experience* (p. 11). Madison, CT: International Universities Press.

Woodham, A., & Peters, D. (1997). *Encyclopedia of healing therapies.* New York: DK Publishing.

Wyandt, C. M., & Williamson, J. S. (1999). For physicians: A comprehensive overview of popular herbs, their pharmacologic activities and potential uses. In *Talking to patients: Excerpts from the physician's guide to alternative medicine.* Atlanta, GA: American Health Consultants.

Wyatt, G. (1989). Holistic care: Linking mind, emotion, and body. *Michigan Hospital Association's Magazine for Health Care Professionals,* May, 5–9.

Wyatt, G. K., Friedman, L. L., Given, C. W., Given, B. A., & Beckrow, K. C.(1999). Complementary therapy use among older cancer patients. *Cancer Practice, 7*, 136–144.

Wyatt, G. K., Given, B. A., Given, C. W., & Beckrow, K. C. (2001). A subacute care intervention for short-stay breast cancer surgery (DAMD17-96-1-6325): Final report to the U.S. Army Medical Research and Materiel Command, Department of Defense.

Xu, S., Liu, Z., Li, Y., & Xu, M. (1995). Treatment of cancerous abdominal pain by acupuncture on zusanli (ST36): A report of 92 cases. *Journal of Traditional Chinese Medicine, 15*, 189–191.

# 11

## Family Caregiving Interventions in Cancer Care

**Barbara Given**
**Charles W. Given**
**Sharon Kozachik**
**Susan Rawl**

<br>

This review examines the intervention research focused on family caregivers responsible for the home care of patients with cancer. Changes in the healthcare system make home care a difficult situation for families; home care for individuals with cancer is increasing in complexity due to shorter stays in the acute care setting and more aggressive treatment. Family members must cope with their emotional responses to the cancer diagnosis and cope with the physical, social, and financial dimensions of providing care. Further, family members are now expected to play a major role in assisting with the management of the disease, treatment, and treatment-related side effects. Cancer and its treatment may alter family identity, roles, communication patterns, and daily functioning. These changes can occur over an extended period of time as family members deal with unfamiliar situations and demands as cancer treatment continues, as the disease progresses, or as patients recover and survive.

Family members indicate they feel ill prepared, have insufficient knowledge, and receive little assistance from the formal healthcare system. Family members may not know how to take on the caregiving role, may be unfamiliar with what care they must provide, and may not utilize available resources (Given & Given, 1992; Oberst, Thomas, Gass, & Ward, 1989). The impact of caregiving on cancer patients can be critical to the health and well-being of the caregiver (Given et al., 1993; McCorkle, 1993; Northouse, 1988; Oberst et al., 1989; Sales, 1991; Schulz & Beach, 1999), and caregivers often neglect their own healthcare needs in order to assist their loved one.

Family caregiving has been conceptualized as the provision of unpaid aid or assistance by one or more family members to another family member related to a healthcare problem (beyond that required as part of normal, everyday life). Caregiving may not always be distinguished from aid and assistance given as a part of the normal family relationship, so caregiving may be difficult for family members to label. Some of the difficulty in defining the family caregiver role exists in the history and nature of the relationship between the caregiver and the care receiver, as well as the ambiguous and evolving demands of care.

The aim of this chapter is to review the literature on interventions directed toward family caregivers that moderate caregiver distress and enable them to provide the needed care. The specific focus of this review is the general literature about caregiving for cancer patients. In addition, an examination of the intervention studies used to help family caregivers with the care process will be provided. Literature was reviewed through a computerized search supplemented by the personal library collection of the authors. Because an interdisciplinary, biobehavioral approach was desired, the databases searched included MEDLINE®, CINAHL®, PsychINFO, and HealthSTAR®. The range for each search was 1990 through 2001, and all searches were completed in English. Key words used included *family caregiver*, *caregiving*, *family*, *cancer*, *clinical trials*, and *interventions*. *Interventions* and *clinical trials* were entered with more specific terms used to sort categories and narrow the topic to relevant articles. Because not enough articles were found to cover the cancer illness trajectory, this search was considered unsuccessful and resulted in a need to return to the larger database. In keeping with the recommendations by Pasacreta and McCorkle (2000), however, this chapter will focus on psychoeducational interventions, support, and counseling. Interventions targeted to caregivers across the cancer care continuum will be included.

Examining the role of family caregivers and the impact of caregiving on family members has been an area of research for the past three decades, primarily for the elderly and those with dementia. Literature related to family involvement in cancer care, however, is limited, although some research has been done on coping and adjustment. Limited and only recent research exists that examines the impact of cancer care on family caregivers.

## THEORETICAL MODELS

A search for theoretical models used to describe the family care of cancer patients resulted only in the work of the chapter authors (Given & Given, 1996). The use of formal theoretical models has not been articulated in caregiver intervention studies. Frameworks implied in the research are most often limited to stress and coping. Prior research has not integrated care demands, levels of involvement in care, or caregiving skills of family members. Intervention models seldom incorporate patient recovery, the course of the illness, or treatment trajectory. Because few models exist to guide this review, the literature will be organized into three primary areas: First, an overview of the impact of care on family caregivers—focusing primarily on the distress, burden, and effects on caregiver physical health—is included. Second, the caregiver characteristics that affect the ability to care and the quality of care provided are described. Third, intervention trials that have been completed to moderate negative caregiver responses to the care they provide are summarized. Finally, current research limitations and suggestions for future research are discussed.

## THE EFFECTS OF CAREGIVING

### Effects on Caregiver Psychological Health

Descriptive studies have provided evidence that family members of patients with cancer experience distress due to their caregiving roles, and this distress continues over time (Given et al., 1993; Given, Stommel, Collins, King, & Given, 1990; Northouse, Mood, Templin, Mellon, & George, 2000; Northouse & Peters-Golden, 1993; Oberst & Scott, 1988; Raveis, Karus & Siegel, 1998; Toseland, Blanchard, & McCallion, 1995). Caregiving distress may be related to direct care tasks, complex medical procedures, the disruption of daily routines, role overload, or the need to provide emotional support. A number of review articles describe the psychological impact of cancer on family caregivers (Cooley & Moriarty, 1997; Kristjanson & Ashcroft, 1994; Laizner, Shegda, Barg, & McCorkle, 1993;

Northouse et al., 2000; Northouse, Dorris, & Charron-Moore, 1995). Depression and anxiety have most often been examined as indicators or symptoms of caregiver distress. Descriptive studies have documented that caregivers experience anxiety and depression, as well as a sense of helplessness and fear (Blank, Clark, Longman, & Atwood, 1989; Nijboer, Tempelaar, Triemstra, Van den Bos, & Sanderman, 2001; Northouse et al., 1995; Oberst et al., 1989; Siegel, Raveis, Mor, & Houts, 1991; Weitzner, Moody, & McMillan, 1997). About 25% to 30% of cancer caregivers are depressed or distressed.

Overall, caregiving is more stressful for women (both wives and daughters) than for men (both husbands and sons; Baider et al., 1996; Nijboer et al., 2001; Northouse et al., 1995; Northouse et al., 2000; Raveis et al., 1998; Sales, Schultz, & Beigel, 1992; Schulz, Visintainer, & Williamson, 1990; Schulz & Williamson, 1991). In addition, wives, husbands, daughters, and sons appear to approach the practice of caregiving in different ways, which may affect caregiver outcomes (Gerstel & Gallagher, 1993; Raveis et al., 1998). In married couples, husbands caring for wives with cancer focus on caregiving tasks while continuing their own activities and interests, such as gardening; they do not expect their wives' needs for care to interfere with these activities. Wife caregivers, however, give priority to their husbands' needs and choices (Miller, 1990b) and may consider their own needs to be secondary. Wives focus attention on the interpersonal aspects of caregiving, such as how their relationships with their husbands are changing, and they find changes to be uncomfortable. They are also more distressed by the caregiving role and care demands.

Nijboer, Triemstra, Tempelaar, Sanderman, and van de Bos (1999) studied colorectal cancer patients and their partners. Caregiver experiences were assessed by the Caregiver Reaction Assessment (CRA) scale, which contains four negative subscales (a disrupted schedule, an impact on finances, a lack of family support, and an impact on health) and one positive subscale (self-esteem). The mental health of caregivers was assessed in terms of depression and quality of life. Although caregiving may lead to depression, especially in those experiencing a loss of physical strength, caregivers may sustain their quality of life through increased self-esteem from caregiving.

Providing emotional support can be as, or more, burdensome than providing direct care (Carey, Oberst, McCubbin, & Hughes, 1991). Changes or restrictions in work roles and career opportunities, increased financial costs and demands, and strain in marital relationships all lead to an increased burden (Stommel, Given, Given, & Collins, 1995; Siegel et al., 1991; Weitzner, Meyers et al., 1997). Raveis et al. (1998) found that care-providing daughters who had an existing health condition themselves reported limitations in their ability to care and reported higher levels of depression.

## Effects on Caregiver Physical Health

Although declines in physical health and premature death have been reported (Schulz, 1999, 2001), little research in cancer care has been conducted on physical health outcomes of family caregivers (Schulz & Beach 1999; Weitzner, Meyers et al., 1997). Given and Given (1992), Given et al. (1993), and Kurtz, Kurtz, Given, and Given (1994) have found that family caregivers experience significant negative physical consequences as patient illness progresses. Beach, Schulz, and Yu (2000) and Schulz (1997) found that increases in patient impairment increased caregiving demands in couples and that caregiver strain was generally related to poor health status, increased health risk behaviors, and higher use of prescription drugs, as well as increased anxiety and depression. In addition to eating disorders and sleep disturbances, other research has reported lower immune functioning (Kiecolt-Glaser, Dura, Speicher, Trask, & Glaser, 1991), altered response to influenza vaccinations (Kiecolt-Glaser, Glaser, Gravenstein, Malarkey, & Sheridan, 1996), slower wound healing (Kiecolt-Glaser, Marucha, Malarky, Mercade, & Glaser, 1995), increased blood pressure (Franklin, Ames, & King, 1994), and altered lipid profiles (Vitaliano, 1995) in family caregivers.

Burton, Bewson, and Schultz (1997) explored the relationships between caregiving and lifestyle health behaviors and the use of preventive services. They found that being a high-level caregiver increased the odds of getting inadequate rest, having insufficient time to exercise, and forgetting to take prescription drugs when compared to noncaregivers. However, caregivers with a strong sense of control over life events had good health-promotive behaviors compared to those with a weak sense of control. Few studies have examined caregiver health behaviors such as routine screening, smoking, or primary care visits.

## General Positive Effects of Caregiving

Although caregiving has negative psychological and physical effects, attending to the needs of a loved one often provides satisfaction and meaning for the caregiver. The extent to which positive results have been disregarded in the caregiving literature is startling. Inattention to the rewards of caregiving is particularly problematic. Some studies have suggested that caregiving can be pleasurable. It is plausible that rewards and satisfaction, with the combinations of other roles, may provide a buffer. However, it is also plausible that studies may have biased samples and have attracted caregivers with a positive sense of well-being and an ability to manage multiple roles (Raveis et al., 1998). A number of investigators have monitored the importance of having positive approaches. Picot et al. (1995, 1997) have developed and used a caregiver rewards scale, and Archbold et al. (1995) described the mutuality between the patient and caregiver. High negative and high positive results may exist simultaneously (Lawton, Rajagopal, Brody, & Kleban, 1992); it is thus imperative that both the rewards and challenges of caregiving be examined (Nijboer et al., 2000).

In the following sections, acknowledging and understanding caregiver stress, including factors that contribute to the caregiver distress, factors that relieve this distress, and patterns of distress (extent and duration), are addressed. Although patterns of distress that occur over the care trajectory have not been well described, studies on family care for cancer demonstrate that distress does occur. Researchers report that caregiver and patient distress are correlated (Given & Given, 1996; Northouse, Templin, Mood, & Oberst, 1998). Therefore, it appears that by moderating caregiver distress it may be possible to affect the distress experienced by both the patient and caregiver.

## CHARACTERISTICS OF AT-RISK CAREGIVERS

Gender, age, financial status, living arrangements, family relationships, family roles, the developmental stage, and care load and demands are related to caregiver distress and should be considered when planning interventions. Each of these characteristics influences caregiver availability, capability, and willingness to assist with cancer care. Further, each of these characteristics intersects with each other in complex ways. For example, higher caregiver distress has been associated with having a lower income, living only with the patient, experiencing lower daily emotional support, having a strained caregiver–patient relationship prior to the illness, experiencing a negative sense of obligation to the patient, having a low mastery of skills, facing high levels of patient dependency, experiencing increased caregiving demands, and engaging in high levels of involvement in caregiving tasks (Nijboer et al., 1998, 2000; Nijboer, Triemstra, Tempelaar, Sanderman, & van den Bos, 1999). Complicating matters further is the fact that research has been directed toward certain risk characteristics (e.g., gender), while little research has been directed toward others (e.g., living arrangements). The complicated dimensions of burden and distress associated with cancer care need to be understood to plan meaningful interventions that will assist family caregivers to continue providing care throughout the cancer treatment and illness trajectory.

## Caregiver Characteristics: Gender

Gender has been shown to be differentially related to caregiver distress. Levels of depression among caregivers are the highest for wives, followed by daughters, then other female caregivers, sons, and finally husband caregivers (Stommel, Given, & Given, 1990). Female caregivers may be more adversely affected by caregiving role functions than male caregivers, a pattern that holds among caregivers of physically impaired, stroke, heart disease, dementia, and cancer patients (Robinson 1990; Siegel et al., 1991). Spousal caregivers appear to be at particular risk for caregiver distress, because they typically provide the most extensive and comprehensive care, maintain their role longer, tolerate greater levels of disability among family members than adult children and other nonspousal caregivers, experience more lifestyle adjustments, and exhibit lower levels of well-being (Siegel et al., 1991).

## Caregiver Characteristics: Age

Age contributes to caregiver distress (Given & Given, 1996; Nijboer et al., 2000). Intergenerational caregivers are often middle-aged (adult caregivers) parents and are more likely to suffer role conflicts due to multiple and competing role demands, whereas intragenerational caregivers suffer from caregiver role entrenchment. Elderly spouse caregivers may have fewer defined roles to perform than adult children caregivers and may respond to the demands of cancer care by isolating themselves from social and family roles to become completely focused on providing care.

Older and aging families living with cancer may have other problems related to care tasks, such as decreased physical abilities that may result from their own frailty and comorbid conditions such as diabetes, cardiovascular disease, social isolation, or diminished family resources. Caregivers of younger patients may report more distress from care than those caring for older patients (Given et al., 1993; Schumacher et al., 1993). Schumacher et al. found that caregivers of young male patients with lower functional status and lower levels of efficacy experienced more strain than caregivers for older patients.

## Caregiver Characteristics: Socioeconomic Status

Cancer care is most burdensome for patients and caregivers with low incomes and limited financial resources if substantial out-of-pocket costs occur. Unemployed or low-income caregivers may experience more distress because they may have fewer resources and less capacity to respond to distress. Davis-Ali, Chesler, and Chesney (1993) concluded that higher-income families may not concern themselves with the financial hardships of cancer care because they are able to purchase or seek resources. However, income and overall financial concerns cause distress for caregivers during long periods of caregiving (Clipp & George, 1992) as resources become depleted. Given, Given, and Stommel (1994) found that substantial out-of-pocket costs, loss of income, and family labor costs may occur and contribute to financial burden. Out-of-pocket expenses for transportation, clothing, and phone bills—as well as wages lost for both patient and caregiver care—may cause substantial burdens and distress for families.

## Caregiver Characteristics: Living Arrangements and Family Relationships

Living arrangements may need to be altered, either temporarily or permanently, to manage the care of cancer patients. The patient may move into the caregiver's home to facilitate care, or family members may move into the home of the patient to provide care. Secondary caregivers are much more involved in parental care than spousal care situations. When a patient is widowed, single, or divorced, more caregivers are involved. Caregivers who live with the person with cancer are found to be more depressed than those who lived in separate households (Stommel & Kingry, 1991). When the caregiver is not the spouse, the obligations and expectations may be lower, and the caregiver may not be willing to accept the personal costs of providing care. The more distant the relative, the less obligated family members feel to provide care (Given et al., 1993; Schumacher, Dodd, & Paul, 1993).

## Caregiver Characteristics: Family Roles and Developmental Stage

Current and previous role relationships between patients and their family caregivers need to be considered when developing interventions to ease the care role for the caregiver. Family caregiving is a stressful normative expectation with feelings of obligation and attachment, and individuals often assume caregiving responsibilities to show that they are committed to supporting the family (Cicirelli, 1992). Family caregiving must be placed within a historic context, because bonds of affection and reciprocity that sustain caregiving take root in past patient–caregiver relationships. Family cohesion or conflict may reflect the way families usually function and can be compounded in response to the challenges of cancer care. Both the recipient and giver of care bring a history of interactions that may enhance or complicate the care process. The social integration of care roles into the usual family role dynamic may influence the lack of resultant strain (Zarit & Pearlin, 1993). Therefore, it is important to consider not only the influence of family relationships, but also the quality of relationships in terms of impact on the evolving care recipient–caregiver relationship.

Adult children providing parental care—often daughters caring for a parent or parent-in-law when a spouse caregiver is not available—may be caught between their work life, professional careers, their own family roles, and caregiving demands. Responsibilities to parents may at times take precedence over responsibilities to their spouses, children, coworkers, and employers because the care of a parent is seen as the more pressing and immediate need. Barnes, Given, and Given (1992) found that working daughters reported less personal time for themselves, less time for social activities, and less privacy than unemployed daughter caregivers.

Caregivers adapt employment obligations to manage and meet caregiving obligations (Anastas, Gibeau, & Larson, 1990; Franklin, Ames, & King, 1994; Neal, Chapman, Ingersol-Dayton, & Emlen, 1993). Family members with other role obligations, including employment, report withdrawals from work, work absences, or reductions in work productivity necessary to control their caregiver burden and distress. Caregivers report difficulty maintaining work roles while assisting family members. For some caregivers, employment provides a respite from ongoing cancer care activities and serves as a buffer to distress. Employment confirms both economic as well as personal benefits. As family members take leaves of absence, miss days of work, or leave work early to provide care, they may be sacrificing economic rewards and benefits, diversion from caring, self-esteem, and personal rewards (Given, Given, & Stommel, 1994).

The family developmental stage may differentially influence family response and availability because roles often conflict, compete with, and are disrupted by care demands (Hileman, Lackey, & Hassanein, 1992; Kristjanson & Ashcroft, 1994). If caregiving is required "off time" in younger families, care challenges are even more burdensome and stressful because not only are they unexpected, but also the needed support may not be available. Kristjanson and Ashcroft described how distress may be greater during a transition from one developmental stage to another and it is during transitions that most family dysfunction is likely to occur.

Middle-aged family caregivers providing care for a family member— usually a spouse—often find cancer care difficult because they have to negotiate their career paths, other family roles, their stage of life, and the implications of widowhood. These caregivers take on the roles vacated by the individual with cancer (Buehler & Lee, 1992). Needs arise from domains in lifestyle functioning and developmental stage, such that more socially active caregivers may require more assistance to compensate for the additional roles they must try to balance.

Northouse et al. (1995, 1998, 2000) found that spouses reported decreases in family functioning and social support combined with increases in emotional distress over time. Strong predictors of role problems were the spouses' own baseline role problems and levels of marital satisfaction. They documented that social support, illness uncertainty, symptom distress, and hopelessness accounted for spousal role problems. Wives who adjusted well to their disease contributed to the positive adjustment of their spouses. Families with better spousal communication may experience less disruption, role conflict, and role strain over time. Nijboer et al. (2001) suggested that social and psychological resources, both mediated by normative and non-normative family roles and the developmental stage, required by caregivers should be considered as the caregivers adopt and adapt to the processes of care.

## Caregiver Characteristics: Care Load and Care Demands

Care load and care demands are two separate yet intricately intertwined concepts. Care load refers to the variation and complexity of care tasks being provided, from providing personal care, providing transportation, assisting with treatment, and attending physician appointments. Care demands, on the other hand, refer to the frequency and intensity level of the care provided.

A relationship between distress and actual care demands has been assumed to exist but has not been systematically examined. The amount of time or hours per day devoted to cancer care, the inability to control the timing of care, the intimacy of care required, and the amount of physical care provided have not been systematically examined. The severity of the illness and the complexity of treatment that make care necessary are integral to determining the risk for negative caregiver reactions and distress. The stage of cancer; length of illness; phase in treatment trajectory; symptom experience; impact of cancer and treatment on functional, psychological, and mobility status; and patient role changes will influence cancer care demands on families (Given et al., 1993). When care requirements are beyond the capacity of the patient, they are translated to the caregiver as care load and care demands. Involvement in care tasks is described in relationship to patient functional disability (activities such as bathing, dressing, and eating) and instrumental activities of daily living such as cleaning, doing laundry, and providing transportation. The care demands take place in the context of the other roles of the family caregiver, adding complexity to the care situation as well as to the family dynamics, hence the potential for caregiver distress.

Family involvement in cancer patient care ranges from providing direct care, performing complex monitoring tasks, interpreting patient symptoms, assisting with decision-making, and providing emotional support and comfort. Each form of involvement demands different skills, organizational capacities, role demands, and psychological strengths from family members (Schmuacher, Stewart, Archbold, Dodd, & Dibble, 2000; Stommel et al., 1995). Families must interact and negotiate with the healthcare system to obtain information, services, and equipment, as well as with family and friends to enlist and mobilize support for assistance. As care demands— along with direct and indirect care requirements—change over time in response to the stage of cancer and cancer treatment, caregivers must be able to adapt the amount and intensity of their assistance.

The severity and duration of a patient's illness, symptoms, and physical decline are thought to be related to caregiver distress. In the terminal stages, families may be overwhelmed with the demands of not only the illness, but also a poor prognosis and the threat of approaching death. Patient reactions to illness appear to influence family member reactions, and at times family member distress equals or exceeds that of the patient (Carey et al., 1991; Given et al., 1990).

Weitzner, McMillan, and Jacobsen (1999) found that family caregivers of patients receiving palliative care had significantly lower caregiver quality of life scores and lower physical health scores than those receiving curative care. After accounting for the caregiver's level of education, the treatment status accounted for no additional significant variability in caregiver physical health. Lower quality of life scores of caregivers was a reflection of the patients' poorer performance status.

Several small-scale studies have shown that recurrent disease may be associated with caregiver distress (Given & Given, 1992; Northouse, 1995). However, Schumacher et al. (1993) found that depression among caregivers of patients with recurrent disease was significantly related to caregiver gender, perceived adequacy of social support, and coping efficacy, rather than the recurrent disease per se.

Reactions of families in the early phase of diagnosis, treatment, and the threat of illness have been documented by Oberst and James (1985) and Oberst and Scott (1988). Constancy in adjustment—that is, change in patient status, or either improvement or deterioration—may influence the family response over time. Given et al. (1993) demonstrated that it was not the care load itself, but the change in care demands (either increased or decreased) that resulted in caregiver distress. When changes in patients' conditions are due to remissions and exacerbations, this necessitates changes in the family caregivers' care responsibilities and role demands. Change adds stress, and constant adaptations require more work, negotiation, and adjustments by family members. Other researchers have indicated that caregiver well-being is unrelated to the care receiver's level of impairment or decline in health (Miller, 1990a; Miller, 1990b).

Family members provide care on demand during the day, at night, and on weekends and holidays, which may continue over a number of years. McCorkle and Wilkerson (1991) found that during a 6-month period, even though patient symptoms and functional abilities improved, caregivers reported that they were continuing to provide assistance to patients. At 6 months, caregivers still had to modify schedules to assist patients to deal with cancer and be available for care 24 hours a day. Caregiver distress may continue even after patient status improves (Given et al., 1993; McCorkle & Wilkerson, 1991; Northouse & Peters-Golden, 1993) or varies with treatment type, phase, and stage of disease.

To measure involvement in care, a number of dimensions must be assessed: (a) the nature of the tasks, (b) the frequency of task performance, (c) the hours of care provided each day, (d) the ability to perform tasks at predictable or set times, and (d) the support received from other family members (McCorkle & Wilkerson, 1991). Tasks of care cover those related to physical care (Given et al., 1990; McCorkle & Wilkerson, 1991); nutrition (Houts et al., 1988); emotional, social, and spiritual support (Given et al., 1990; Houts et al., 1988); housekeeping (Oberst et al., 1989); transportation (Blank et al., 1989; Oberst et al., 1989); and financial assistance (Blank et al., 1989; Given et al., 1990; Mor, Masterson-Allen, Houts, & Siegel, 1992). Involvement often depends on disease status, placement in the cancer care trajectory, and the level of physical function. Symptom management and control become a major focus for both the patient and the family as they struggle to manage the symptoms of disease and side effects from surgery, chemotherapy, and/or radiation therapy (Dodd, 1984a, 1984b; Given & Given, 1991; Given, Given, Stommel, & Lin, 1994; McCorkle & Wilkerson, 1991; Nail, Jones, Greene, Schipper, & Jensen, 1991). Symptom distress influences the social and physical functions of the family caregiver and curtails caregiver–patient role interaction. Patient symptom distress may also lead to caregiver distress, which may be manifested as anger, anxiety, frustration, or depression. This distress affects the demands on family caregivers' ability to provide care, or even to care for themselves.

Care for difficult symptoms, such as pain management, influences the level of caregiver strain (Miaskowski et al., 1997; Musci & Dodd, 1990). Ferrell, Wisdom, Rhiner, and Alletto (1991) and Ferrell, Ferrell, Rhiner, and Grant (1991) have studied pain management as one of the most intractable problems for family caregivers that accounts for substantial anxiety, distress, and frustration. Family caregivers assist with both nonpharmacologic and pharmacologic pain-management strategies. Miaskowski et al. (1997) reported that caregivers of patients with pain scored higher on anxiety and depression subscales of the Profile of Mood (POM) states and had significantly higher total mood disturbance scores than those caregivers caring for patients without pain. Ferrell and colleagues have reported that the reactions of caregivers of patients with pain include feeling inadequate, helpless, angry, and worried about the future; further, these caregivers are willing to engage in self-sacrifice that may, perhaps, benefit the patient, but may have negative effects on themselves (Ferrell et al., 1991; Ferrell & Rhiner, 1991; Ferrell, Taylor, Grant, Fowler, & Corbisiero, 1993).

Research on the effects of patient functional status on caregiver distress has been mixed. The severity of the functional impairment (e.g., the activities of daily living and cognitive and social functioning) and the severity of symptoms are significantly related to caregiver distress (Clipp & George, 1992; Given et al., 1993; Oberst et al., 1989). An impaired patient cognitive function produces higher caregiver distress than impaired physical functioning. Family caregivers may adapt to the demands that impaired physical functioning places upon them, but caring for patients with cognitive deficits produces high and sustained levels of caregiver burden (Carey et al., 1991).

## FAMILY CAREGIVER INTERVENTIONS

Despite all the work on caregiving, few attempts have been made to describe how families acquire the skills they need to provide the required patient care. Archbold et al. (1995) are among the first researchers who studied how nursing interventions affect caregiver preparedness, enrichment, and predictability.

### Complications Related to Intervention Efforts

The definition and assessment of caregiver activities are complicated by the variety, complexity, and skill level required for the care tasks. All activities are not direct care or psychomotor tasks such as dressing changes, injections, catheter care, or assistance with dependencies. Monitoring and surveillance, the coordination of care, supervision, and the provision of emotional support are care responsibilities that require different skills, such as skills in decision-making and judgment. Classifying these diverse care activities is complex because they are multidimensional. In addition, at some points in the care trajectory, the caregiver role may require observation and supervision only, while at other points (e.g., end of life) total physical care may be needed. Further, the caregiving role may be assumed for only a few weeks by some caregivers but for many months by others, with greatly varying demands in intensity across these diverse caregiving situations as the patient disease and treatment status changes.

Schumacher et al. (2000) elucidated a beginning categorization of skills needed in the family care process. They proposed nine categories including monitoring, interpreting, making decisions, taking action, making adjustments, accessing resources (includes coordinating care), providing hands-on care (direct care), working with the ill person, and negotiating the healthcare system for care needs. These categories encompass the more "direct" care tasks usually described, including administering medications and injections, providing wound care and catheter care, helping with activities of daily living, and providing transportation. However, these categories go well beyond direct tasks to include areas where judgment and decision-making become pivotal in providing quality care. The early work of Schumacher et al. (1993, 1996) describes the role-acquisition process. Both psychomotor and cognitive (decision-making) skills are important for interventions. We may need to tailor the intervention based on the number and types of skills needed. Schumacher's work strongly suggests that attention to caregiver role acquisition is needed as family members take on the complex responsibilities of cancer care. Through intervention research we can test ways to deliver support to caregivers and moderate caregiver distress.

Research on responses to caring for a family member with cancer has relied heavily on negative variables such as caregiver burden, depression, or stress. We know little about those caregivers who are not distressed and who are not at risk for becoming distressed. The vast majority of caregivers do not have depression scores at levels suggestive of clinical depression, nor are their burden scores high. Longitudinal data suggest that most caregivers learn to adapt, cope, and adjust to their caregiving role over time (Schulz & Williamson, 1991; Williamson & Schulz, 1990). Few intervention studies to facilitate adaptation for family caregivers have been found. Given the extensive descriptive literature, it is important to consider intervention studies in which positive outcomes are reported.

Several factors have to be considered as limitations in the descriptive studies, which may bias the results. Researchers have used convenience samples and have not included comparison groups. Many studies limited their samples to include only patients with breast cancer or some other single cancer. Furthermore, researchers have given limited attention to the context of caregiving tasks. Although studies have included caregiver gender and race (or ethnicity), socioeconomic status and caregiver competing roles, obligations, and commitments (such as employment) have not been routinely examined. Intimate partnerships and the quality of the prior relationship between the caregiver and the care receiver have only been examined in the breast cancer literature. Personality factors or dispositions of caregivers have also received limited attention (Hooker, Frazier, & Monchan, 1994; Moen, Robinson, & Fields, 1994). Most of the descriptive studies suffer from small sample sizes and often from using nonstandardized measures with untested psychometric properties. Without better methodology in descriptive work and more representative samples, it is difficult to envision the nature of intervention studies designed to impact family caregiver health status.

## Summary of Intervention Studies Supporting Family Caregivers

Few intervention studies have been conducted using psychosocial or behavioral interventions designed to enhance caregiver well-being. Here, the focus is primarily on caregiver studies with randomized trials. The work summarized is limited to studies since 1990, but a few frequently cited studies also deserve discussion (see Table 11.1 for summaries). (The annual review chapter by Pasacreta & McCorkle, 2000, is an important intervention review; readers are referred to that review.)

FAMILY CAREGIVER INTERVENTIONS: COUNSELING

Goldberg and Wool (1985) conducted a 12-session intervention of social support counseling over 6 months with spouses and adult children of newly diagnosed lung cancer patients in treatment, using a randomized control group design. No conceptual framework was described. Fifty-three caregivers were assigned to the counseling intervention or to usual treatment, and approximately half of the patients in each group dropped out over time. Caregivers and patients were assessed at initial treatment, prior to implementing the intervention, and again at 8 and 16 weeks. The support functions of the intervention were to help maintain the social support system, to promote the patient's sense of autonomy, to be an advocate in the care system, to encourage communication between the patient and family, and to facilitate mutual expressions of feeling. No changes were found on measures of psychosocial or physical functioning for the caregiver. The interventionists were social workers and psychologists. These investigators did not describe the details of the intervention and attributed their lack of findings to the subjects who did not really have needs but participated anyway. They recommended screening so interventions can be targeted to those who need it. Caregivers were doing well and thus caregivers experienced limited or no distress.

In a randomized control design, Blanchard, Toseland, and McCallion (1996) implemented a coping with cancer (CWC) intervention for spouses of cancer patients. A conceptual framework was not included. Thirty

**TABLE 11.1 Intervention Studies of Family Caregiving with Cancer Patients**

| | Theoretical/ conceptual framework | Design | Sample | Measures | Results |
|---|---|---|---|---|---|
| Barg, Pasacreta, Nuamah, and Robinson (1998) | Given Family Caregiver Model, Psycho-educational | Group format caregiver education session, one to three sessions; symptom management and psychosocial support and resources identification | $N = 150$, primarily female over the age of 50 | CRA Caregiver Demands Scale, health status, confidence in care | Caregiver reported family conflict and was overwhelmed with role; at follow-up, burden did not rise although intensity did; own health improved, confidence in care increased |
| Blanchard, Toseland, and McCallion (1996) | None reported | Psychosocial intervention with social worker; six coping-with-cancer sessions | $N = 30$ spouses, $M$ age $= 50$ | Health status, psychological well-being, social support, Index of Coping, SF-20, Functional Living Index, CESD, State Trait Anxiety, Zarit Burden Scale | No impact on caregiver depression |

| Reference | Theoretical/conceptual framework | Design | Sample | Measures | Results |
|---|---|---|---|---|---|
| Bultz, Speca, Brasher, Geggie, and Page (2000) | Psycho-educational | Psycho-educational support group for partners of cancer patients | $N = 36$ breast cancer patients | POMS, MAC, index of martial satisfaction; Duke-UNC Functional Support Scale | Men and women in intervention group had reduced mood disturbance; more confident in providing support; increased martial satisfaction; POMS high for control group |
| Ferrell, Grant, Chan, Ahn, and Ferrell (1995) | None reported | Pain education intervention including pain assessment, pharmacological interventions, nonpharmacological interventions; measured prior to intervention and one and three weeks following | $N = 50$ patients, primarily solid tumors; caregiver $M$ age $= 61$, 66% spouses | Burden, quality of life, attitudes about pain, knowledge about pain | Improved knowledge and attitudes about pain; improved overall quality of life and improved quality of life in psychological and social areas |

*(continued)*

**TABLE 11.1** Intervention Studies of Family Caregiving with Cancer Patients *(continued)*

| | Theoretical/ conceptual framework | Design | Sample | Measures | Results |
|---|---|---|---|---|---|
| Goldberg and Wool (1985) | None reported | Twelve-session counseling with social worker and psychologist; social-support intervention | $N$ = 53 lung cancer patients currently in treatment | Psychological functioning, POMS, PAIS, physical functioning, Karnofsky | No differences found on POMS, PAIS |
| Jepson, McCorkle, Adler, Nuamah, and Lusk (1999) | None reported | Longitudinal, six-month clinical trial; home-care approach; measures taken at discharge, three and six months after discharge by OCNs | $N$ = 161, $M$ age = 62; solid tumors, surgical patients, mostly spouses, 84% white, 35% stage III and IV | CESD Depression, CRA | No difference between groups; psychosocial status improved between baseline and three months; psychosocial status declined for caregivers with physical problems |

| | Theoretical/ conceptual framework | Design | Sample | Measures | Results |
|---|---|---|---|---|---|
| Kozachik et al. (2001) | Given Family Caregiver Model | Psychosocial intervention; nine sessions with nurse specialist (five in-person, four phone) | $N = 120$ with solid tumors | CESD, SF-36, Speilberger anxiety, CRA, SF-36, patient symptom experience | Baseline depression and number of patient symptoms predicted caregiver depression at waves II and III; main effect for patient symptoms on caregiver depression at waves II and III; trend toward intervention affecting caregiver depression |
| Pasacreta, Barg, Nuamah, and McCorkle (2000) | Given Family Caregiver Model, psycho-educational | Caregiver education, one to three sessions, measured at pre-intervention and four months later | $N = 187$ | CRA, perceived health status | Caregiver health status improved; confidence in providing care improved |

*(continued)*

**TABLE 11.1  Intervention Studies of Family Caregiving with Cancer Patients** *(continued)*

| | Theoretical/ conceptual framework | Design | Sample | Measures | Results |
|---|---|---|---|---|---|
| Sabo, Brown, and Smith (1986) | None reported | Nonrandom, support-group approach; 24 points over 10 weeks | Breast cancer patients | Martial relationship concerns, fears, support, and networks; self-esteem, depression, sexual compatibility | Increased communication between husband and wife |
| Smeenk et al. (1998) | None reported | Quasi-experimental; home care intervention with nurse coordinator, 24-hour phone consult and home care dossier; care-delivery approach with communication | $N = 106$ lung, colon, and breast cancer patients | Overall quality of life index | Quality of life improved in the intervention group at one week and three months after patient death |

| Theoretical/<br>conceptual | Design | Sample | Measures | Results |
|---|---|---|---|---|
| None reported | Psychosocial intervention to help spouse cope with stress of partner's cancer; six sessions, problem-solving/ coping approach by social worker | $N = 40$ in each group, spouses of solid tumor (mostly breast and lung) patients, $M$ age $= 50$ | CESD, Spielberger state trait anxiety, SF20, health status, Index of Coping, Zarit Burden Inventory, Functional Living Index, Social Support, Caregiver problems, index of coping, dyadic adjustment | Intervention differentially effective for distressed caregivers; in experimental group, better physical, social, and role functioning; ability to cope with problems; no depression effect |

Toseland,
Blanchard, and
McCallion (1995)

spouses were randomized to the CWC group and 36 to usual services. The intervention was a problem-solving approach to reduce or manage problems underlying caregiver distress. An experienced oncology social worker conducted six 1-hour individual counseling sessions. Measures included the SF-20, Functional Living Index—Cancer QOL, Perceived Health Status, and Centers for Epidemiological Studies on Depression. The State-Trait Anxiety Inventory was used to measure anxiety and the Zarit Burden Inventory was used to measure burden. Pressing problems from the Smith, Smith, and Toseland (1991) measure were used. Dyadic adjustment and social functioning were also used, as was the Index of Coping Responses (MOOS).

Assessments occurred at baseline, after completing the 6-week intervention, and again at 6 months. The mean caregiver age was 55 years in the control group and 50 years in the experimental group. The average length of caregiving time was 21 months for the intervention group and 31 months for the control group. The number of hours of care provided per week was 2.7 for the experimental and 3.1 for the control group. The two most common cancer diagnoses were breast, followed by lung. The intervention did not impact caregiver depression, but did decrease patient depression.

The only significant intervention effect for spouses was the effect of time on the psychosocial well-being variable and on coping behavior. An univariate follow-up revealed significantly reduced depression in both groups as well as reduction in avoidance coping in both groups. Qualitatively, spouses and patients reported that the intervention helped to improve their communication.

FAMILY CAREGIVER INTERVENTIONS: PROVIDING INFORMATION AND EDUCATION

Family members continue to report that the uncertainty in care expectations and the disease and treatment status of the patient add to their distress (Blanchard, Albrecht, & Ruckdeschel, 1995, Given & Given, 1996; Northouse et al., 2000; Oberst & Scott, 1988; Oberst et al., 1989). Ongoing informational needs include updates on clinical status, prognosis, and treatment expectations. Providing information (educational interventions) has been reported in the literature as a useful way of reaching family caregivers (Northouse & Wortman, 1995; Zahlis & Shands, 1991). In the work of Northouse and Peters-Golden (1993) and Oberst and Scott (1988), family caregivers indicated that they need information not only about physical tasks of caregiving activities, but also on how to manage patients' emotional needs (such as depression, anxiety, or anger).

Ferrell, Grant, Chan, Ahn, and Ferrell (1995) examined the impact of pain education on family members providing home care to elderly patients with cancer. Fifty family caregivers of patients experiencing cancer-related pain were included. Patient diagnoses were primarily solid tumor cancers with the cancer diagnosed in the previous year. Caregivers had a mean age of 61 years; 66% were spouses. The pain education program included three components: pain assessment, pharmacologic interventions, and nonpharmacologic interventions. Patients and their family caregivers were evaluated prior to initiation of the program and at 1 and 3 weeks following the intervention. Quality of life, knowledge and attitudes about pain, and caregiver burden were the primary study variables. Findings based on measures of quality of life and caregiver burden demonstrated the physical and psychological impact of family caregiving and pain management. The patients' pain experience had a significant impact on family members. The pain education program was effective in improving knowledge and attitudes regarding pain management for the caregiver. Quality of life improved in psychological and social areas and overall scores.

Caregivers report that their information needs persist and change over the cancer illness trajectory as the illness and treatment change. At points of transition, caregivers need new information to deal with these changes, yet healthcare providers expect caregivers to sort out the relevant information. Pasacreta and McCorkle (2000) suggested that results of educational interventions have neither been clearly described nor consistently measured.

Despite research that indicates the importance of information to help patients and family caregivers, few randomized clinical trials of educational interventions directed toward family caregivers have been tested; most existing studies have focused on pain management. This lack of research limits our understanding. Caregivers assist with a general but largely unstudied set of tasks, but little other work demonstrates effects on patients and their family caregivers.

FAMILY CAREGIVER INTERVENTIONS: DEVELOPING PROBLEM-SOLVING SKILLS

Toseland, Blanchard, and McCallion (1995) implemented a randomized trial for psychosocial interventions for spouses of cancer patients diagnosed with solid tumors, primarily breast and lung. A six-session problem-solving intervention was implemented by an experienced oncology social worker. This intervention included support, problem-solving, and coping skills, and was designed to help spouses cope with the stress of caring for their partners. Spouses were interviewed prior to the intervention and within two weeks after the intervention using a battery of assessments, including demographic variables, psychological variables (CES-D and State-Trait Anxiety), health status (SF-20), and social support (social functioning subscale of the health and daily living form). Toseland et al. assessed pressing problems (adapted from Northouse & Wortman, 1990), stressful caregiver problems, help-seeking behaviors, coping skills, the Zarit Burden Inventory, and marital satisfaction. Participants attended at least four sessions and were encouraged to discuss their own and their partners' reactions to the cancer. Participants were found to be more psychologically distressed than the general population, but were not as distressed as psychiatric outpatients. Caregiver levels of involvement in care were low (about 3 to 4 hours per week), although they had been providing care, on average, for about 2 years. Most of the care provided was emotional support with little personal care or household management.

Toseland et al. (1995) used repeated measures of multivariate analysis of variance. I found little change over time for the caregivers in either the control or the intervention groups. These investigators also performed analyses to examine whether the intervention program was differentially effective for distressed caregivers. Toseland et al. studied 24 caregivers— 13 from the intervention group and 11 from the control group—who scored one standard deviation below the mean score on the dyadic adjustment. This analysis revealed that caregivers in the intervention group showed significant improvements in physical, role, and social functioning on the SF-20. Examining the moderately burdened caregivers revealed that they did show improvement in their ability to cope with pressing problems. At 6 months, caregivers experienced no significant effects. Targeting interventions to distressed caregivers may result in the most effective, efficient, and cost-effective use of the interventions.

FAMILY CAREGIVER INTERVENTIONS:
EXAMINING CAREGIVER PSYCHOSOCIAL STATUS

A randomized clinical trial was conducted by Kozachik et al. (2001) to test the effects of a psychoeducational intervention for patients with newly diagnosed cancer who had recently initiated chemotherapy and their family caregivers (59 dyads in the control group and 61 dyads in the experimental group). The intervention focused on symptom management, patient and family education, the coordination of resources, emotional support, and caregiver preparation. At intake, nurses assessed the caregivers' and patients' physical (SF-36) and emotional health status (CES-D), symptom experience, knowledge deficits, and resource needs. Nurses and caregivers collaboratively designed a supportive plan of care for the patient by selecting intervention strategies for the caregiver to implement. At subsequent encounters, the nurse evaluated the current status and efficacy of the intervention strategies used.

Follow-up data collection occurred at 9 and 24 weeks after entry into the study. In addition, caregiver depression was assessed at each wave; results indicated that baseline caregiver depression and the number of patient symptoms at baseline and wave 2 were significant predictors of caregiver depression at wave 2. Caregiver depression at baseline and the number of patient symptoms at baseline, wave 2, and wave 3 were significant predictors of caregiver depression at wave 3. A main effect existed for the number of symptoms reported by patients and the level of caregiver depression at baseline on caregiver depression at waves 2 and 3. However, number of patient symptoms did not appear to affect caregiver depression for either of the intervention groups. This finding makes it difficult to argue that number of patient symptoms predict or moderate the effects of caregiver depression. Final data suggested that nursing interventions were beginning to positively affect caregiver depression, but the data were not strong enough to be significant.

Barg, Pasacreta, Nuamah, and Robison (1998) implemented a 6-hour psychoeducational Caregiver Cancer Education Program (CCEP) that addressed symptom management, psychosocial support, and resource identification. A convenience sample of 150 caregivers attended sessions. The majority of caregivers were female and cared for patients over 50 years of age. Sixty-one percent of the caregivers assumed the caregiver role less than 6 months previously. Twenty-two percent provided under 5 hours of care per week, while 32% provided 6 to 20 hours per week. Thirty-eight percent of the caregivers reported that their health suffered due to caregiving and 20% reported being very stressed. The majority of patients received assistance, and 70% reported that their families were not working well together. Forty-six percent reported inadequate financial resources. Thirty-five percent were overwhelmed with caregiver roles; 61% reported that all their activities centered around caregiving, requiring them to adjust their schedules and relinquish other activities. Psychosocial issues, such as watching the patient become more ill and not knowing what to do, were reported as the most difficult issues they faced. Many caregivers were ambivalent in the role, but saw it as an important task.

A longitudinal study utilizing a convenience sample of 187 cancer caregivers who attended the CCEP was reported by Pasacreta, Barg, Nuamah, and McCorkle (2000). Data were collected before attendance of the CCEP and at 4 months later. Findings confirmed the chronic and consuming nature of cancer caregiving. However, data indicated that the perception of burden did not worsen when caregiving tasks increased in intensity. Caregiver perceptions of their own health improved over time. In addition, the number of caregivers who reported being well informed and confident about caregiving increased after participating in the CCEP. Further study that randomizes caregivers is needed to substantiate the role of similar programs in enhancing caregiver skills and minimizing caregiver distress (Pasacreta et al., 2000).

Jepson, McCorkle, Adler, Nuamah, and Lusk (1999) examined changes in the psychosocial status of caregivers ($N = 161$) of postsurgical patients with cancer. In a longitudinal randomized trial, these investigators analyzed how caregiver distress was affected by whether caregivers had physical problems of their own and whether patients received a home-care intervention. Half the patients were randomly assigned to receive a standardized home-care nursing intervention in which 32% were referred to home care. The other half received a standardized intervention over a 4-week period consisting of three home visits and six phone calls from an oncology clinical nurse specialist. The intervention focused on assessing and monitoring problems, helping with symptom management, teaching self-care, and coordinating resources. The population of interest was caregivers of patients who (a) were diagnosed with a solid-tumor cancer within the past 2 months; (b) were age 60 or older; (c) were hospitalized for surgical treatment of the cancer and expected to live at least 6 months; and (d) had a complex problem at hospital discharge. Data were collected at the time of the patients' discharge and approximately 3 and 6 months later. Psychosocial status was measured using the Caregiver Reaction Assessment (CRA) and the CESD scales. A repeated measure analysis of variance was performed for each psychosocial measure. The factors used included time (i.e., interview 1, 2, or 3), the group (treatment versus control), and the caregivers' physical problems. Overall, psychosocial status improved from baseline to 3 months and was about the same at 6 months. Among caregivers with physical problems, the psychosocial status of those in the treatment group declined compared to those in the control groups in the 3 months after discharge; an opposite pattern was observed during the following 3 months. Results indicated that caregivers who have physical problems of their own are at risk for psychological morbidity, which may have a delayed effect. This delay may reflect the replacement of initial optimism with discouragement as caregivers face the reality of long-term illness.

Bultz, Speca, Brasher, Geggie, and Page (2000) found that partners of breast cancer patients provided support at a time when their own coping abilities were taxed by the challenge of cancer. Of 118 consecutive patients approached, 36 patients and their partners participated in a randomized controlled trial of a brief psychoeducational group intervention for partners only. Instruments included the Profile of Mood States (POMS), the Index of Marital Satisfaction (IMS) and the DUKE-UNC Functional Social Support Scale (FSSS), which were administered pre-intervention, postintervention, and at the 3-month follow-up. Patients also completed the Mental Adjustment to Cancer Scale (MAC). Patients whose partners received the intervention at 3 months reported less mood disturbance, greater confidant support, and increased marital satisfaction.

FAMILY CAREGIVER INTERVENTIONS: EXAMINING THE EFFECTS
OF INTERVENTION DELIVERY SYSTEMS

Smeenk et al. (1998) investigated the effects of a transmural home care intervention for terminal cancer patients on the quality of life of family caregivers. The intervention was designed to optimize cooperation and coordination between the "intramural" and "extramural" healthcare organizations. The intervention consisted of four elements: (a) a specialist nurse coordinator, (b) a 24-hour telephone service operated by nurses with access to a home care team, (c) a collaborative home care dossier and case file, and (d) protocols designed for specific care. The home care dossier was developed to improve communication between caregivers and to enhance the coordination of patient care. The dossier consisted of consents, a list of caregivers involved, discharge reports for the doctor, nursing transfer reports for patient care, medication lists, dietician reports, and multidisciplinary reports. The care protocols were developed, standardized, and included intravenous therapy, epidural and spinal pain relief, and the pharmaceutical trajectory. Overall, there were 34 intervention patients and 11 control patients with primary diagnoses of lung, colon, or breast cancer; most patients had metastatic disease. Participants had a mean age of 63 years. Caregiver quality of life was measured 1 week before, 1 week after, and 4 weeks after the patient was discharged from the hospital, and again 3 months after the patient's death. Multiple regression showed that compared to standard care, the intervention significantly improved the caregiver quality of life at 1 week after and 3 months after the death of the patient compared to standard care. Enhanced coordination and cooperation between intramural and extramural care led to improved supportive care for caregivers. Multiple regression analysis showed that the intervention contributed significantly to caregivers' overall quality of life compared to standard care.

## SUMMARY AND CONCLUSIONS

Several factors cast limitations on how to interpret the findings of the studies summarized here and prevent any comparison or ability to pool data. The studies reviewed here differed in design and/or results. Descriptions of conceptual frameworks upon which interventions were based were basically absent. The interventions summarized here included support groups, psychoeducational approaches, and problem-solving support; counselors, nurses, and social workers implemented the interventions, which ranged from 6 to 12 sessions covering 2 to 6 months. Although we reviewed the factors from descriptive studies associated with caregiver distress, most of the intervention studies did not consider variables such as prior family relations, caregiver health, skills required to provide care, hours of care, competing role demands, or caregiver age. Further, little detail was provided about the intervention used in the studies. The stage of disease or location in the treatment cycle was not uniformly described for understanding the nature of care requirements for the caregiver.

Few studies described the nature of care tasks for the caregiver: We do not know if caregivers were managing symptoms, providing direct care, monitoring patient status, or performing a combination of these tasks. The measures used for outcomes were primarily the CES-D, Speilberger State-Trait Anxiety, PAIS, and POMS for emotional distress; the Karnofsky Performance Scale, SF-20, or SF-36 for physical functions; and the CRA or Zarit Caregiver Burden for the measurement of the burden experienced. Marital satisfaction, marital relationships, and sexual functions were measured in only two of the studies. Lacking common measures makes drawing conclusions about the impact of behavioral and psychoeducational interventions on caregiver outcomes difficult.

Unfortunately, the healthcare system gives priority to the urgent problems of patients and often takes little time to identify the healthcare needs of caregivers, which leads to delays in the detection of caregiver distress or declining health status due to irregular, incomplete, or no health assessments. Few studies consider health-promotion strategies as mediating factors of the negative effects of providing care. Jepson et al. (1999) found that those caregivers with physical health problems had a *decline* in physical status as a result of caregiving, and Toseland et al. (1995) found that the intervention tested *differentially* affected distressed caregivers. Several investigators have suggested that interventions might have an effect with caregivers at a higher risk for burden and distress, but no one has tested interventions targeted to such a group. Thus, few intervention studies, and even fewer randomized trials with clear and significant findings were found. At this point, not enough evidence exists to identify a clear direction for research, but successful interventions should help caregivers assume and master their role in the care of cancer patients.

## DIRECTIONS FOR FUTURE RESEARCH

Future intervention studies need to identify at-risk cancer caregivers and to broaden research populations. This recommendation was initially suggested by Goldberg and Wool (1985), but seems to not yet have been heeded. At-risk caregivers may have limited coping resources, poor mental and physical health, or a prior history of poor adjustment. Virtually no intervention studies focus on variations or adaptations needed in interventions related to ethnic, racial, cultural, or socioeconomic diversity. Different sampling strategies that target minority populations, the economically distressed, and caregivers other than those who are middle-aged are needed. In addition, researchers need to begin studying the care processes of cancers other than breast, lung, and prostate to see how caregiving varies among cancer sites.

It is essential that descriptive—and preferably longitudinal—designs be fit to the course of the disease and treatment. Beginning with the initial treatment and proceeding through adjuvant and palliative therapy, researchers must appreciate the variation patients experience in the severity, types, and/or duration of needs; how needs evolve over time; and the resulting impact on family caregivers. More aggressive cancer treatments over a shorter period of time are likely to produce greater patient needs, resulting in greater short-term demand for care from family caregivers. The stage of disease and the aggressiveness of therapy could prove to be important variables signaling the intervals between measurement observations. Without information as to how the course of disease and associated treatment influence the provision of care, it is difficult to understand patient and family needs and the extent to which care needs drive the dynamics of family accommodation to caregiving. Intervention studies are needed that target each phase of caregiving in an effort to not only influence the negative responses of caregivers, but to also improve the clinical outcomes of patients. To successfully evaluate the impact of interventions on caregiver distress, research must be oriented toward understanding the consequences of the caregiving role over the cancer care trajectory. By fitting designs to the site, stage, and treatment modalities of the disease, and to the age and/or developmental stage of the dyad, researchers can specify more precisely the optimum observation intervals for measures in order to better specify when patients and their families are more likely to need assistance or have negative responses.

Along with identifying the complex factors that create potentially negative situations, research much focus on identifying cues for potentially positive situations. Targeting the time and context of care in which caregivers become more optimistic, gain personal satisfaction from their caregiving role, and/or experience relief from the burden of care will help develop interventions to enhance the caregiving role and moderate caregiver burden. Identifying how and when positive caregiver outcomes affect positive patient outcomes should also be a future research focus.

More research is needed to understand the *quality* of care that family members are able to provide and then to understand how that care impacts the overall patient clinical outcome and therapeutic plan. Future research can identify and test patient- and family-directed interventions. Such research can then chart the interventions' impact upon the quality of care and clinical outcomes for patients and the health (both mental and physical) of family caregivers. The results of these interventions should preserve normal functioning for patients and their families, and shorten the negative impact of cancer upon the family.

Longitudinal studies of caregiver adaptation to the caregiving role over time are needed to explore the complex interactions of caregiver physical health, mental health, and how usual self-care and health-promotion practices are altered, given the continuous and ever-evolving role of caregiving. Caregivers are called upon to make pivotal decisions on behalf of their patients, and research must respond to the question of whether or not caregiver distress affects decision-making and judgment about patient care. To answer the question of whether the negative health effects of caregiving occur differentially among groups, health-promotion behavior studies should be targeted to specific subgroups of caregivers: by relationship to patient, by gender, by age group, by income status, by racial and ethnic groups, and by cultural affiliation. Further, factors that influence caregivers' abilities to successfully adopt new health and self-care practices need to be described. Knowledge of which self-care practices (nutrition, exercise, sleep, stress management, preventive healthcare, or illness care visits) change or are ignored and which remain stable given increasing care demands is essential. Interventions and clinical trials that assist the caregiver to engage in activities that promote health and build physiological resilience must be explored, including exercise programs, good nutrition guidance, social activation, regular sleep, and monitoring his or her own physical and emotional health.

Many, if not most, research studies are completed in cancer centers, so we know little about patients who do not receive care in major centers. Many caregivers are overwhelmed with the care demands they face and choose not to participate in the intervention studies. Perhaps these are the at-risk caregivers who could benefit most from interventions. Building multidisciplinary, multisite research alliances can facilitate the process of accruing more diverse samples of caregivers, thereby fostering the generalizability of research findings.

Family caregivers must be equipped to adequately implement complex therapeutic regimens, manage home-care technology, meet patient needs for symptom management, help patients follow prescribed dietary regimens, and maintain and facilitate patient emotional health. Interventions must recognize professional or formal caregivers and family caregivers as partners in healthcare, partners who offer unique and vital skills and resources. To better understand the effects of care dynamics on family caregivers and on patient outcomes, terms such as *caregiver responsibilities*, *caregiver roles*, and *tasks of care* need to be more rigorously explored and defined.

Current intervention research into the demands of care and the burden felt by family caregivers is in its infancy. Here we hope to have demonstrated the need for future research and we hope to have offered challenges and goals for current—and future—scholars and researchers in this important aspect of the cancer experience.

# REFERENCES

Anastas, J. W., Gibeau, J. L., & Larson, P. J. (1990). Working families and eldercare: A national perspective in an aging America. *Social Work, 35,* 405–411.

Archbold, P., Stewart, B., Miller, L., Harvath, T., Greenlick, M., Van Buren, L., et al. (1995). The PREP system of nursing interventions: A pilot test with families caring for older members. *Research in Nursing and Health, 18,* 3–16.

Baider, L., Kaufman, B., Peretz, T., Manor, O., Ever-Hadani, P., & De Nour, A. K. (1996). Mutuality of fate: Adaptation and psychological distress in cancer patients and their partners. In L. Baider, C. Cooper, and A. Kaplan De-Nour (Eds.), *Cancer and the family* (pp. 187–224). New York: John Wiley & Sons.

Barg, F., Pasacreta, J., Nuamah, R., & Robinson, K. (1998). A description of a psychoeducational intervention for family caregivers of cancer patients. *Journal of Family Nursing, 4*, 394–413.

Barnes, C. L., Given, B. A., & Given, C. W. (1992). Caregivers of elderly relatives: Spouses and adult children. *Health and Social Work, 17*, 282–289.

Blanchard, C., Albrecht, T., & Ruckdeschel, J. (1997). The crisis of cancer: Psychological impact of family caregivers. *Oncology, 11*, 189–194.

Blanchard, C. G., Albrecht, T., Rucksdeschel, J., Grant, D., & Hammick, R. (1995). The role of social support in adaptation to cancer and to survival. *Journal of Psychosocial Oncology, 13*, 75–95.

Blanchard, C., Toseland, R., & McCallion, P. (1996). The effects of a problem solving intervention with spouses of cancer patients. *Journal of Psychosocial Oncology, 14*, 1–21.

Blank, J., Clarke, L., Longman, A., & Atwood, J. (1989). Perceived home care needs of cancer patients and their caregivers. *Cancer Nursing, 12*, 78–84.

Bodnar, J., & Kiecolt-Glaser, J. (1994). Caregiver depression after bereavement: Chronic stress isn't over when it's over. *Psychology and Aging, 9*, 322–380.

Buehler, J. A., & Lee, H. J. (1992). Exploration of home care resources for rural families with cancer. *Cancer Nursing, 15*, 299–308.

Bultz, B., Speca, M., Brasher, P., Geggie, P., & Page, S. (2000). A randomized controlled trial of a brief psychoeducational support group for partners of early stage breast cancer patients. *Psycho-oncology, 9*, 303–313.

Burton, L. C., Newsom, J. T., Schulz, R., Hirsch, C. H., & German, P. S. (1997). Preventive health behaviors among spousal caregivers. *Preventative Medicine, 26*, 162–169.

Carey, P., Oberst, M., McCubbin, M., & Hughes, S. (1991). Appraisal and caregiving burden in family members caring for patients receiving chemotherapy. *Oncology Nursing Forum, 18*, 1341–1348.

Carlson, L., Bultz, B., Speca, M., & St-Pierre, M. (2000). Partners of cancer patients: Part I. Impact, adjustment, and coping across the illness trajectory. *Journal of Psychosocial Oncology, 18*(2), 39–63.

Carlson, L., Bultz, B., Speca, M., & St-Pierre, M. (2000). Partners of cancer patients: Part II. Current psychosocial interventions and suggestions for improvement. *Journal of Psychosocial Oncology, 18*(3), 33–43.

Cicirelli, V. G. (1992). *Family caregiving: Autonomous and paternalistic decision making*. Newbury Park, CA: Sage.

Clark, N., & Rakowski, W. (1983). Family caregivers of older adults: Improving helping skills. *Gerontologist, 23*, 637–642.

Clipp, E., & George, L. (1992). Patients with cancer and their spouse caregivers. *Cancer, 69*, 1074–1079.

Cooley, M., & Moriarty, H. (1997). An analysis of empirical studies examining the impact of the cancer diagnosis and treatment of an adult on family functioning. *Journal of Family Nursing, 3*, 318–347.

Davis-Ali, S. H., Chesler, M. A., & Chesney, B. K. (1993). Recognizing cancer as a family disease: Worries and support reported by patients and spouses. *Social Work in Health Care, 19*, 45–65.

Dodd, M. J. (1984a). Measuring informational intervention for chemotherapy knowledge and self-care behavior. *Research in Nursing and Health, 7*, 43–50.

Dodd, M. J. (1984b). Patterns of self care in cancer patients receiving radiation therapy. *Oncology Nursing Forum, 11*(3), 23–27.

Ferrell, B. R., Cohen, M., Rhiner, M., & Rozek, A. (1991). Pain as a metaphor for illness: Family caregivers' management of pain—part 2. *Oncology Nursing Forum, 18*, 1315–1321.

Ferrell, B. R., Ferrell, B. A., Rhiner, M., & Grant, M. (1991). Family factors influencing cancer pain management. *Postgraduate Medicine Journal, 67*(Suppl. 2), 64–69.

Ferrell, B. R., Grant, M., Chan, J., Ahn, C., & Ferrell, B. A. (1995). The impact of cancer pain education on family caregivers of elderly patients. *Oncology Nursing Forum, 22*, 1211–1218.

Ferrell, B. R., & Rhiner, M. (1991). High-tech comfort: ethical issues in cancer pain management for the 1990s. *Journal of Clinical Ethics, 2*, 108–112.

Ferrell, B. R., Taylor, E. J., Grant, M., Fowler, M., & Corbisiero, R. (1993). Pain management at home: Struggle, comfort, and mission. *Cancer Nursing, 16*, 169–178.

Ferrell, B. R., Wisdom, C., Rhiner, M., & Alletto, J. (1991). Pain management as a quality of care outcome. *Journal of Nursing Quality Assurance, 5*, 50–58.

Franklin, S. T., Ames, B. D., & King, S. (1994). Acquiring the family elder care role: Influence on female employment adaptation. *Research on Aging, 16*, 27–42.

Gerstel, N., & Gallagher, S. (1993). Kinkeeping and distress: Gender, recipients of care, and work-family conflict. *Journal of Marriage and Family, 55*, 598–607.

Given, B., & Given, C. (1991). Family caregivers of cancer patients. In S. Molly Hubbard, T. Greene, & T. Knobf (Eds.), *Current practice in cancer nursing* (pp. 1–9). Philadelphia: J. B. Lippincott Co.

Given, B., & Given, C. (1992). Patient and family caregiver reaction to new and recurrent breast cancer. *Journal of the American Medical Women's Association, 47*, 201–212.

Given, B., Stommel, M., Collins, C., King, S., & Given, C. (1990). Responses of elderly spouse caregivers. *Research in Nursing and Health, 13*, 73–85.

Given, B. A., & Given, C. W. (1996). Family caregiver burden from cancer care. *Cancer nursing: A comprehensive textbook* (2nd ed., pp. 93–104). New York: Harcourt Brace.

Given, B. A., Given, C. W., & Stommel, M. (1994). Family and out-of-pocket costs for women with breast cancer. *Cancer Practice, 2*, 187–193.

Given, B. A., Given, C. W., Stommel, M., & Lin, C. S. (1994). Predictors of use of secondary carers used by the elderly following hospital discharge. *Journal of Aging and Health, 6*, 353–376.

Given, C., Given, B., Stommel, M., Collins, C., King, S., & Franklin, S. (1992). The Caregiver Reaction Assessment (CRA) for caregivers of persons with chronic physical and mental impairments. *Research in Nursing and Health, 15*, 271–283.

Given, C., Stommel, M., Given, B., Osuch, J., Kurtz, M., & Kurtz, J. (1993). The influence of the cancer patient's symptoms, functional states on patient's depression and family caregiver's reaction and depression. *Health Psychology, 12,* 277–285.

Goldberg, R., & Wool, M. (1985). Psychotherapy for the spouses of lung cancer patients: Assessment of an intervention. *Psychotherapy and Psychosomatics, 43,* 141–150.

Heinrich, R., & Schag, C. (1985). Stress and activity management: Group treatment for cancer patients and spouses. *Journal of Consulting and Clinical Psychology, 53,* 439–446.

Hileman, J. W., Lackey, N. R., & Hassanein, R. S. (1992). Identifying the needs of home caregivers of patients with cancer. *Oncology Nursing Forum, 19,* 771–777.

Hong, J., & Steller, M. (1995). The psychological consequences of multiple roles: The non-normative case. *Journal of Health and Social Behavior, 36,* 386–392.

Hooker, K., Frazier, L., & Monchan, D. (1994). Personality and coping among caregivers of spouses with dementia. *The Gerontologist, 34,* 386–392.

Houts, P., Nezu, A., Nezu, C., & Bucher, J. (1989). The prepared family caregiver: A problem-solving approach to family caregiver education. *Patient Education and Counseling, 27,* 63–73.

Houts, P. S., Yasko, J. M., Kahn, S. B., Schelzel, G. W., & Marconi, K. M. (1986). Unmet psychological, social, and economic needs of persons with cancer in Pennsylvania. *Cancer, 58,* 2355–2361.

Houts, P. S., Yasko, J. M., Simmonds, M. A., Kahn, S. B., Schelzel, G. W., Marconi, K. M., et al. (1988). A comparison of problems reported by persons with cancer and their same sex siblings. *Journal of Clinical Epidemiology, 41,* 875–881.

Jepson, C., McCorkle, R., Adler, D., Nuamah, I., & Lusk, E. (1999). Effects of home care on caregivers' psychological status. *Image: Journal of Nursing Scholarship, 31,* 115–120.

Johnson, E., & Stark, D. (1980). A group program for cancer patients and their family members in an acute care teaching hospital. *Social Work Health Care, 5,* 335–349.

Kiecolt-Glaser, J. K., Dura, J. R., Speicher, C. E., Trask, O. J., & Glaser, R. (1991). Spousal caregivers of dementia victims: Longitudinal changes in immunity and health. *Psychosomatic Medicine, 53,* 345–362.

Kiecolt-Glaser, J. K., Glaser, R., Gravenstein, S., Malarkey, W. B., & Sheridan, J. (1996). Chronic stress alters the immune response to influenza vaccine in older adults. *Proceedings of the National Academy of Sciences of the United States of America, 93,* 3043–3047.

Kiecolt-Glaser, J. K., Marucha, P. T., Gravenstein, S., Malarkey, W. B., Mercado, A. M., & Glaser, R. (1995). Slowing of wound healing by psychological distress. *Lancet, 346,* 1194–1196.

Kleban, M., Brody, E., Schoonover, C., & Hoffman, C. (1989). Family help to the elderly: Perception of sons-in-law regarding parent care. *Journal of Marriage and the Family, 51,* 303–312.

Kozachik, S. L., Given, C. W., Given, B. A., Pierce, S. J., Azzouz, F., Rawl, S. M., et al. (2001). Improving depressive symptoms among caregivers of patients with cancer: Results of a randomized clinical trial. *Oncology Nursing Forum, 28,* 1149–1157.

Kristjanson, L., & Ashcroft, T. (1994). The family's cancer journey: A literature review. *Cancer Nursing, 17*, 1–17.

Kristjanson, L., Nikoletti, S., Porock, D., Smith, M., Lobchuk, M., & Pedler, P. (1998). Congruence between patients' and family caregivers' perceptions of symptom distress in patients with terminal cancer. *Journal of Palliative Care, 14*(3), 24–32.

Kuhlman, G., Wilson, H., Hutchinson, S., & Wallhagen, M. (1991). Alzheimer's Disease and family caregiving: Critical synthesis of the literature and research agenda. *Nursing Research, 40*, 331–337.

Kurtz, M., Kurtz, J., Given, C., & Given, B. (1995). Relationship of caregiver reactions and depression to cancer patients' symptoms, functional states and depression—A longitudinal view. *Social Science and Medicine, 40*, 837–846.

Kurtz, M., Kurtz, J., Given, C., & Given, B. (1997). Predictors of post bereavement depressive symptomatology among family caregivers of cancer patients. *Supportive Care for Cancer, 5*, 53–60.

Laizner, A., Shegda, L., Barg, F., & McCorkle, R. (1993). Needs of family caregivers of persons with cancer: A review. *Seminars in Oncology Nursing, 9*, 114–120.

Lawton, M., Rajagopal, D., Brody, E., & Kleban, M. (1992). The dynamics of caregiving for a demented elder among Black and White families. *Journal of Gerontology: Psychological Sciences, 47*(Suppl.), 156–164.

Lewis, F., Hammond, M., & Woods, N. (1993). The family's functioning with newly diagnosed breast cancer in the mother: The development of an explanatory model. *Journal of Behavioral Medicine, 16*, 351–370.

McCorkle, R., Yost, L., Jepson, C., Malone, D., Baird, S., & Lusk, E. (1993). A cancer experience: Relationship of patient psychosocial responses to care-giver burden over time. *Psycho-oncology, 2*, 21–32.

Miaskowski, C., Kragness, L., Dibble, S., & Wallhagen, M. (1997) Differences in mood states, health status, and caregiver strain between family caregivers of oncology outpatients with and without cancer-related pain. *Journal of Pain and Symptom Management, 13*, 138–147.

Miller, B. (1990a). Gender differences in spouse caregiver strain: Socialization and role expectations. *Journal of Marriage and the Family, 52*, 311–321.

Miller, B. (1990b). Gender differences in spouse management of the caregiving role. In E. K. Abel & M. K (Eds.), *Circles of care: Work and identity in women's lives* (pp. 92–104). Nelson. Albany, NY: State University of New York Press.

Moen, P., Robinson, J., & Fields, V. (1994). Women's work and caregiving roles: A life course approach. *Journal of Gerontology: Psychological Sciences, 49*(Suppl.), 176–186.

Mor, V., Masterson-Allen, S., Houts, P., & Siegel, K. (1992). The changing needs of patients with cancer at home. A longitudinal view. *Cancer, 69*, 829–838.

Musci, E. C., & Dodd, M. J. (1990). Predicting self-care with the patients and family members after the states and family functioning. *Oncology Nursing Forum, 17*, 393–400.

Nail, L. M., Jones, L. S., Greene, D., Schipper, D. L., & Jensen, R. J. (1991). Use and perceived efficacy of self-care activities in patients receiving chemotherapy. *Oncology Nursing Forum, 18*, 883–887.

Neal, M. B., Chapman, N. J., Ingersoll-Dayton, B., & Emlen, A. C. (1993). *Balancing work and caregiving for children, adults, and elders.* Newbury Park, CA: Sage.

Nijboer, C., Tempelaar, R., Sanderman, R., Triemstra, M., Spruijt, R., &van den Bos, G. (1998). Cancer and caregiving: The impact on the caregiver's health. *Psychooncology, 7,* 3–13.

Nijboer, C., Tempelaar, R., Triemstra, M., van den Bos, G., & Sanderman, R. (2001). The role of social and psychological resources in caregivers of cancer patients. *Cancer, 89,* 1029–1039.

Nijboer, C., Triemstra, M., Tempelaar, R., Sanderman, R., & van den Bos, G. (1999). Determinants of caregiving experiences and mental health of partners of cancer patients. *Cancer, 86,* 577–588.

Nijboer, C., Triemstra, M., Tempelaar, R., Mulder, M., Sanderman, R., & van den Bos, G. (2000). Patterns of caregiver experiences among partners of cancer patients. *The Gerontologist,. 40,* 738–746.

Northouse, L. (1988). Social support in patients' and husbands' adjustment to Breast Cancer. *Nursing Research, 37,* 91–95.

Northouse, L., Cracchiolo-Caraway, A., & Pappas, C. (1991). Psychologic consequences of breast cancer on partner and family. *Seminars in Oncology Nursing, 7,* 216–223.

Northouse, L., Dorris, G., & Charron-Moore, C. (1995). Factors affecting couples' adjustment to recurrent breast cancer. *Social Science and Medicine, 41,* 69–76.

Northouse, L., Mood, D., Templin, T., Mellon, S., & George, T. (2000). Couples' patterns of adjustment to colon cancer. *Social Science and Medicine, 50,* 271–284.

Northouse, L., & Peters-Golden, H. (1993). Cancer and the family: Strategies to assist spouses. *Seminars in Oncology Nursing, 9,* 74–82.

Northouse, L., Templin, T., Mood, D., & Oberst, M. (1998). Couples' adjustments to breast cancer and benign breast disease: A longitudinal analysis. *Psycho-oncology, 7,* 37–48.

Northouse, L. L., & Wortman, C. B. (1990). Models of helping and coping in cancer care. *Patient Education and Counseling, 15,* 49–64.

Oberst, M., & James, R. (1985). Going home: Patient and spouse adjustments following cancer surgery. *Topics in Clinical Nursing, 7,* 46–57.

Oberst, M., & Scott, D. (1988). Post-discharge distress in surgically treated cancer patients and their spouses. *Research in Nursing and Health, 11,* 223–233.

Oberst, M., Thomas, S., Gass, K., & Ward, S. (1989). Caregiving demands and appraisal of stress among family caregivers. *Cancer Nursing, 12,* 209–215.

Pasacreta, J., Barg, F., Nuamah, I., & McCorkle, R. (2000). Participant characteristics before and 4 months after attendance at a family caregiver cancer education program. *Cancer Nursing, 23,* 295–303.

Pasacreta, J., & McCorkle, R. (2000). Cancer care: Impact of interventions on caregiver outcomes. In J. Fitzpatrick & J. Goeppinger (Eds.), *Annual review of nursing research* (Vol. 19, pp. 127–148). New York: Springer Publishing Co.

Picot, S. (1995). Rewards, costs, and coping of African American caregivers. *Nursing Research, 44,* 147–152.

Picot, S., Youngblut, J., & Zeller, R. (1997). Development and testing of a measure of perceived caregiver or adults. *Journal of Nursing Measurement, 5,* 33–52.

Plant, H., Richardson, J., Stubbs, L., Lynch, D., Ellwood, J., Slevin, M., et al. (1987). Evaluation of a support group for cancer patients and their families and friends. *British Journal of Hospital Medicine, 38,* 317–322.

Pruchno, R., & Resch, N. (1989). Husbands and wives as caregivers: Antecedents of depression and burden. *The Gerontologist, 29,* 159–165.

Raveis, V., Karus, D., & Siegel, K. (1998). Correlates of depressive symptomatology among adult daughter caregiver of a patient with cancer. *Cancer, 83,* 1652–1663.

Robinson, K. M. (1990). Predictors of burden among wife caregivers. *Scholarly Inquiry for Nursing Practice, 4,* 189–203.

Russo, J., & Vitaliano, P. P. (1995). Life events as correlates of burden in spouse caregivers of persons with Alzheimer's disease. *Experimental Aging Research, 21,* 273–294.

Sabo, D., Brown, J., & Smith, C. (1986). The male role and mastectomy: Support groups and men's adjustment. *Journal of Psychosocial Oncology, 4*(1/2), 19–31.

Sales, E. (1991). Psychosocial impact of the phase of cancer on the family: An updated review. *Journal of Psychosocial Oncology, 9,* 1–18.

Sales, E., Schulz, R., & Beigel, D. (1992). Predictors of strain in families of cancer patients: A review of the literature. *Journal of Psychosocial Oncology, 10,* 1–26.

Schulz, R., & Beach, S. R. (1999). Caregiving as a risk factor for mortality: The caregiver health effects study. *Journal of the American Medical Association, 282,* 2215–2219.

Schulz R., & Williamson, G. (1991). A 2-year longitudinal study of depression among Alzheimer's caregivers. *Psychology and Aging, 6,* 569–578.

Schulz, R., Visintainer, P., & Williamson, G. (1990). Psychiatric and physical morbidity effects of caregiving. *Journal of Gerontology: Psychological Sciences, 45,* P181–P191.

Schumacher, K. (1996). Reconceptualizing family caregiving: Family-based illness care during chemotherapy. *Research in Nursing and Health, 19*(4), 261–271.

Schumacher, K., Dodd, M., & Paul, S. (1993). The stress process in family caregivers of persons receiving chemotherapy. *Research in Nursing and Health, 16,* 395–404.

Schumacher, K., Stewart, B., Archbold, P., Dodd, M., & Dibble, S. (2000). Family caregiving skill: Development of the concept. *Research in Nursing and Health, 23,* 191–203.

Siegel, K., Raveis, V., Mor, V., & Houts, P. (1991). The relationship of spousal caregiver burden to patient disease and treatment-related conditions. *Annals of Oncology, 2,* 511–516.

Smeenk, F., de Witte, L., van Haastregt, J., Schipper, R., Viezemans, H., & Crebolder, H. (1998). Transmural care of terminal cancer patients: Effects of the quality of life of direct caregivers. *Nursing Research, 47,* 129–136.

Smith, G. C., Smith, M. F., & Toseland, R. W. (1991). Problems identified by family caregivers in counseling. *Gerontologist, 31,* 15–22.

Staller, E., & Palzliski, K. (1989). Other roles of caregivers: Competing responsibilities or supportive resources. *Journal of Gerontology, 44,* 5231–5238.

Stommel, M., Given, C. W., & Given, B. (1990). Depression as an overriding variable explaining caregiver burdens. *Journal of Aging and Health, 2,* 81–102.

Stommel, M., Given, B. A., Given, C. W., & Collins, C. E. (1995). The impact of frequency of care activities on the division of labor between primary caregivers and other care providers. *Research on Aging, 17*, 412–433.

Stommel, M., & Kingry, M. (1991). Support patterns for spouse-caregivers of cancer patients. The effect of the presence of minor children. *Cancer Nursing, 14*, 200–205.

Theorell, T., Haggmark, C., & Eneroth, P. (1987). Psycho-endocrinological reactions in female relatives of cancer patients: Effects of an activation programme. *Acta-oncologica, 26*, 419–424.

Toseland, R., Blanchard, C., & McCallion, P. (1995). A problem solving intervention for caregivers of cancer patients. *Social Science in Medicine, 40*, 517–528.

Vachon, M., Freedman, K., Formo, A., Rogers, J., Lyall, W., & Freeman, S. (1977). The final illness in cancer: The widow's perspective. *Canadian Medical Association, 117*, 1151–1154.

Walker, A., Pratt, C., & Eddy, L. (1995). Informal caregiving to aging family members: A critical review. *Family Relations, 44*, 402–411.

Weitzner, M., Jacobsen, P., Wagner, H. Jr., Friedland, J., & Cox, C. (1999). The Caregiver Quality of Life Index-Cancer (CQOLC) scale: Development and validation of an instrument to measure quality of life of the family caregiver of patients with cancer. *Quality of Life Research, 8*, 55–63.

Weitzner, M., McMillan, S., & Jacobsen, P. (1999). Family caregiver quality of life: Differences between curative and palliative cancer treatment settings. *Journal of Pain and Symptom Management, 17*, 418–428.

Weitzner, M., Meyers, C., Steinbruecker, S., & Jacobsen, J. (1996). Family caregiver quality of life (QOL): A preliminary report of a validational study. *Supportive Care in Cancer, 4*, 232.

Weitzner, M., Meyers, C., Stuebing, K., & Saleeba, A. (1997). Relationship between quality of life and mood in long-term survivors of breast cancer treated with mastectomy. *Supportive Care in Cancer, 5*, 241–248.

Weitzner, M., Moody, L., & McMillan, S. (1997). Symptom management issues in hospice care. *American Journal of Hospice and Palliative Care, 14*, 190–195.

Weitzner, M. A., Haley, W. E., & Chen, H. (2000). Cancer in the elderly: The family caregiver of the older cancer patient. *Hematology/Oncology Clinics of North America, 14*, 1–14.

Wellisch, D. K., Fawzy, F. I., Landsverk, J., Pasnau, R. O., & Wolcott, D. L. (1989). An evaluation of the psychosocial problems of the home-bound cancer patient: Relationship of patient adjustment to family problems. *Journal of Psychosocial Oncology, 7*, 55–76.

Williamson, G., & Schulz, R. (1990). Relationship orientation, quality of prior relationship, and distress among caregivers of Alzheimer's patients. *Psychology and Aging, 5*, 502–509.

Zahlis, E., & Shands, M. (1991). Breast cancer: Demands of the illness on the patient's partner. *Journal of Psychosocial Oncology, 9*, 75–93.

Zarit, S., Todd, P., & Zarit, J. (1986). Subjective burden of husbands and wives as caregivers: A longitudinal study. *The Gerontologist, 26*, 260–266.

# 12

---

# Interventions at the End of Life

---

## Betty Ferrell
## Barbara Hastie

In classical behavioral theory, death, like any behavior, would be considered a learned experience or a stimulus-response. However, strict
behavioral theories are challenged in end-of-life care because death is
an individualized, ever-changing, nonreproducible, unalterable event that is
typically not a "learned" experience. The lack of behavioral intervention
research in end-of-life care may be, in part, because many behavioral interventions have been based on strict principles of behavior therapy, including
self-monitoring the occurrence of a particular problem or behavior, functional analysis of the relevant antecedent and consequent variables, cognitive-behavioral analyses of compliance, and many behavior-modification
techniques such as modeling, reinforcement, and self-control. The declining stamina, changing cognitive ability, and limited availability of the
terminally ill patient make engagement exceptionally challenging. Moreover, the hallmark of many behavioral interventions is mutually contracted
treatment goals. In a terminally ill population, waning health and declining
cognitive ability make validation and compliance exceptionally difficult.
Research-related issues such as competency, informed consent, recruitment,
and attrition acquire new ethical dimensions when attempting to study terminally ill populations.

The research on behavioral interventions with terminally ill cancer
patients has focused on the type and location of disease (Champion, 2001),
genetic predispositions and risk factors, the stage of disease progression

(Holland, 1998), and treatments, including surgical interventions. Predictions on outcomes of various disorders based on psychological and personality features, and options for physical as well as psychological illness recovery, have also been topics of interest. Little research has been conducted to assess options, interventions, and outcomes for terminally ill cancer patients as a compromised population. Despite the limited research on behavioral interventions in end-of-life care for cancer patients, this chapter will evaluate relevant studies as they pertain to various symptoms, disease trajectories, and results, and it will also include and appraise systematic reviews, the quality of evidence, and relevant meta-analyses.

Important aspects to consider at the end of life are settings of care, unique patient considerations, patient variables unique to cancer populations, and behavioral interventions designed for physical symptoms as well as those aimed at psychological symptoms. All these factors have significant influence on the type, ability, and results of the intervention employed. This chapter will explore the interrelationships of these elements on the role and outcome of behavioral interventions in terminally ill cancer populations. Data were drawn for this chapter from several sources, including PsychINFO and MEDLINE®; various scientific journals covering the fields of medicine, psychology, nursing, and palliative care; book chapters; and government agency reports. Searches were done for studies published between 1990 and 2001; the keywords used included various combinations of *cancer, palliative care, end of life, terminally ill, life-threatening illness, behavioral interventions, psychological interventions, therapy, psychological symptoms, physical symptoms, caregivers, outcomes, hospice,* and *death.*

## THE CHALLENGE OF BEHAVIORAL INTERVENTIONS AT THE END OF LIFE

### Settings of Care Provided at the End of Life

*Where* care is provided affects the results of care, and affects the design, measurement, and results of interventions. Much end-of-life care is now provided in the home. Elderly patients are likely to experience end-of-life care in nursing homes or other long-term care settings, and terminally ill patients are treated within outpatient hospital settings and intensive care units (ICUs). In this section, the provision of care in different contexts is explored. How the settings of care influence and affect behavioral interventions for patients and family caregivers is also examined.

## CARE IN THE HOME

Over the past two decades, major changes in healthcare have replaced long hospital stays with early discharges, leading to a dramatic increase in care provided within the home. This trend has been especially true for terminally ill cancer patients. Family members and home care nurses must assume care for patients with complex and highly technical treatment plans. Home care is characterized by an intensive management of symptoms and by the needs for supportive care of both the patient and the family caregivers who assume the burdens of the illness and its treatment (Bentur, 2001; Ferrell, Ferrell, Ahn, & Tran, 1994; Ferrell, Virani, & Grant, 1998). In the home environment, family members typically become the primary caregivers (Aneshensel, Pearlin, Mullan, Zarit, & Whitlatch, 1995).

Patients, families, and healthcare professionals often prefer care at home rather than in institutional settings, assuming that patients are more comfortable there, especially as physical needs and the desire for comfort increase as cancer advances (see Chapter 11, "Family Caregiving Interventions in Cancer Care"). With attention on critical physical symptoms, little focus is given to behavioral interventions for symptom management and, typically, families are not equipped to assess patient preferences or institute such care (Payne, Smith, & Dean, 1999).

Recent research has also demonstrated that barriers in home care settings may exist that actually hinder cancer symptom management. These barriers may be especially evident in the area of pain management, including patient and family fears of addiction, failure of the patient to report pain, and limited access to needed services (Berry & Ward, 1995; Ersek, Kraybill, & DuPen, 1999; Ferrell, Grant, Borneman, Juarez, & ter Veer, 1999; Paice, Toy, & Shott, 1998). The heavy reliance on unlicensed family members, coupled with decreased access to diagnostic facilities and limited pharmacy services, can influence the effectiveness of symptom management at home. Personality and psychological characteristics of patients and caregivers, in addition to family dynamics, may also pose additional barriers to introducing behavioral interventions in the home setting (Gatchel & Turk, 1999; Given et al., 1993). Meeting the goal of managing symptoms effectively and addressing psychological distress may be particularly challenging in the home environment.

Interventions intended for patients indirectly (and sometimes directly) can benefit family members as well. In the home environment, this "residual" effect may be especially beneficial not only in educating family caregivers, but ultimately in addressing their own psychosocial and spiritual needs. Reduced caregiver distress likely leads to an increased efficacy in communicating treatment modalities and behavioral strategies to the patient (McCorkle, Robinson, Nuameh, Lev, & Benoliel, 1998; Payne et al., 1999). However, although the need is well documented, and strong evidence exists in interventions for caregivers across the disease trajectory, little evidence exists to evaluate outcomes in the home environment for end-of-life caregiver populations.

Thus, the home care setting maintains a balance of advantages and disadvantages. The potential benefits, however, may outweigh the cost and necessity of increased training for professionals and families, especially in addressing behavioral interventions in end-of-life care. Augmenting the training and interventions in home care may offer opportunities for increased efficacy in behavioral assessment and treatment, as well as enhanced quality of life in this growing realm of healthcare and caregiving.

## CARE IN HOSPICE

Hospice care seeks to provide physical, social, spiritual, and emotional care while protecting patient and family choice (Byock, 2000; Egan & Labyak, 2001; Lynn, 2001). In contrast to the problem-oriented curative model, the palliative/hospice model is quality of life and closure oriented, embodying the full scope of the patient and family dying experience (Block, 2001; Byock, 2000; Field & Cassell, 1997). Hospice and end-of-life care pose additional challenges to behavioral interventions, given waxing and waning symptoms and the uniqueness of the death experience to any other life event. A further complication is the typical brevity of hospice; treatment outcomes are evaluated in terms of the initial induction of behavior change, generalization to a "real-life setting," and changes maintained over time.

Despite the lack of studies, a viable approach to behavioral interventions in the hospice context is a cognitive-behavioral approach that combines Social Learning Theory but focuses more on the ways an individual perceives, interprets, and relates an event to other life circumstances. The patient is educated about the process by which thoughts, beliefs, and behaviors are interactive and can influence the current situation. These techniques have been used extensively in chronic and cancer pain populations (Fordyce, 1994; Syrjala, 1993; Syrjala & Chapko, 1995). Cognitive-behavioral approaches may increase understanding, enhance communication, and manage bereavement for the family in hospice (Loscalzo & Jacobsen, 1990; Manetto & McPherson, 1996; Syrjala & Chapko, 1995; Turk, 1996).

Hospice often symbolizes an approaching end to life, and the notion of hospice often exacerbates anxieties and maladaptive coping patterns as the patient and family members recognize their limited remaining time together. A cognitive-behavioral approach would address family anxieties at the last stage of life as hospice does: Rather than view the *quantity* of time remaining, the *quality* of time and life would be the focus (Herbst, Lynne, Mermann, & Rhymes, 1995). Rather than focusing on past events of hurtful relationship issues in the family, cognitive restructuring (a behavioral intervention) would employ techniques to question the validity of interpretations made at those points in time and would address new interactions. Behaviors would follow based on these restructured interpretations, allowing for a revised approach to the relationship, possibly creating better relationship quality in the last stage of life.

## CARE IN NURSING HOMES AND LONG-TERM CARE FACILITIES

Nursing homes have increasingly become a venue for the dying (Wilson, 2001). Although nursing homes have no age restrictions, data demonstrate that older individuals are more likely to die in nursing homes than in any other setting (Alliance of Aging Research, 1998). The nursing home setting has its own set of unique challenges and special needs (Baer & Hanson, 2000). Besides enormous bureaucratic barriers, physical, psychosocial, and spiritual complications resound among the terminally ill in nursing homes (Weissman & Matson, 1999; Wilson & Daley, 1997). Attention to the psychological, social, and spiritual problems of residents are often relegated to an already overburdened nursing staff (Ferrell, Ferrell, & Osterweil, 1990; Foley & Gelband, 2001). Reimbursement issues are problematic in nursing home settings, causing the care of nonphysical problems to be exceptionally challenging (Wilson, 2001).

Research regarding death in nursing homes has evolved to examine the predictors of bereavement outcomes, including family perceptions of care, educational needs of the staff, and issues of pain management (Ferrell, Taylor, Sattler, Fowler, & Cheyney, 1993; Kelly et al., 1999; Ryan & Scullion, 2000; Weissman, Griffie, Gordon, & Dahl, 1997). The Institute of Medicine recommended enhanced research in nursing homes to identify who is responsible for care, what care residents can expect, what practice guidelines are used to guide care, how adequate physician and nursing support is for dying residents, how quality of care for the dying resident is assessed, how family and patient preferences are assessed and determined, and whether dying residents are segregated from the general population (Foley & Gelband, 2001).

## INPATIENT HOSPITAL CARE

Although a majority of Americans would prefer to die at home, only a small percentage actually have their wishes granted as they spend their last days in hospital settings (Whedon, 2001). The hospital environment may be especially challenging for the terminally ill cancer patient. Once admitted to the hospital, staff availability is generally predicated on the degree of immediate need. In addition, institutional budgets rarely afford health professionals for general behavioral interventions. However, with the adoption of the National Comprehensive Cancer Network Guidelines for Psychosocial Care (NCCN, 1999), the assessment and treatment of psychological symptoms may become more integrated into oncology (Holland & Chertkov, 2001). Currently, insufficient funding exists for standard psychosocial care along with the reluctance of healthcare staff to request such consults, mostly due to the stigma associated with mental healthcare (Whedon, 2001).

Hospital settings may actually provide opportunities for research and institutional change, primarily through readily available data, regulatory efforts, and access to consultation team members (Whedon, 2001). Given the increased societal attention to enhanced end-of-life care, the resources for assisting clinicians or teams in quality-improvement efforts have increased, which may translate into the inclusion of research and behavioral interventions for end-of-life care (Cleeland, 2001).

## INTENSIVE CARE UNIT (ICU) HOSPITAL CARE

ICUs represent the most aggressive form of care, generally focused on life preservation, constant care, and stabilization. Staff members in the ICU are generally caught between the goal of preserving life and the reality of having to prepare the family for possible death (Puntillo & Stannard, 2001). Research has demonstrated that when communication between clinicians and patients is poor, patients and families may have unrealistic expectations, and physicians may be reluctant to adhere to patient refusals for care (Lynn et al., 1997).

No studies have examined cancer patient behavioral interventions in an ICU. Depending on patients' levels of consciousness and degrees of impairment, mental health professionals could be of assistance, especially in preparation for painful procedures or when various pharmacological interventions may not be beneficial. Thus, mental health professionals may be of benefit to family members *and* staff. Although the aura of crisis does not lend itself to behavioral interventions, it may be possible to create prospective interventions and train hospital staff on stress management, thereby ultimately affecting the quality of care.

OUTPATIENT HOSPITAL CARE

Outpatient settings may provide more amenable opportunities for behavioral interventions in end-of-life care. As the length of hospital stays decreases, an increasing amount of care occurs within the outpatient setting for young patients and for older patients, for relatively healthy patients and for terminally ill patients. As a result, staff may develop long-term relationships with patients along with an understanding of family and the personal dynamics of care (DuPen & Robinson, 2001). In addition, outpatient clinics augment patient autonomy and flexibility, and they allow for family involvement in care and interventions. Staff training and time restrictions, however, may preclude clinics from offering optimum palliative care.

Outpatient settings have clear advantages when it comes to behavioral interventions. Given the emphasis on environmental factors in behavioral theory, family, formal providers, and the patient's community can become involved in the intervention. After learning an intervention from an outpatient care setting, patients can implement strategies in their natural settings. Preparing the patient through behavioral interventions to be used outside the treatment setting may further enhance patient efficacy and mastery, and likely lead to adopted, maintained behaviors by repeated reinforcements in multiple settings (Bandura, 1986). Because of the significant and changing limitations of terminally ill patients, behavioral interventions need to become more flexible, and protocols need to be adapted to this population. Nonetheless, with the increasing number of outpatient comprehensive cancer centers managing patient symptoms over the disease trajectory, more and more research on terminally ill patients is taking place in outpatient settings.

## Unique Considerations at the End of Life

Care settings obviously affect behavioral interventions with end-of-life populations. Further complications related to the characteristics and experiences of patients requiring end-of-life care are explored in this section.

PATIENT AND CAREGIVER AGE

Age complicates approaching, assessing, treating, and managing symptoms at the end of life as the valence placed on and the understanding of issues of death are often moderated by patient age and developmental stage (Abeles, Gift, & Ory, 1994). Historically, attention to age at the end of life has focused on the elderly (Derby & O'Mahoney, 2001). However, with increased public attention to quality of life up to the time of death, treatment programs and care strategies are being developed to address the needs of various age cohorts at the end of life (Balducci & Entermann, 2000). As such, behavioral assessment and treatment vary in different stages of the life span (Resnick & Rozensky, 1996).

Ferrell et al. (Ferrell & Ferrell, 1996, 1998; Ferrell, Ferrell, & Rivera, 1995; Ferrell, Grant, et al., 1995) highlighted the relevance and unique nature of caring for the aging with cancer and dealing with complicated accompanying symptoms such as pain. Even within the geriatric population, variances exist such that the young-old (i.e., those 60–75 years old) have very different needs than the old-old (i.e., those 75 years and older) patient cohort (Abeles et al., 1994). Additionally, the ways of expressing symptoms and distress vary within this cohort and may be far more diverse than anticipated by investigators and clinicians (Balducci 1994; Kahn, Houts, & Harding, 1992). Researchers have asserted several critically important behavioral questions related to work on the cognitive function and understanding of older adults facing the end of life, including how older adults make treatment decisions, what information they retain in an encounter with a physician, and how information can be structured to maximize comprehension (Zauszniewski, Chung, & Krafcik, 2001). Moreover, family dynamics, burden of care, cognitive status, and economic issues have a potentially profound influence on end-of-life care for the elderly (Weitzner, Haley, & Chen, 2000). Special attention should be given to the needs and the communication styles of older adults in considering assessing and tailoring behavioral interventions in cancer populations (Mantovani et al., 1996; Rodriguez, 2001).

PATIENT AND CAREGIVER CULTURAL BACKGROUND

Health beliefs are strongly influenced by cultural factors (Koenig, 1997; Koenig & Gates-Williams, 1995), and this is especially poignant in interpreting how patients and family caregivers understand cancer treatment and respond to illness-related death (Braun, Pietsch, & Blanchette, 2000). Cultural factors include, but are not limited to, ethnic identity, gender, age, differing abilities, sexual orientation, religion and spirituality, financial status, place of residency, employment, and educational level (Moadel et al., 1999; Zoucha, 2000). Even within the same culture, differences exist across gender, caste, and class, but more profound variations exist in a cross-cultural context. Culture affects every aspect of quality of life as well as end-of-life care.

Cultural factors are particularly relevant in defining, assessing, and implementing behavioral interventions in end-of-life care (Gerrish, 2000). Cultural biases of healthcare providers and public-policy agencies often result in underserved populations having less access to services. Further, among minorities, symptoms are often misunderstood, misinterpreted, and undertreated (Ng, Dimsdale, Shragg, & Deutsch, 1996; Payne, Smith, & Dean, 1999; Underwood, 1994). Language barriers may play a significant role in how behavioral strategies are relayed and interpreted. The diversity of world views, corresponding biases, and training in end-of-life care suggest the need for the careful consideration of cultural factors in behavioral interventions at the end of life (Becker, 1999).

## PATIENT COGNITIVE AND PSYCHOLOGICAL STATUS

The changing cognitive status of patients at the end of life presents special challenges to the implementation of various psychological interventions. Behavioral and cognitive-behavioral approaches presuppose cognitive intactness. The requirement of cognitive involvement needed to assess, plan, and implement strategies to address maladaptive beliefs and behaviors presents a barrier to traditional behavioral interventions in a terminally ill population. Recognizing this barrier provides much-needed information on adapting treatment modalities that recognize the fluid state of cognitive status. It is possible to address less severe psychological symptoms, such as adjustment disorders, with behavioral interventions. Such approaches may be useful in moving toward life closure and addressing familial relationships (Gavrin & Chapman, 1995).

Literature documents the psychiatric and neuropsychological effects of illness and treatment, especially with advanced disease (Breitbart & Cohen, 1998; Bruera et al., 1992). Neurotic and psychotic disorders are reported, and metabolic disturbances, chemotherapy, or other treatments have neuropsychiatric effects (Breitbart & Wein, 1998; Passik and Breitbart, 1993; Pereira, Hanson, & Bruera, 1997). Delirium is among the most common psychiatric symptom prevalent in hospital settings and has been shown to reach up to 85% prevalence among terminally ill cancer patients (Lipowski, 1990). The behaviors exhibited in a state of delirium are neurobiological and not necessarily environmental, thereby mitigating the theoretical underpinnings of employing behavioral interventions in this population. Delirium further complicates behavioral intervention.

Most patients facing the end of life have significant anxiety or depression at some point. The need to identify and manage anxiety and depression cannot be overemphasized because ongoing symptoms have been shown to significantly affect general emotional well-being, adjustment to illness, cognition, pain perception, and overall treatment outcome (Breitbart, Jaramillo, & Chochinov, 1998; Massie & Popkin, 1998). Formal assessment-screening instruments for functional and psychological impairments are helpful to evaluate and minimize the possibility that detectable problems will be missed (Cella, 1998).

Anxiety, depression, and dementia may become more prevalent with advancing cancer. Though the former may be treatable through behavioral interventions, the severity of the psychological state and the waning stamina of the patient must be taken into account before introducing any behavioral strategy. Severe depression may preclude retention and participation in an intervention, and clinicians must be mindful of the fragile status of the terminally ill patient as well as recognize the possible need for the inclusion of psychopharmacologic management of severe symptoms.

Patient emotional status may increase vulnerability, which may mitigate against achieving mastery and behavior change—essential goals of interventions. Motivational aspects are especially important for integrating behavioral strategies, and the emotional state of the terminally ill patient may preclude any interest in or positive results of such interventions.

The measurement of patient status poses additional challenges; the majority of contemporary psychometric instruments (e.g., MMPI-2, SCL-90, and MCMI-III) requires patient stamina, fairly intact cognitive function, and adequate literacy skills (Butcher, Dahlstrom, Graham, Tellegen, & Kaemmer, 1989; Derogatis, 1994; Millon, 1994). Some psychometric instruments are shorter and thus less taxing (e.g., SF-36, BDI, and BAI), although they present more of a checklist of symptoms rather than a psychological or personality assessment tool (Ware & Sherbourne, 1992). Recognition of the burden of such tools on patients, along with the advent of addressing quality of life, has led to the development of instruments more amenable to the vulnerable physical and psychological states of cancer patients at the end of life (Kornblith & Holland, 1994; Spilker, 1996).

Constantly changing symptoms leading to decreased physical functions make an assessment of behavioral intervention results at the end of life especially complicated. Although investigators assert the need for standardized instruments with significant validation and quantitative power, the clinical environment and aspects of employing such data-gathering methods may be nearly impossible for the terminally ill without placing an undue burden on them. Some researchers utilize family members as proxies for gathering information, but this practice may also place additional hardship on already overburdened caregivers and may be viewed as taking away limited time. Qualitative techniques, on the other hand, have shown to be especially valuable in identifying patient themes, and this method has seemed to be far less taxing to the patient and the caregiver.

CAREGIVER AND FAMILY STATUS

As mentioned earlier, the fragility and ever-changing physical and psychological status of the terminally ill cancer patient create special challenges when considering behavioral interventions. Increasing symptoms lead to increased dependence, making individual participation in behavioral strategies difficult, at times impossible. Options may be available for more cognitive strategies, but clinicians and researchers must be especially mindful of the physical status of the patient and family caregivers who also typically experience significant burden (Ferrell, 1998; Ferrell & Coyle, 2001; see also Chapter 11).

Studies have revealed the profound economic, physical, and psychological toll of caregiving for family members (Arno, Levine, & Memmott, 1999; Ferrell, 1996; Ferrell, Grant et al., 1999). The enormity of problems and how these problems complicate bereavement have been recognized, and support programs for caregivers are growing. Literature consistently supports the importance of family members during advanced illness. Caregivers' own health, attitudes, and knowledge have a profound effect on the successful management of patient symptoms (Steinhauser et al., 2000).

Caregiving affects not only the individual, but all family members. Likewise, the death and serious illness of a family member leads to the disruption of family system equilibrium (Herz-Brown, 1989). The homeostasis of the family unit is profoundly affected by a number of factors including (a) the social and ethnic context of death, (b) the history of previous losses, (c) the timing of the death in the life cycle, (d) the nature of the death, (e) the position and function of the person in the family system, and (f) the openness of the family system (Herz-Brown, 1989). Moreover, death threatens to disrupt the entire family's notion of development, marriage, child-bearing, and career development (Gibson-Hunt, 2000). Symptom management and family perceptions of healthcare providers have been shown to profoundly affect bereavement (Levine, 2000; Schachter & Coyle, 1998; Steinhauser et al., 2000). Thus, behavioral approaches may be especially important for caregivers to address maladaptive beliefs, coping strategies, and cognitions about death and care.

PATIENT AND CAREGIVER SOCIAL ISOLATION

Care at the end of life often results in social withdrawal and isolation, the transformation of family relationships and roles, and new burdens on both patients and family caregivers. Difficulties arise when, for various reasons, patients withdraw from the relational and social interactions. Such a response may be needed to preserve previous and limited resources. However, healthcare professionals and even family members could be trained to assess such a retreat as necessary rather than maladaptive. This point may actually prove beneficial in bereavement care, and in fact most studies address interventions after death rather than during the last days and months.

Social psychologists have demonstrated that group and situational forces are considerably more powerful predictors of behavior than the assessment of individual differences. Interestingly enough, research has indeed revealed the importance of individual differences with regard to depression as well as in predicting survival rates. This supports behavioral interventions that tailor and target treatments to specific individuals' behavior and environments. Conversely, Christensen, Wiebe, Smith, and Turner (1994) showed that perceived family social support, not depression or other psychological factors, predicts adjustment in the bereavement stage. Such results lend credence to the impact of family dynamics and personal environments as they impact behavior and interventions aimed at addressing psychosocial distress at the end of life.

# BEHAVIORAL INTERVENTIONS FOR PHYSICAL SYMPTOMS AT THE END OF LIFE

## Patient Physical Symptoms Common at the End of Life

A plethora of research has reported the physical symptoms common at the end of life. Symptoms are often classified according to biological system or neurological involvement (Holland, 1998). Common symptoms of patients nearing the end of life include anorexia and cachexia; bowel management, including constipation and diarrhea; dyspnea, death rattle, and cough; dysphagia, dry mouth, and hiccups; fatigue; hydration, thirst, and nutrition problems; lymphedema; nausea and vomiting; neurological disturbances; and pain (see also Chapters 6, 7, 8, and 9).

## Existing Evidence and Gaps in the Literature

Most healthcare professionals addressing end-of-life care will assert the critical importance of complex symptoms that often appear simultaneously and to varying degrees throughout the course of disease progression (Bruera & Neumann, 1998). Enormous amounts of time and attention are placed on addressing and managing symptoms, but less time is spent studying behavioral intervention options for those approaching death. Behavioral intervention studies are targeted toward specific symptoms experienced by individuals with terminal cancer, although many of the interventions involve pharmacological treatments (Bruera & Fainsinger, 1998; Jackson & Lipman, 2000a, 2000b; Lloyd-Williams, Freidman, & Rudd, 1999; Tyler, 2000). Some investigators and clinicians have demonstrated positive effects from certain behavioral techniques tailored to terminal cancer patients' symptoms and disease stages, and some symptoms have been more widely studied than others (Fawzy, Fawzy, Arndt, & Pasnau, 1995; Sryjala & Chapko, 1997; Turk & Feldman, 1992).

Increased research and clinical attention has been given to studying interventions and treatments for pain and fatigue, but most of these studies capture participants at a time in their treatment when death is not imminent (Bruera & Lawlor, 1997; Curt, 2000; Holzheimer, 2000; Loscalzo & Jacobsen, 1990; Paice & Fine, 2001; Portenoy & Lesage, 1999). The increased attention to symptoms may be due in part to the heightened public attention to the issue of pain management, the new pain standards that require pain assessment and treatment, and the dramatic increase in chronic pain populations. The World Health Organization, the National Comprehensive Cancer Network of the American Cancer Society (ACS), and the American Pain Society have each developed guidelines and algorithms for managing cancer pain, and some address pain management for the terminally ill (APS, 1998; NCCN/ACS, 2001; WHO, 1993, 1996, 1998). Many of the published guidelines offer limited information on behavioral interventions for cancer-related symptoms at the end of life. Despite increased recognition by professional organizations to address end-of-life care, evidence suggests that symptom relief at the end of life continues to be a major problem in healthcare.

Within the guidelines and published research on pain management and on other medically related symptoms, cognitive-behavioral techniques are reported as important noninvasive interventions (Cleeland, 2001) and are listed in Table 12.1. Cognitive-behavioral therapy techniques are effective for patients with cancer, predominantly for cancer-related pain and other

**TABLE 12.1   Behavioral Interventions for Psychological Symptoms at the End of Life**

| Intervention | Resource | Type of resource or approach and population |
|---|---|---|
| Art therapy | Connell (1992) | • Review and descriptive study with palliative care population |
| | Luzatto and Gabriel (1998) | • Review and instructional chapter with oncology patients |
| | Riley (1995) | • Review and interventions-based book with families in various settings |
| | Scudder-Teufel (1995) | • Clinical application study with terminally ill leukemia patients |
| Autogenic training | Linden (1993) | • Review of training and specific theory; general population stress management |
| | Lehrer and Woolfolk (1993) | • Principles and techniques training; general population stress management |
| Biofeedback | Basmijian (1989) | • Principles, theory, and training book aimed at various patient populations |
| Cognitive distraction or focusing | Cleeland (2001) | • Government report with recommendations for cancer patients |
| | Lambert (1999) | • Clinical study focused on pain in pediatric patients |
| | McCarthy, Cool, Petersen, and Bruene (1996) | • Clinical study focused on pediatric pain, cancer, and bone marrow transplant patients |
| | Vaserling, Jenkins, Tope, and Burish (1993) | • Clinical study focused on general cancer population side effects |

| Intervention | Resource | Type of resource or approach and population |
|---|---|---|
| Cognitive restructuring/ cognitive modifications | Turk and Feldman (1992) | • Cognitive-behavioral resource book specific for terminally ill patients |
| | Beck, Rush, Shaw, and Emery (1979) | • Theory and instructional book applicable across patient populations |
| | Meichenbaum (1977) | • Theory and instructional book not specific for terminally ill populations |
| Group therapy | Blake-Mortimer, Gore-Felton, Kimerling, Turner-Cobb, and Spiegel (1998) | • Review article of group therapy specific to cancer patient populations |
| | Spiegel and Claussen (2000) | • Research-based handbook specific to oncology patients |
| | Spira (1998) | • Review and clinical chapter specific to cancer patient populations |
| Diaphragmatic breathing/ relaxation response | Benson (1996) | • Review and training book for various patient populations although predominantly those with chronic illnesses |
| Hypnosis | Barber (1993) | • Theory and clinical applications chapter for general stress management |
| | Hammond (1990) | • Theory and instructional book for various patient populations |
| | Liossi and Hatira (1999) | • Clinical study for pediatric cancer population |
| Meditation | Benson (1996) | • Review book for cardiac and chronic illness patients |
| | Kabat-Zinn (1994) | • Experiential book predominantly for pain patients |
| | Kabat-Zinn, Ohm-Massion, Hebert, and Rosenbaum (1998) | • Review, training, and theoretical chapter specific for cancer patient populations, not necessarily terminally ill |

*(continued)*

**TABLE 12.1    Behavioral Interventions for Psychological Symptoms at the End of Life (continued)**

| Intervention | Resource | Type of resource or approach and population |
|---|---|---|
| Music therapy | Hanser (1999) | • Descriptive and instructional chapter for geriatric patients |
| | Lane (1993, 1994) | • Review and descriptive resources for medically ill and oncology populations |
| | Martin (1991) | • Review and instructional book for terminally ill patients |
| | Trauger-Querry & Haghighi (1999) | • Descriptive article for hospice patient populations |
| | Lehrer & Woolfolk (1993) | • Guidebook applicable across patient populations |
| Spiritual interventions/ prayer | Cole & Pargament (1999) | • Description of pilot clinical study with diagnosed oncology patients |
| | Fitchett & Handzo (1998) | • Clinical application chapter with various cancer patient populations |
| | Johnston-Taylor (2001b) | • Review and clinical chapter with cancer patients in palliative care |
| | Kemp (2001) | • Instructional chapter of interventions with cancer patients in palliative care |
| Storytelling/ life review | McFadden & Atchley (2001) | • Multidisciplinary instructional book for aging populations |
| | Johnston-Taylor (2001b) | • Review and instructional book with various patient populations |
| Stress inoculation training | Meichenbaum (1993) | • Instructional resource books, not specifically for terminally ill |

physical symptoms, although prevailing research has studied patients at various stages of the disease and active treatment trajectories rather than at life's end (Breitbart & Payne, 1998; Cleeland 2001; Holland & Chertkov, 2001). Scant research exists specifically studying behavioral interventions for terminal cancer patients, although one book is specifically tailored to address potential interventions rooted in cognitive-behavioral theories

(Turk & Feldman, 1992). No evidence exists from randomized, clinical trials or other similarly tested designs as they pertain to behavioral intervention outcomes except for one chapter on perceptions and therapies for pain control. Research conducted in the area of the terminally ill has been limited, empirical, anecdotal, or in small, descriptive studies in hospice. Such work has focused primarily on pain and physical symptoms and does not specifically study behavioral interventions.

## Methodological Issues in Behavioral Interventions for Physical Symptoms

Depending on the type of cancer, the treatment effects, the progression of the illness, and symptom severity vary considerably at the end of life (Ferrell & Coyle, 2001). With these constantly changing and often increasing symptoms, onset, duration, and severity are often unpredictable, making timing and observation for intervention results extremely challenging. One of the core characteristics of behavior therapy states that treatment methods are specified, replicable, and objectively evaluated. With the continual development and change of symptoms, interventions may not be replicable and the same intervention that works on one symptom for one patient may be contraindicated for another or may be inappropriate for that same patient later in the disease trajectory. Further, most evaluations of symptoms at the end of life are subjective. That is, patients relay their symptoms—including pain, fatigue, bowel management, and other complications—and, thus, symptom experience cannot always be objectively measured. A completely objective evaluation, such as with standard, validated psychometric instruments, would be difficult.

Moreover, many of the treatment outcome measures of terminally ill populations are reported by family members *after* the death of their loved one (McCorkle et al., 1998; Payne et al., 1999). This posthumous approach makes validating the technique as well as the assessment difficult, and it raises methodological and psychometric questions. Assessing the intervention outcome can be differentially biased. A negative situation, coupled with strong emotional valence, often produces an unfavorable recall (Reeves & Graber, 1993). In hospice literature, family members who have experienced the death of a loved one who had inadequate symptom management have increased psychological distress, prolonged and complicated bereavement, and often report negatively on treatment and care (Hickman, Tilden, & Tolle, 2001). These factors highlight the necessity of determining sound, valid ways of capturing important intervention and treatment outcome data without subjecting the patient to undue hardship and without requiring the family caregiver to disengage emotionally for the sake of objectivity.

Another area of methodological concern involves attrition rates and the capacity of the intervention to achieve a significant outcome. Clearly, in a terminally ill cancer population, attrition may be unpredictable or it may significantly increase with increased symptoms, rendering the patient unable to engage in any interventions. On the other hand, the augmentation of symptoms at the end of life has allowed important information to be gathered regarding symptom control, treatment, and quality as well as quantity of intervention (Block, 2000; Gavrin & Chapman, 1995; Ingham & Portenoy, 1998). Moreover, the problem-at-hand may be clinically relevant (i.e., the significant clinical outcome as determined by the patient, such as decreased physical symptoms) rather than statistically significant. This shift in focus may indeed require a paradigm shift for traditional research approaches; virtually nothing has been done to adequately address the research needs in terminally ill cancer populations.

A patient or family goal of physical comfort is quite different from a "traditional" goal of a behaviorist to extinguish a certain behavior in exchange for a more optimal, socially learned one. Thus, not only must assessment be taken into consideration, but the end goal and desired behavior change must be considered.

Research addressing physical symptoms in terminally ill cancer patients typically involves a qualitative assessment or a very brief, targeted assessment of quality of life (Ferrell, Hassey-Dow, & Grant, 1995). Traditionally, qualitative assessment has not been a standard evaluation technique utilized in the behavioral or cognitive-behavioral realm; however, such assessment may offer important and useful information on outcomes at the end of life.

## Implementation and Outcome Effects on Caregiver

The health, knowledge, attitude, and psychological well-being of the caregiver have been shown to have an enormous impact on the successful management of patient symptoms as well as compliance with behavioral interventions (Carlson, Bultz, Speca, & St. Pierre, 2000). Identifying caregiver psychological needs early in their loved one's illness develops a foundation for interventions to improve the long-term psychological outcome and bereavement after the death of the loved one (Kelly et al., 1999).

Caregivers need education and support to cope with the myriad physical demands of end-of-life care. Few studies have addressed behavioral interventions for families, although several studies have asserted dire need (Hull, 1993; Levine, 2000; Payne et al., 1999). In reviewing the literature from 1975 to 1999, Pasacreta and McCorkle (2000) found a limited number of well-designed training programs for caregivers of patients in palliative care. Despite the fact that most of those programs were limited in scope and often represented selection bias in well-adjusted caregivers, results demonstrated favorable outcomes, particularly for managing grief and bereavement.

In their training programs for caregivers and healthcare professionals, Ferrell et al. aimed to turn caregiver helplessness into helpfulness (Ferrell, Grant et al., 1999; Ferrell & Rivera, 1995; Juarez & Ferrell, 1996). Equipping the caregiver not only helps to decrease their sense of distress, but the ill family member also benefits. If caregivers learn and can implement the behaviors, patients may be more likely to engage in the behaviors (Bandura, 1986; Jacobsen & Hann, 1998). These external events of newly learned behaviors may serve as cues to action for patients and may offer a modified approach to the Health Belief Model, which typically has not been applied in terminally ill populations (Gochman, 1997; Steptoe & Wardle, 1995). Newly learned behaviors may also enhance the sense of self-efficacy, important in behavior modification and influenced by the individual's perception of their ability to control and determine their behavior.

## BEHAVIORAL INTERVENTIONS FOR PSYCHOLOGICAL SYMPTOMS COMMON AT THE END OF LIFE

Although several studies have addressed psychological factors present in the face of terminal illness, the literature is scant for reports on implementing behavioral interventions at the end of cancer patients' lives. As in the realm of physical symptoms, the timing and dose of interventions are especially complicated given the constantly changing symptom presentation. In the psychological domain, symptoms may change as a result of disease progression; treatment; environmental factors, including setting and family dynamics; and the nearness and recognition of impending death.

### Patient and Caregiver Psychological Symptoms Common at the End of Life

Studies abound highlighting the myriad psychological symptoms related to medical illness (see Chapter 6), and how those dramatically escalate when one realizes that an illness is, or has the potential to be, terminal (Cleeland,

2001; Fishman, 1992; Holland, 1998). Characterological disorders can be exacerbated, and maladaptive behavior and coping patterns often become more entrenched when illness threatens life. Nevertheless, psychological reactions influence physical symptoms and mediate the effectiveness of various interventions, specifically behavioral techniques and treatment compliance (Fordyce, 1994; Gatchel & Turk, 1999). Conversely, physical symptoms have been shown to significantly affect general emotional well-being, adjustment to illness, cognition, pain perception, and overall treatment outcomes (Fox, 1998; Loscalzo, 1996; Zabora et al., 2001).

Common psychological symptoms at the end of life include agitation, anxiety, confusion, delirium, depression, fear, restlessness, terminal agitation, and uncertainty. The tendency is to unintentionally relegate symptoms that cause distress into the realm of "psychological disturbance" without a clear differentiation between psychiatric symptoms versus those psychological or psychosocial in nature. Psychiatric disturbances can often be managed with psychotropic medications, whereas psychological distress can be effectively addressed through nonpharmacological means. Notably, more research exists addressing psychiatric complications such as delirium, reduced capacity for attention and problem-solving, and dementia in patients with end-stage disease (Kuebler, English, & Heidrich, 2001).

Importantly, research has demonstrated strong evidence that behavioral interventions can effectively manage certain medical symptoms and change behavior related to medical problems and disease, specifically targeted at physical symptoms (Owen, Klapow, Hicken, & Tucker, 2001; Sryjala & Chapko, 1995; Turk, 1996; Turk & Okifuji, 1997; Zabora & Loscalzo, 1996). Behavioral interventions for psychological symptoms are similar to those employed for physical complications, and most techniques are aimed at stress and anxiety reduction. Commonly applied behavioral interventions researched in medical populations are listed in Table 12.2.

## Spiritual Dimension and Interventions

In recent years, the inclusion of spiritual issues in medicine and psychological care has increased (Jenkins & Pargament, 1995; Matthews & Larson, 1995). In 1975, Benson found a strong link between mind and body, and became one of the leaders in addressing this interaction. Later, the addition of the spiritual dimension became especially important in working with patients who had terminal diseases. Researchers further asserted the power and biology of belief and how belief can influence recovery, healing, and moving into death (Koenig et al., 1999). Behaviorists were, and in some

## Table 12.2 Behavioral Interventions for Physical Symptoms at the End of Life

| Intervention | Resources |
|---|---|
| Aroma therapy | Buckle (1999, 2001)<br>National Hospice and Palliative Care Organization (2001)<br>Osterlund & Beirne (2001)<br>Snyder & Lindquist (1998) |
| Art therapy | Luzatto & Gabriel (1998) |
| Biofeedback | Basmijian (1989)<br>Burish & Jenkins (1992) |
| Cognitive-behavioral therapy | Turk & Feldman (1992) |
| Cognitive distraction or focusing | Jacobsen & Hann (1998)<br>Vaserling, Jenkins, Tope, & Burish (1993) |
| Cutaneous modalities | Ferrell-Tory & Glick (1993)<br>Giasson & Bouchard (1998)<br>Krieger (1993)<br>Mackey (1995, 2001)<br>McCaffery & Wolff (1992)<br>National Institutes of Health (1997) |
| Diaphragmatic breathing/relaxation response | Benson (1996) |
| Hypnosis | Hammond (1990)<br>Lambert (1999)<br>Liossi & Hatira (1999)<br>Spira & Speigel (1992)<br>Syrjala, Cummings, & Donaldson (1992) |
| Meditation | Forker (2001)<br>Kabat-Zinn (1994)<br>Kabat-Zinn, Ohm-Massion, Hebert, & Rosenbaum (1998) |
| Music therapy | Lane (1993, 1994)<br>Schroeder-Sheker (1993)<br>Snyder & Chlan (1999)<br>Trauger-Querry & Haghighi (1999) |
| Passive relaxation with guided imagery | Eller (1999)<br>Syrjala, Donaldson, Davis, Kippes, & Carr (1995) |
| Progressive muscle relaxation | Baider, Uziely, & De-Nour (1994)<br>Bernstein and Carlson (1993) |

cases continue to be, suspicious of integrating any notion of spirituality in psychomedical care. Interestingly, although general medicine and psychology were just beginning to include spiritual care in end-of-life treatment, it was a core foundation of the hospice movement as a critical element to approaching death. In addition, for nurses and chaplains, addressing spiritual needs became vital to a comprehensive assessment and treatment at life's end (Cairns, 1999).

Many investigators tend to merge spiritual issues into the realm of psychology. This may be due to the fact that spiritual distress is not easily quantifiable and often overlaps with psycho-existential anguish. Moreover, "meaning in illness" corresponds to both the spiritual dimension of life as well as the psychological. As such, many of the interventions that manage spiritual distress are behavioral in nature and correspondingly address psychological angst (Fitchett & Handzo, 1998; Johnston-Taylor, 2001a, 2001b). Ferrell et al. have demonstrated the important role of the spiritual realm in the quality of life for both patient and family caregiver (Ferrell, 1998; Ferrell & Borneman, 1999). Specific interventions for spiritual care have included life review and storytelling, journal writing, engaging in the arts, utilizing dreams as a window to the spirit, grief therapy, and family counseling.

## Measurement and Outcomes Issues

Psychological symptoms and psychosocial complications can include general distress and often involve nontangible and difficult-to-measure symptoms such as spiritual angst, uncertainty, hope, and meaning in illness. Fear, anxiety, and depression are more "measurable" symptoms, but the question remains whether established psychometric instruments are applicable, useful, and sensitive to the fragile and complex populations of the terminally ill. Likewise, the goals for treatment and outcomes established for nonlife-threatening illnesses are likely to be considerably different for terminally ill individuals. The behavioral approach must adopt some flexibility if such research is to be viable, valid, and applicable. The method and theoretical foundation of tailoring interventions must be reviewed when considering work with a terminally ill population. The behavioral approach necessitates that cognitive changes lead to behavioral changes; the naturally changing cognitive status of the terminally ill creates limitations in the interventions and treatment approaches. A paradigm shift must occur within the strict behavioral underpinnings.

# SYNTHESIS OF THE LITERATURE: LOGICAL NEXT STEPS

The context of care is extremely relevant to the type, nature, and intensity of the behavioral treatment provided. In addition, the fragility and constantly changing status of the terminally ill patient make the establishment and implementation of behavioral treatments enormously difficult. However, a profound lack of research exists on the tailoring, targeting, and outcomes of behavioral interventions at the end of life. This chapter has highlighted the complexities and raised issues for future research.

No behavioral studies specifically within a terminally ill cancer hospice population have been reported in the literature. More common are studies with cancer patients who are recently diagnosed, undergoing treatment, or who are survivors of cancer. Depending on the study design as well as the tailoring and targeting of the intervention, particularly in a population of the imminently dying, the efficacy of the intervention and outcome varies. It is important to consider what essential elements should be reviewed and studied to determine efficacy and outcome in a palliative care cancer population receiving behavioral interventions.

Increased research addressing the various psychological and behavioral assessments and interventions as options for care across various settings, including long-term care facilities, is needed. In recent years, psychologists, neuropsychologists, and psychiatrists have increasingly served as consultants to nursing homes, offering assessments, group and family therapy, and limited cognitive and behavioral interventions. However, limited reimbursement, time restrictions, and failing conditions of patients have precluded treatment. Research addressing the need for such specialized assessments and treatments may highlight the value of making such care a part of reimbursement and public-policy priorities.

At present, insufficient funding exists for standard psychosocial care and healthcare staff are reluctant to request such consults, mostly due to the stigma associated with mental health care. However, with the adoption of the NCCN (1999), the assessment and treatment of psychological symptoms may become more integrated into oncology. Whedon (2001) highlighted that inpatient and outpatient settings may actually provide opportunities for research and institutional change primarily through readily available data, regulatory efforts, and access to consultation team members.

Although evidence supports the benefits of behavioral interventions in medical conditions, a tremendous need remains for improved research techniques, assessments, instruments, and treatments for the population approaching life's end. Establishing a "gold standard" that addresses the physical, psychological, social, and spiritual needs during advanced illness is absolutely necessary.

## REFERENCES

Abeles, H., Gift, H. C., & Ory, M. G. (1994). *Aging and quality of life*. New York: Springer.

Alliance of Aging Research. (1998). *Seven deadly myths: Uncovering the facts about the high costs of the last year of life*. Washington DC: Alliance for Aging Research.

American Pain Society (APS) Quality Care Committee. (1998). Quality improvement guidelines for the treatment of acute pain and cancer pain. *Journal of the American Medical Association, 274*, 1874–1880.

American Pain Society (APS). (1999a). *Guidelines for the management of acute and chronic sickle-cell disease*. Glenview, IL: American Pain Society.

American Pain Society (APS). (1999b). *Guidelines for the management of HIV/AIDS pain*. Glenview, IL: American Pain Society.

Aneshensel, C. S., Pearlin, L. I., Mullan, J. T., Zarit, S. H., & Whitlatch, C. J. (1995). *Profiles in caregiving: The unexpected career*. San Diego: Academic Press.

Arno, P. S., Levine, C., & Memmott, M. M. (1999). The economic value of informal caregiving. *Health Affairs, 18*, 182–188.

Baer, W. L., & Hanson, J. C. (2000). Families' perception of the added value of hospice in the nursing home. *Journal of American Geriatric Society, 48*, 879–882.

Baider, L., Uziely, B., & De-Nour, A. K. (1994). Progressive muscle relaxation and guided imagery in cancer patients. *General Hospital Psychiatry, 16*, 340–347.

Balducci, L. (1994). Perspectives on quality of life of older patients with cancer. *Drugs and Aging, 4*, 313–324.

Balducci, L., & Entermann, M. (2000). Cancer and aging: An evolving panorama. *Hematology Oncology Clinics of North America, 14*, 1–16.

Bandura, A. J. (1986). *Social foundations of thought and action: A social cognitive theory*. Englewood Cliffs, NJ: Prentice Hall, Inc.

Barber, T. X. (1993). Hypnosuggestive approaches to stress reduction: Data, theory, and clinical applications. In P. M. Lehrer & R. L. Woolfolk (Eds.), *Principles and practice of stress management* (pp. 169–204). New York: Guilford Press.

Basmajian, J. V. (Ed.). (1989). *Biofeedback: Principles and practice for clinicians* (3rd ed.). Baltimore: Williams & Wilkins.

Bates-Jensen, B. M., Early, L., & Seaman, S. (2001). Skin disorders. In B. R. Ferrell & N. Coyle (Eds.), *Textbook of palliative nursing* (pp. 204–244). New York: Oxford University Press.

Beck, A. T. (1976). *Cognitive therapies and emotional disorders*. New York: Guilford Press.

Beck, A. T., Rush, A. J., Shaw, B. F., & Emery, G. (1979). *Cognitive therapy for depression*. New York: Guilford Press.

Becker, R. (1999). Teaching communication with the dying across cultural boundaries. *British Journal of Nursing, 8*, 938–942.

Benson, H. (1996). *Timeless healing: The power of biology and belief*. New York: Simon and Shuster.

Bentur, N. (2001). Hospital at home: What is its place in the health system? *Health Policy, 55*, 71–79.

Bernstein, D. A., & Carlson, C. R. (1993). Progressive relaxation: Abbreviated methods. In P. M. Lehrer & R. L. Woolfolk (Eds.), *Principles and practice of stress management* (pp. 53–88.) New York: Guilford Press.

Berry, P. E., & Ward, S. E. (1995). Barriers to pain management in hospice: A study of family caregivers. *Hospice Journal, 10*(4), 19–33.

Blake-Mortimer, J., Gore-Felton, C., Kimerling, R., Turner-Cobb, J., & Spiegel, D. (1999). Improving the quality and quantity of life among patients with cancer: A review of the effectiveness of group psychotherapy. *European Journal of Cancer, 35*, 1581–1586.

Block, S. D. (2000). Assessing and managing depression in the terminally ill: ACP-ASIM End-of-Life Care Consensus Pane. *Annals of Internal Medicine, 132*, 209–218.

Block, S. D. (2001). Psychological considerations, growth, and transcendence at the end of life: The art of the possible. *Journal of the American Medical Association, 285*, 2898–2905.

Braun, K. L., Pietsch, J. H., & Blanchette, P. L. (Eds.). (2000). *Cultural issues in end-of-life decision making*. Thousand Oaks, CA: Sage Publications.

Breitbart, W., Jaramillo, J. R., & Chochinov, H. M. (1998). Palliative and terminal care. In J. C. Holland (Ed.), *Psycho-oncology* (pp. 437–449). New York: Oxford University Press.

Breitbart, W., & Payne, D. K. (1998). Pain. In J. C. Holland (Ed.), *Psycho-oncology* (pp. 450–467). New York: Oxford University Press.

Breitbart, W. C., & Cohen, K. R. (1998). Delirium. In J. C. Holland (Ed.), *Psycho-oncology* (pp. 564–575). New York: Oxford University Press.

Breitbart, W. C., & Wein, S. E. (1998). Metabolic disorders and neuropsychiatric symptoms. In J. C. Holland (Ed.), *Psycho-oncology* (pp. 639–652). New York: Oxford University Press.

Bruera, E., & Fainsinger, R. L. (1998). Clinical management of cachexia and anorexia. In D. Doyle, G. W. C. Hanks, & N. MacDonald (Eds.), *Oxford textbook of palliative medicine* (pp. 548–557). New York: Oxford University Press.

Bruera, E., & Lawlor, P. (1997). Cancer pain management. *Acta Anaesthesiologica Scandinavica, 41*, 146–153.

Bruera, E., Miller, L., McCallion, J., Macmillan, K., Krefting, L., & Hanson, J. (1992). Cognitive failure in patients with terminal cancer: A prospective study. *Journal of Pain and Symptom Management, 7,* 192–195.

Bruera, E., & Neumann, C. M. (1998). Management of specific symptom complexes in patients receiving palliative care. *Canadian Medical Association Journal, 158,* 1717–1726.

Buckle, J. (1999). Use of aromatherapy as a complementary treatment for chronic pain. *Alternative Therapies in Health and Medicine, 5*(5), 42–51.

Buckle, J. (2001). The role of aromatherapy in nursing care. *Nursing Clinics of North America, 36,* 57–72.

Burish, T. G., & Jenkins, R. A. (1992). Effectiveness of biofeedback and relaxation training in reducing side effects of cancer chemotherapy. *Health Psychology, 11,* 17–23.

Butcher, J. N., Dahlstrom, W. G., Graham, J. R., Tellegren, A., & Kaemmer, B. (1989). *MMPI-2 (Minnesota Multiphasic Personality Inventory-2): Manual for administration and scoring.* Minneapolis: University of Minnesota Press.

Byock, I. (2000). Completing the continuum of cancer care: Integrating life-prolongation and palliation. *Cancer Journal and Clinics, 50,* 123–132.

Cairns, A. B. (1999). Spirituality and religiosity in palliative care. *Home Healthcare Nurse, 17,* 450–455.

Carlson, L. E., Bultz, B. D., Speca, M., & St. Pierre, M. (2000). Partners of cancer patients: Part II. Current psychosocial interventions and suggestions for improvements. *Journal of Psychosocial Oncology, 18*(3), 33–43.

Carpenter, R. (1998). Fever. In C. C. Chernecky & B. J. Berger (Eds.), *Advanced and critical care oncology nursing: Managing primary complications* (pp. 156–171). Philadelphia: W. B. Saunders.

Cella, D. F. (1998). Quality of life. In J. C. Holland (Ed.), *Psycho-oncology* (pp. 1135–1146). New York: Oxford University Press.

Champion, V. L. (2001). Behavioral oncology research: A new millennium. *Oncology Nursing Forum, 28,* 975–982.

Christensen, A. J., Wiebe, J. S., Smith, T. W., & C. W. Turner. (1994). Predictors of survival among hemodialysis patients: Effect of perceived support. *Health Psychology, 13,* 521–525.

Cleeland, C. S. (2001). Cross-cutting research issues: A research agenda for reducing distress of patients with cancer. In K.M. Foley & H. Gelband (Eds.), *Institute of medicine and national research council: Improving palliative care for cancer summary and recommendations* (pp. 8–85). Washington, D.C.: National Academy Press.

Cole, B., & Pargament, K. (1999). Re-creating your life: A spiritual/psychotherapeutic intervention for people diagnosed with cancer. *Psycho-oncology, 8,* 395–407.

Connell, C. (1992). Art therapy as part of a palliative care programme. *Palliative Medicine, 6,* 18–25.

Curt, G. A. (2000). Impact of fatigue on quality of life in oncology patients. *Seminars in Hematology, 37*(4 Suppl. l6), 14–17.

Davies, B. (2001). Supporting families in palliative care. In B. R. Ferrell & N. Coyle (Eds.), *Textbook of palliative nursing* (pp. 363–373). New York: Oxford University Press.

Derby, S., & O'Mahoney, S. (2001). Elderly patients. In B. R. Ferrell & N. Coyle (Eds.), *Textbook of palliative nursing* (pp. 435–449). New York: Oxford University Press.

Derogatis, L. R. (1994). *SCL-90-R (symptom checklist 90-revised): Administration, scoring, and procedures manual.* Minneapolis: National Computer Systems.

DuHamel, K. N., Johnson-Vickberg, S. M., & Redd, W. H. (1998). Behavioral interventions in pediatric oncology. In J. C. Holland (Ed.), *Psycho-oncology* (pp. 962–980). New York: Oxford University Press.

DuPen, A. R, & J. Robinson, J. (2001). The outpatient setting. In B. R. Ferrell & N. Coyle (Eds.), *Textbook of palliative nursing* (pp. 622–631). New York: Oxford University Press.

Egan, K. A., & Labyak, M. J. (2001). Hospice care: A model for quality end of life care. In B. R. Ferrell & N. Coyle (Eds.), *Textbook of palliative nursing* (pp. 7–26). New York: Oxford University Press.

Eller, L. S. (1999). Guided imagery interventions for symptom management. *Annual Review of Nursing Research, 17,* 57–84.

Emanuel, E. J., Fairclough, D. L., Slutsman, J., & Emanuel, L. L. (2000). Understanding economic and other burdens of terminal illness: The experience of patients and their caregivers. *Annals of Internal Medicine, 132,* 451–459.

Ersek, M., Kraybill, B. M., & DuPen, A. (1999). Factors hindering patients use of medications for cancer pain. *Cancer Practice, 7,* 226–232.

Ferrell, B. R. (1995). The impact of pain on quality of life: A decade of research. *Nursing Clinics of North America, 30,* 609–624.

Ferrell, B. R. (1996). Pain: how patients and families pay the price. In M. J. M. Cohen & J. N. Campbell (Eds.), *Pain treatment at a crossroads* (Vol. 7). Seattle, WA: International Association for the Study of Pain (IASP).

Ferrell, B. R. (1998). The family. In D. Doyle, G.W.C. Hanks, & N. MacDonald (Eds.), *Oxford textbook of palliative medicine* (2nd ed.). New York: Oxford University Press.

Ferrell, B. R., & Borneman, T. (1999). Pain and suffering at the end of life (EOL) for older patients and their families. *Generations, XXIII,* 12–17.

Ferrell, B. R., & Coyle, N. (2001). *Textbook of palliative nursing.* New York: Oxford University Press.

Ferrell, B. R., & Ferrell, B. A. (1996). *Pain in the elderly.* London: International Association for the Study of Pain (IASP).

Ferrell, B. R., & Ferrell, B. A. (1998). The older patient. In J.C. Holland (Ed.), *Psycho-oncology* (pp. 839–844). New York: Oxford University Press.

Ferrell, B. R., Ferrell, B. A., Ahn, C., & Tran, K. (1994). Pain management for elderly patients with cancer at home. *Cancer, 74,* 2139–2146.

Ferrell, B. A., Ferrell, B. R., & Osterweil, D. (1990). Pain in the nursing home. *Journal of the American Geriatric Society, 38,* 409–414.

Ferrell, B. R., Ferrell, B. A., & Rivera, L. M. (1995). Pain in cognitively impaired nursing home patients. *Journal of Pain Symptom Management, 10*, 591–598.

Ferrell, B. R., Grant, M., Borneman, T., Juarez, G., & ter Veer, A. (1999). Family caregiving in cancer pain management. *Journal of Palliative Medicine, 2*, 185–195.

Ferrell, B. R., Grant, M., Chan, J., Ahn, C., & Ferrell, B. A. (1995). The impact of cancer pain education on family caregivers of elderly patients. *Oncology Nursing Forum, 22*, 1211–1218.

Ferrell, B. R., Grant, M., Rhiner, M., & Padilla, G. V. (1992). Home care: Maintaining quality of life for patient and family. *Oncology, 6*, 136–140.

Ferrell, B. R., & Griffith, H. (1994). Cost issues related to pain management: Report from the Cancer Pain Panel of the Agency for Health Care Policy and Research. *Journal of Pain and Symptom Management, 9*, 221–234.

Ferrell, B. R., Rhiner, M., Shapiro, B., & Dierkes, M. (1993). The experience of pediatric cancer pain. Part I: Impact of pain on the family. *Journal of Pediatric Nursing, 9*, 368–379.

Ferrell, B. R., & Rivera, L. M. (1995). Cancer pain: Impact on elderly patients and their family caregivers. In R. Roy (Ed.), *Chronic pain in old age: An integrated biopsychosocial perspective* (pp. 103–126). Toronto: University of Toronto Press.

Ferrell, B. R., Taylor, E. J., Sattler, G. R., Fowler, M., & Cheyney, B. L. (1993). Searching for the meaning of pain: Cancer patients', caregivers', and nurses' perspectives. *Cancer Practice, 1*, 185–194.

Ferrell, B. R., Virani, R., & Grant, M. (1998). Home care outreach for palliative care education. *Cancer Practice, 6*, 79–85.

Ferrell-Tory, A. T., & Glick, O. J. (1993). The use of therapeutic massage as a nursing intervention to modify anxiety and the perception of cancer pain. *Cancer Nursing, 16*, 93–101.

Field, M. J., & Cassel, C. K. (Eds.). (1997). *Approaching death: Improving care at the end of life*. Washington, D.C.: Institute of Medicine, National Academy Press.

Fishman, B. (1992). The cognitive behavioral perspective on pain management in the terminally ill. In D. C. Turk & C. S. Feldman (Eds.), *Noninvasive approaches to pain management in the terminally ill* (pp. 73–88). Binghamton, NY: The Haworth Press.

Fitchett, G., & Handzo, G. (1998). Spiritual assessment, screening, and intervention. In J. C. Holland (Ed.), *Psycho-oncology* (pp. 790–808). New York: Oxford University Press.

Fleischer, A. B., Jr., & Michaels, J. R. (1998). Pruritis. In J. A. Billings, A. Berger, R. Portenoy, & D. Weissman (Eds.), *Principles and practice of supportive oncology* (pp. 245–250). Philadelphia: Lippincott-Raven.

Foley, K. M., & Gelband, H. (Eds.). (2001). Institute of Medicine and National Research Council: Improving palliative care for cancer summary and recommendations. Washington, D.C.: National Academy Press.

Fordyce, W. E. (1994). Pain and suffering: What is the unit? *Quality of Life Research, 3*(Suppl. 1), 51–56.

Forker, A. D. (2001). Transcendental meditation and hypertension. *Alternative Medicine Alert, 4*, 61–65.

Fox, B. H. (1998). Psychosocial factors in cancer incidence and prognosis. In J. C. Holland (Ed.), *Psycho-oncology* (pp. 110–124). New York: Oxford University Press.

Frager, G., & Shapiro, B. (1998). Pediatric palliative care and pain management. In J. C. Holland (Ed.), *Psycho-oncology* (pp. 907–922). New York: Oxford University Press.

Franks, P. J., Salisbury, C., Bosanquet, N., Wilkinson, E. K., Kite, S., Naysmith, A., et al. (2000). The level of need for palliative care: a systematic review of the literature. *Palliative Medicine, 14,* 93–104.

Gatchel, R. J, & Turk, D. C. (Eds.). (1999). *Psychosocial factors in pain: Critical perspectives.* New York: The Guilford Press.

Gavrin, J., & Chapman, C. R. (1995). Clinical management of dying patients. *Western Journal of Medicine, 163,* 268–277.

Gerrish, K. (2000). Individualized care: Its conceptualization and practice within a multiethnic society. *Journal of Advanced Nursing, 32,* 91–99.

Giasson, M., & Bouchard, L. (1998). Effect of therapeutic touch on the well being of persons with terminal cancer. *Journal of Holistic Nursing 16,* 383–389.

Gibson-Hunt, G. (2000). Caregiving and the workplace. In C. Levine (Ed.), *Always on call: When illness turns families into caregivers.* New York: United Hospital Fund of New York.

Given, C. W., Stommel, M., Given, B., Osuch, J., Kurtz, M. E., & Kurtz, J. C. (1993). The influence of cancer patients, symptoms, and functional state on patients' depression and family caregivers' reaction and depression. *Health Psychology, 12,* 277–285.

Gochman, D. S. (1997). *Handbook of health behavior research 1: Personal and social determinants.* New York: Plenum Press.

Grant, M., & Rivera, L. (1995). Pain education for nurses, patients, and families. In D. B. McGuire, C. H. Yarbro, & B. R. Ferrell (Eds.), *Cancer pain management* (2nd ed., pp. 289–320). Boston: Jones & Bartlett Publisher.

Gray, M., & Campbell, F. G. (2001). Urinary tract disorders. In B. R. Ferrell & N. Coyle (Eds.), *Textbook of palliative nursing* (pp. 175–191). New York: Oxford University Press.

Hammond, D. C. (1990). *Handbook of hypnotic suggestions and metaphors.* New York: W. W. Norton & Company.

Hanser, S. B. (1999). Using music therapy in treating psychological problems in older adults. In M. Duffy (Ed.), *Handbook of counseling and psychotherapy with older adults* (pp. 197–213). New York: John Wiley & Sons, Inc.

Herbst, L. H., Lynn, J., Mermann, A. C., & Rhymes, J. (1995, February). What do dying patients want and need? *Patient Care,* pp. 27–39.

Herz-Brown, F. (1990). The impact of death and serious illness on the family life cycle. In B. Carter & M. McGoldrick (Eds.), *The changing family life cycle* (2nd ed.). Boston: Allyn and Bacon.

Hickman, S. E., Tilden, V. P., & Tolle, S. W. (2001). Family reports of dying patients' distress: The adaptation of a research tool to assess global symptom distress in the last week of life. *Journal of Pain and Symptom Management, 22,* 565–574.

Holland, J. C. (Ed.). (1998). *Psycho-oncology.* New York: Oxford University Press.

Holland, J. C., & Chertkov, L. (2001). Clinical practice guidelines for the management of psychosocial and physical symptoms of cancer. In K. M. Foley & H. Gelband (Eds.), *Institute of Medicine and National Research Council: Improving palliative care for cancer summary and recommendations* (pp. 7–60). Washington, D.C.: National Academy Press.

Holzheimer, A. (2000). The essentials of pain management for cancer patients receiving home care. *Home Care Providers, 5,* 120–125.

Hull, M. M. (1993, February). Coping strategies of family caregivers in hospice home care. *Caring,* pp. 78–88.

Ingham, J., & Portenoy, R. K. (1998). Pain and physical symptom assessment. In J. C. Holland (Ed.), *Psycho-oncology* (pp.1147–1164). New York: Oxford University Press.

Jacobsen, P. B., & Hann, D. M. (1998). Cognitive behavioral interventions. In J. C. Holland. (Ed.), *Psycho-oncology* (pp. 717–729.) New York: Oxford University Press.

Jackson, K. C., & Lipman, A. G. (2000a). Anxiety in palliative care patients. In A. G. Lipman, K. C. Jackson, & L. S. Tyler (Eds.), *Evidenced-based symptom control in palliative care: Systematic reviews and validated clinical practice guidelines for 15 common problems in patients with life-limiting disease* (pp. 23–35). Binghamton, NY: Pharmaceutical Products Press.

Jackson, K. C., & Lipman, A. G. (2000b). Delirium in palliative care patients. In A. G. Lipman, K. C. Jackson, & L. S. Tyler (Eds.), *Evidenced-based symptom control in palliative care: Systematic reviews and validated clinical practice guidelines for 15 common problems in patients with life-limiting disease* (pp. 59–70). Binghamton, NY: Pharmaceutical Products Press.

Jenkins, R. A., & Pargament, K. I. (1995). Religion and spirituality as resources for coping with cancer. *Journal of Psychosocial Oncology, 13,* 51–74.

Johnston-Taylor, E. (2001a). Spiritual assessment. In B. R. Ferrell & N. Coyle (Eds.), *Handbook of palliative nursing* (pp. 397–406). New York: Oxford University Press.

Johnston-Taylor, E. (2001b). *Spiritual care: Nursing theory, research, and practice.* Upper Saddle River, NJ: Prentice Hall.

Juarez, G., & Ferrell, B. R. (1996). Family and caregiver involvement in pain management. *Clinics in Geriatric Medicine, 12,* 531–547.

Kabat-Zinn, J. (1994). *Wherever you go, there you are: Mindfulness meditation in everyday life.* New York: Hyperion.

Kabat-Zinn, J., Ohm-Massion, A., Hebert, J. R., & Rosenbaum, E. (1998). Meditation. In J. C. Holland (Ed.), *Psycho-oncology* (pp. 767–779). New York: Oxford University Press.

Kahn, S. B., Houts, P. S., & Harding, S. P. (1992). Quality of life and patients with cancer: A comparative study of patients versus physician perceptions and its implications for cancer education. *Journal of Cancer Education, 7,* 241–249.

Kelly, B., Edwards, P., Synott, R., Neil, C., Baillie, R., & Battistutta, D. (1999). Predictors of bereavement outcome for family carers of cancer patients. *Psycho-oncology, 8,* 237–249.

Kemp, C. (2001). Spiritual care interventions. In B. R. Ferrell & N. Coyle (Eds.), *Handbook of palliative nursing* (pp. 407–414). New York: Oxford University Press.

Koenig, B. A. (1997). Cultural diversity in decision making about care at the end of life. In M. J. Field & C. K. Cassel (Eds.), *Approaching death: Improving care at the end of life* (pp. 363–382). Washington, D.C.: Institute of Medicine, National Academy Press.

Koenig, B. A., & Gates-Williams, J. (1995). Understanding cultural differences in caring for dying patients. *Western Journal of Medicine, 157*, 316–322.

Koenig, H., Idler, E., Kasl, S., Hays, J. C., George, L. K., Musick, M., et al. (1999). Religion, spirituality, and medicine: A rebuttal to skeptics. *International Journal of Psychiatry Medicine, 29*, 123–131.

Kornblith, A. B., & Holland, J. C. (1994). *Handbook of measures of psychological, social, and physical function in cancer.* New York: Memorial Sloan Kettering Cancer Center.

Kreiger, D. (1993). *Accepting your power to heal: The personal practice of therapeutic touch.* Santa Fe, NM: Bear & Co.

Kuebler, K. K., English, N., & Heidrich, D. E. (2001). Delirium, confusion, agitation, and restlessness. In B. R. Ferrell & N. Coyle (Eds.), *Textbook of palliative nursing* (pp. 290–308). New York: Oxford University Press.

Lambert, S. A. (1999). Distraction, imagery, and hypnosis: Techniques for management of children's pain. *Journal of Child and Family Nursing, 2*, 5–15.

Lane, D. (1993, January/February). Music therapy: Gaining an edge in oncology management. *Journal of Oncology Management*, pp. 42–46.

Lane, D. (1994). *Music as medicine.* Grand Rapids, MI: Zondervan Publishing House.

Lederberg, M. S. (1998). The family of the cancer patient. In J. C. Holland (Ed.), *Psycho-oncology* (pp. 981–993). New York: Oxford University Press.

Lehrer, P. M., & Woolfolk, R. L. (Eds.). (1993). *Principles and practice of stress management.* New York: Guilford Press.

Levine, C. (Ed.). (2000). *Always on call: When illness turns families into caregivers.* News York: United Hospital Fund of New York.

Linden, W. (1993). The autogenic training method of J. H. Schultz. In P. M. Lehrer & R. L. Woolfolk (Eds.), *Principles and practice of stress management* (pp. 205–230). New York: Guilford Press.

Lipowski, Z. J. (1990). *Delirium: Acute confusional states.* New York: Oxford University Press.

Lloyd-Williams, M., Friedman, T., & Rudd, N. (1999). A survey of antidepressant prescribing in the terminally ill. *Palliative Medicine, 13*, 243–248.

Loscalzo, M. (1996). Psychological approaches to the management of pain in patients with advanced cancer. *Hematology/Oncology Clinics of North America, 10*, 139–155.

Loscalzo, M., & Jacobsen, P. B. (1990). Practical behavioral approaches to effective management of pain and distress. *Journal of Psychosocial Oncology, 8*, 139–169.

Luzatto, P., & Gabriel, B. (1998). Art psychotherapy. In J. C. Holland (Ed.), *Psycho-oncology* (pp. 743–757). New York: Oxford University Press.

Lynn, J. (2001). Serving patients who may die soon and their families: The role of hospice and other services. *Journal of the American Medical Association, 285,* 925–932.

Lynn, J., Teno, J. M., Phillips, R. S., Wu, A. W., Desbiens, N., Harrold, J., et al. (1997). Perceptions of family members of the dying experience of older and seriously ill patients. *Annals of Internal Medicine, 126,* 97–106.

Mackey, B. T. (1995). Discovering the healing power of therapeutic touch. *American Journal of Nursing, 4,* 27–32.

Mackey, B. T. (2001). Massage therapy and reflexology awareness. *Nursing Clinics of North America, 39,* 159–169.

Manetto, C., & McPherson, S. E. (1996). The behavioral-cognitive model of pain. *Clinics in Geriatric Medicine, 12,* 461–471.

Mantovani, G., Astara, G., Lampis, B., Bianchi, A., Curreli, L., Orru, W., et al. (1996). Evaluation by multidimensional instruments of health-related quality of life of elderly cancer patients undergoing three different "psychosocial" treatment approaches: A randomized clinical trial. *Supportive Cancer Care, 4,* 129–140.

Massie, M. J., & Popkin, M. K. (1998). Depressive disorders. In J. C. Holland (Ed.), *Psycho-oncology* (pp. 518–540). New York: Oxford University Press.

Matthews, D. A., & Larson, D. B. (1995). *The faith factor: An annotated bibliography of clinical research on spiritual subjects* (Vol. 3). Bethesda, MD: National Institute for Healthcare Research.

McCaffrey, M., & Wolff, M. (1992). Pain relief using cutaneous modalities, positioning, and movement. In D. C. Turk & C. S. Feldman (Eds.), *Noninvasive approaches to pain management in the terminally ill* (pp. 121–154). Binghamton, NY: The Haworth Press.

McCorkle, R., Robinson, L., Nuameh, I., Lev, E., & Benoliel, J. Q. (1998). The effects of home nursing care for patients during terminal illness on the bereaved's psychological distress. *Nursing Research, 47,* 2–10.

McFadden, S. H., & Atchley, C. (2001). *Aging and the meaning of time: A multidisciplinary exploration.* New York: Springer Publishing Company.

Meichenbaum, D. (1993). Stress inoculation training: A 20-year update. In P. M. Lehrer & R. L. Woolfolk (Eds.), *Principles and practice of stress management* (pp. 373–406). New York: Guilford.

Millon, T. (1994). *Millon clinical multiaxial inventory-III (MCMI-III).* Minneapolis: National Computer Systems.

Moadel, A., Morgan, C., Fatone, A., Grennan, J., Carter, J., Laruffa, G., et al. (1999). Seeking meaning and hope: Self-reported spiritual and existential needs among an ethnically-diverse cancer patient population. *Psycho-Oncology, 8,* 378–385.

National Comprehensive Cancer Network (NCCN). (1999, February 26–March 2). *Fourth Annual Conference. Practice Guidelines and outcomes data in oncology. Update: NCCN distress management guidelines,* Ft. Lauderdale, FL.

National Comprehensive Cancer Network and American Cancer Society (NCCN/ACS). (2001). *Patient guidelines for the treatment of cancer pain.* Atlanta, GA: ACS.

National Hospice and Palliative Care Organization (NHPCO). (2001). *Complementary therapies in end of life care.* Alexandria, VA: NHPCO.

National Institutes of Health. (1997). NIH consensus statement: Acupuncture. Nov. 3–5, 1997; 15(5), 1–34. Bethesda, MD: NIH.

Ng, B., Dimsdale, J. E., Shragg, P., & Deutsch, R. (1996). Ethnic differences in analgesic consumption for postoperative pain. *Psychosomatic Medicine, 58,* 125–129.

Norman, R. W. (1998). Genitourinary disorders. In D. Doyle, G. W. C. Hanks, & N. MacDonald (Eds.), *Oxford textbook of palliative medicine* (2nd ed., pp. 667–676). New York: Oxford University Press.

O'Connell, L. J. (1996). Changing the culture of dying. A new awakening of spirituality in America heightens sensitivity to the needs of dying persons. *Health Progress, 77*(6), 16–20.

Osterlund, H. & Beirne, P. (2001). Complementary therapies. In B. R. Ferrell & N. Coyle (Eds.), *Textbook of palliative nursing* (pp. 374–381). New York: Oxford University Press.

Owen, J. E., Klapow, J. C., Hicken, B., & Tucker, D. C. (2001). Psychosocial interventions for cancer: Review and analysis using a three-tiered outcomes model. *Psycho-oncology, 10,* 218–230.

Paice, J. A., & Fine, P. G. (2001). Pain at the end of life. In B. R. Ferrell & N. Coyle (Eds.), *Textbook of palliative nursing* (pp. 76–90). New York: Oxford University Press.

Paice, J. A., Toy, C., & Shott, S. (1998). Barriers to cancer pain relief: Fear of tolerance and addiction. *Journal of Pain and Symptom Management, 16,* 1–9.

Pasacreta, J. V., Barg, F., Nuamah, I., & McCorkle, R. (2000). Participant characteristics before and after attendance at a family caregiver cancer education program. *Cancer Nursing, 23,* 295–303.

Pasacreta, J. V., & McCorkle, R. (2000). Cancer care: Impact of interventions on caregiver outcomes. *Annual Review in Nursing Research, 18,* 127–148.

Passik, S. D., & Breitbart, W. (1993). Psychiatric and psychological approaches to cancer pain. In E. Arbit (Ed.), *Management of cancer pain.* Mount Kisko, NY: Futura Publishing Company.

Payne, S., Smith, P., & Dean, S. (1999). Identifying the concerns of informal carers in palliative care. *Palliative Medicine, 13,* 37–44.

Pereira, J., Hanson, J., & Bruera, E. (1997). The frequency and clinical course of cognitive impairment in patients with terminal cancer. *Cancer, 69,* 835–841.

Pittelkow, M. R., & Loprinski, C. L. (1998). Pruritis and sweating. In D. Doyle, G. W. C. Hanks, & N. MacDonald (Eds.), *Oxford textbook of palliative medicine,* (2nd ed., pp. 627–642). New York: Oxford University Press.

Portenoy, R. K., & Lesage, P. (1999). Management of cancer pain. *Lancet, 353,* 1695–1700.

Puntillo, K., & Stannard, D. (2001). The intensive care unit. In B. R. Ferrell & N. Coyle (Eds.), *Textbook of palliative nursing* (pp. 609–621). New York: Oxford University Press.

Reeves, J. L., & Graber, L. M. (1993). Is pain memory state dependent? Symposium: Memory and pain. In R. N. Jamison, S. Pearce, S. Morley, J. L. Reeves, L. M. Graber, J. Lander, et al. (Eds.), *Proceedings of the 7th world congress on pain* (p. 354). Seattle, WA: International Association for the Study of Pain.

Resnick, R. J., & Rozensky, R. H. (1996). *Health psychology through the life span: Practice and research opportunities*. Washington, D.C.: American Psychological Association.

Riley, S. (1995). *Integrative approaches to family art therapy*. Chicago: Magnolia Street Publishers.

Rodriguez, C. S. (2001). Pain measurement in the elderly: A review. *Pain Management Nursing, 2*(2), 38–46.

Ryan, A. A., & Scullion, H. F. (2000). Nursing home placement: An exploration of the experiences of family carers. *Journal of Advanced Nursing, 32*, 1187–1195.

Schachter, S. R., & Coyle, N. (1998). Palliative home care—Impact on families. In J. C. Holland (Ed.), *Psycho-oncology* (pp. 1016–1034). New York: Oxford University Press.

Schroeder-Sheker, T. (1993). Music for the dying: A personal account of the new field of music thanatology—history, theories, and clinical narratives. *Advances: The Journal of Mind-Body-Health*, Winter, pp. 29–33.

Scudder-Teufel, E. (1995). Terminal stage leukemia: Integrating art therapy and family process. *Art Therapy, 12*, 51–55.

Snyder, M., & Chlan, L. (1999). Music therapy. *Annual Review of Nursing Research, 17*, 3–25.

Snyder, M., & Lindquist, R. (Eds.). (1998). *Complementary/alternative therapies in nursing* (3rd ed.). New York: Springer Publishing Company.

Spiegel, D., & Claussen, C. (2000). *Group therapy for cancer patients: A research-based handbook of psychosocial care*. New York: Basic/Pegasus Books.

Spilker, B. (1996). *Quality of life and pharmacoeconomics in clinical trials*. New York: Raven Press.

Spira, J. L. (1998). Group therapies. In J. C. Holland (Ed.), *Psycho-oncology* (pp. 701–716). New York: Oxford University Press.

Spira, J. L., & Spiegel, D. (1992). Hypnosis and related techniques in pain management. In D. C. Turk & C. S. Feldman (Eds.), *Noninvasive approaches to pain management in the terminally ill* (pp. 89–120). Binghamton, NY: The Haworth Press.

Steinhauser, K. E., Christakis, N. A., Clipp, E. C., McNeilly, M., McIntyre, L., & Tulsky, J. A. (2000). Factors considered important at the end of life by patients, family, physicians, and other care providers. *Journal of the American Medical Association, 284*, 2476–2482.

Steptoe, A., & Wardle, J. (1995). *Psychosocial processes and health: A reader*. New York: Cambridge University Press.

Syrjala, K. L. (1993). Integrating medical and psychological treatments for cancer pain. In C. R. Chapman & K. M. Foley (Eds.), *Current and emerging issues in cancer pain research* (pp. 393–409). New York: Raven Press.

Syrjala, K. L., & Chapko, M. E. (1995). Evidence for a biopsychosocial model of cancer treatment-related pain. *Pain, 61*, 69–79.

Syrjala, K. L., Cummings, C., & Donaldson, G. (1992). Hypnosis or cognitive-behavioral training for the reduction of pain and nausea during cancer treatment: A controlled clinical trial. *Pain, 48*, 137–146.

Syrjala, K. L., Donaldson, G. W., Davis, M. W., Kippes, M. E., & Carr, J. E. (1995). Relaxation and imagery and cognitive-behavioral training reduce pain during cancer treatment: A controlled clinical trial. *Pain, 63*, 189–198.

Trauger-Querry, B., & Haghighi, K. R. (1999). Balancing the focus: Art and music therapy for pain control and symptom management in hospice care. *The Hospice Journal, 14*, 25–38.

Turk, D. C. (1996). Biopsychosocial perspective on chronic pain. In R. J. Gatchel & D. C. Turk (Eds.), *Psychological approaches to pain management: A practitioner's handbook* (pp. 3–32). New York: Guilford Press.

Turk, D. C., & Feldman, C. S. (1992). *Noninvasive approaches to pain management in the terminally ill.* Binghamton, NY: The Haworth Press.

Turk, D. C., & Okifuji, A. (1997). Evaluating the role of physical, operant, cognitive and affective factors in the pain behaviors of chronic pain patients. *Behavior Modification, 21*, 259–280.

Tyler, L. S. (2000). Nausea and vomiting in palliative care. In A. G. Lipman, K. C. Jackson, & L. S. Tyler (Eds.), *Evidenced-based symptom control in palliative care: Systematic reviews and validated clinical practice guidelines for 15 common problems in patients with life-limiting disease* (pp. 163–182). Binghamton, NY: Pharmaceutical Products Press.

Underwood, S. (1994). Access to heath care in America: the dilemma faced by the poor in seeking cancer care. *Seminars in Oncology Nursing, 10*, 89–95.

Vaserling, J., Jenkins, R. A., Tope, D. M., & Burish, T. G. (1993). Cognitive distraction and relaxation training for the control of side-effects due to cancer chemotherapy. *Journal of Behavioral Medicine, 16*, 65–80.

Ware, J. E., & Sherbourne, C. D. (1992). The MOS 36-item short form health survey (SF-36): Conceptual framework and item selection. *Medical Care, 30*, 473–486.

Weissman, D. E., Griffie, J., Gordon, D. B., & Dahl, J. L. (1997). A role model program to promote institutional changes for management of acute and cancer pain. *Journal of Pain and Symptom Management, 14*, 274–279.

Weissman, D. E., & Matson, S. (1999). Pain assessment and management in the long-term care setting. *Theories and Medical Bioethics, 20*, 31–43.

Weitzner, M. A., Haley, W. E., & Chen, H. (2000). The family caregiver of the older cancer patient. *Hematology and Oncology Clinics in North America, 14*, 269–281.

Weitzner, M. A., & McMillan, S. C. (1999). The Caregiver Quality of Life Index-Cancer (CQOLC) Scale: revalidation in a home hospice setting. *Journal of Palliative Care, 15*(2), 13–20.

Whedon, M. B. (2001). Hospital care. In B. R. Ferrell & N. Coyle (Eds.), *Textbook of palliative nursing* (pp. 584–608). New York: Oxford University Press.

Wilson, S. A. (2001). Long-term care. In B. R. Ferrell & N. Coyle (Eds.), *Textbook of palliative nursing* (pp. 531–542). New York: Oxford University Press.

Wilson, S. A., & B. J. Daley (Eds.). (1997). *Fostering humane care of dying person in long-term care: A guidebook for staff development instructors.* Milwaukee, WI: Marquette University Press.

World Health Organization, Division of Mental Health. (1993). *WHO-QOL Study protocol: The development of the World Health Organization quality of life assessment instrument* (MNG/PSF/93.9). Geneva, Switzerland: WHO.

World Health Organization. (1996). *Report of the WHO expert committee on cancer pain relief and active supportive care: Cancer pain relief with a guide to opioid availability* (Technical series 804, 2nd ed.). Geneva: World Health Organization.

Zabora, J., Brintzenhofeszoc, K., Curbow, B., Hooker, C., & Piantadosa, S. (2001). The prevalence of psychological distress by cancer site. *Psycho-oncology, 10,* 19–28.

Zabora, J. R., & Loscalzo, M. J. (1996). Comprehensive psychosocial programs: A prospective model of care. *Oncology Issues, 1,* 14–18.

Zauszniewski, J. A., Chung, C. W., & Krafcik, K. (2001). Social cognitive factors predicting the health of elders. *Western Journal of Nursing Research, 23,* 490–503.

Zoucha, R. (2000). The keys to culturally sensitive care. *American Journal of Nursing, 100,* 24GG–24II.

# 13

## Conclusion: The Future of Behavioral Intervention Research in Cancer Care

**Charles W. Given**
**Dànielle Nicole DeVoss**
**Barbara Given**

A n estimated 1,284,900 new cancer diagnoses will be made in 2002 (*ACS Cancer Facts & Figures*, 2002). Deaths from cancer are declining among the majority, but continue to rise among minority populations (*CDC Morbidity and Mortality Weekly*, January 25, 2002). Prevention through healthy diet continues to lose ground as Americans become more obese. Screening practices for the early detection of breast, cervical, and colon cancer have succeeded for families with insurance, but remain a challenge for persons without insurance and/or of low socioeconomic status. New cancer treatments emerge almost monthly, each with their own adverse effects. End-of-life care for those with advanced disease too often fails to meet the needs and wishes of patients and their families, and patients still die in pain. With shifts toward outpatient diagnosis and treatment, families continue to be a primary source of care for patients during diagnosis, during treatment, and toward the end of life. Patients continue to utilize complementary and alternative therapies often without the knowledge of their oncologists or primary care physicians with both positive and negative results. These are sobering facts; however, behavioral interventions offer a perspective from which cancer-related healthcare can be improved. In this concluding chapter, we explore some priority directions that we believe might help to more effectively establish behavioral interventions as part of standard practice in cancer prevention, screening, treatment, and end-of-life care.

In this conclusion chapter, we expand upon several issues that, if given priority in future research, could hasten the dissemination and adoption of behavioral interventions. The first issue relates to recruitment and the inclusion of patients into clinical trials. A second issue relates to how research can identify and test personal and clinical risk factors that place patients at risk for poor outcomes. A related issue is how behavioral interventions can be adjusted to respond to and accommodate patients at a higher risk in order to achieve an adequate outcome. A final issue is the theoretical approaches that underlie the delivery of behavioral interventions and the outcomes that are produced.

## RECRUITMENT ISSUES

Cancer does not spare any one gender, age group, or socioeconomic class. However, the chapters in this collection reveal that participants in behavioral intervention research undertaken in the past 10 to 15 years are comprised of relatively homogeneous groups. Overwhelmingly, participants have been female and middle-aged; further, participants have primarily been diagnosed with breast, colorectal, or lung cancer. Often, cancer centers treat patients who are predominantly middle-class and not vulnerable to certain sociodemographic barriers. Authors of the chapters urge researchers to diversify their study samples.

However, examples of studies that targeted diverse socioeconomic and ethnic samples are included in this book. For example, Haire-Joshu and Nanney summarized the results of dietary and physical activity intervention studies focusing on African-American families, Mexican-American and African-American women, low-income women, and participants recruited from African-American rural churches. Champion discussed recent cancer-screening intervention studies that included culturally and racially diverse older women, African-American women, African-American women residing in a low-income housing project, Vietnamese-American women, and Cherokee Indian women.

To better understand the barriers to participation, future research must consider how age, gender, cultural beliefs, geographic location, sociodemographic variables, and psychological states shape whether or not patients and/or their family caregivers participate in intervention studies. Health-related practices and beliefs—social, psychological, and biological factors—are complex, connected, and related to risk factors, and they may be closely linked to barriers to study participation. Casting rigid frameworks for indicating who participates and who refuses using specific categories such as age or gender may be inaccurate or ineffective. Perhaps it is not a person's age or cultural beliefs, but a sense of exploitation, a lack of social skills, a mistrust of trials, the added time an intervention requires, or how participation places the person in a specific situational relationship that potential participants prefer to avoid, such as having to talk to people with whom they are uncomfortable or who make them feel inferior. Although white middle-class women with breast cancer do represent a dominant group, substantial numbers of these women still refuse to participate. Future work needs to develop more sophisticated frameworks for explaining participation in behavioral interventions. Conventional explanations have focused on probabilistic models to account for variations in participation. For example, racial and ethnic minorities are less likely to participate, as are persons of lower socioeconomic status.

However, a crucial question to address is whether or not majority patients of a higher socioeconomic status who refuse to participate share any characteristics with minorities and those of a lower socioeconomic status. The answer to this query might more adequately explain participation refusal among the latter group. Moreover, it remains to be determined if such shared characteristics—if they are demonstrated to exist—account for a lack of participation in clinical trials or in any activities that involve uncertain outcomes.

A particularly important set of characteristics that might differentiate those who accept from those who refuse enrollment into behavioral interventions might be the site or stage of disease. Refusal to enroll could also be related to patients' views as to whether they were responsible for bringing the disease upon themselves, their level of emotional distress, or their admissions of weakness. These and other factors should be examined. The extent to which risk and situational factors (e.g., the place where patients are accrued) differentiate those who enroll and those who refuse enrollment into behavioral trials is a variable that should also be considered in future research. A necessary step in diversifying patient study populations is to see how spaces of recruitment may affect the entire intervention and study process—from patient accrual to responses to interventions, and to the outcomes achieved. Many patients seek care at centers where randomized control trials (RCTs) are not offered, where behavioral trials are low priority, or where other care and/or trials are privileged (e.g., drug trials).

Whether or not certain characteristics such as gender, race, and/or psychological characteristics affect enrollment should be explored across the cancer trajectory. They deserve, however, to be linked and analyzed with respect to perceptions of disease, preferences not to be involved in research, or considerations that interventions are not priority activities. Characteristics more closely related to disease or treatment, such as the severity of the disease and the complexity of treatment protocols—which may differentiate patient and family enrollment in behavioral interventions at various points along the disease trajectory—should be studied. For example, Ferrell suggested in Chapter 12 that few RCTs are done with those who are at the end of life; future research should seek to determine whether this is a provider or a patient and family issue.

An interesting question not addressed is how participation among those with more risk and situational factors is related to poorer outcomes. An existing assumption is that patients who choose not to participate (for example, older patients, minorities, or economically disadvantaged individuals) are all at a potentially higher risk for poorer outcomes and thus could benefit more from behavioral interventions. Studies cited by Haire-Joshu and Nanney (in Chapter 2) and by Champion et al. (in Chapter 3) have been the only ones that have conducted careful tests of this supposition. Far less is known about how characteristics of participation define the risk of poor outcome among symptom management and supportive care interventions.

## ADJUSTMENT VARIABLES

Including diverse populations and enrolling individuals from different healthcare and community institutions are crucial first steps for future behavioral intervention cancer care research. Once patients enroll in behavioral interventions, the next step is for researchers to consider how and when to adjust both intervention intensity and duration (i.e., the dose) based on patient and family characteristics or need. Adjustment itself is a complicated variable; adjustment may mean more intensity over a shorter period of time, or less intensity over a longer period of time. The implications of adjustment approaches are crucial; a variety of factors and possible results affect the conditions that allow for intervention adjustment.

Depending upon the intended outcome or patient status, the duration of interventions is varied across the studies summarized in these chapters. For example, the duration of interventions with end-of-life patients is often truncated. The duration of exercise interventions with patients under hospital care is limited by the length of the patient's stay in the hospital. The duration of herbal therapy interventions is guided by per-gram intake and intake over time. Overall, in the studies summarized here, the duration of interventions has spanned from a 2- to 5-minute counseling session or a 5- to 10-minute telephone call to an intervention of 9 therapy hours over 6 weeks, or to interventions that spanned 3 years in monthly and quarterly increments. Other durations included exercise sessions 4 to 5 times a week for 30 minutes each, 90-minute guided imagery sessions once a week, or a 45-minute music therapy cassette twice daily. The effectiveness of the variations in intervention duration for specific patient populations merits additional study.

Interventions sometimes started with a rigorous biweekly schedule for one month, and then continued with monthly sessions for 8 months. Obviously, a variety of variables shaped the duration and mode of the interventions, including the type of intervention (e.g., guided imagery or screening education) and the context for the intervention (e.g., immediately following CT or RT sessions in group formats). The follow-up durations reported in the studies summarized in this book range from 4 weeks to 6 weeks to 3 months, up to survey follow-ups every 2 years for 7 years.

Here, again, a variety of factors have influenced the follow-up time. For example, in end-of-life interventions, the follow-up time may be quite limited; in studies that took place in workplace settings, employee participants may only be available for a set amount of time. In none of the chapters did the authors discuss any interventions where content was held constant and the duration or intensity was varied. Also, no discussion was made as to how these differences might correspond with certain risk factors of patients and, in turn, to the outcomes that were achieved. More work will need to be done to develop the optimal intensity and/or duration for different classes of patients and different degrees of patient problems, and how these variations are related to one or more risk factors in order to achieve the desired outcome. Whether or not vigor is maintained and/or if an attention to protocol is adhered to over the intervention duration deserves further exploration. It is hard to believe that every person in a study would need the same dose and the same duration, as many problems are resolved through other means and problems are all experienced at different intensities.

Another aspect of interventions that has not received attention is the modes of delivery. A variety of intervention delivery methods and approaches were explored in this book and include media approaches with scripted and nonscripted telephone contact, videotapes and audiotapes (general and/or culturally tailored), slide presentations, and interactive computer media (e.g., CD-ROM). Print media information included pamphlets, brochures, illustrated booklets, newsletters, signs and posters, church bulletins, cookbooks, handouts, letters (general and tailored), physician office reminders, and patient-conducted food and pain diaries. A variety of intervention studies compared approaches using mixed media, such as the use of a letter; a letter and a brochure; or a letter, a brochure, and a videotape. Important comparisons among modes of delivering interventions remain to be explored.

Initial questions that require attention include the following: Do persons who present with certain personal or disease-related risk factors appear to do better with certain modes of behavioral intervention delivery? How should doses be designated depending on variations in and the severity of problems experienced by patients? Do persons of lower socioeconomic status fair better when interventions are presented in person? Do highly educated patients prefer more compressed approaches, such as CD-ROMs, or text-based interventions they can read at their convenience? Further, how do modes of delivery relate in systematic ways to the intensity and duration of the intervention? For example, can a greater number of interventions be delivered by telephone during a given interval than can be delivered in person? How much more or less effective is an intervention conducted by phone rather than in person? Are the outcome effects similar across variations in socioeconomic status and race or among patients at greater or lesser emotional or physical distress? How much more effective is a tailored than a general intervention for a given patient problem, and what is the increment of difference in outcomes?

The studies summarized in the chapters do not address how variations in the severity of the problem being addressed might influence the intensity, duration, or modes of delivery of the interventions. Little was said in the discussions about mixed modes of delivery, such as whether or not a mixed-mode intervention delivery is more effective for patients more compromised due to disease or number of symptoms. These are interrelated issues that will have to be addressed to optimize interventions according to the mode of delivery, the content of the intervention, personal characteristics of the target audience, and the outcome achieved. As research addresses these issues, a primary goal is to bring the correct intervention to a specific group of persons in a way that is optimally acceptable to them so that the most desirable outcome can be achieved.

Delivery systems varied across studies, including interventions delivered by Registered Dieticians, aerobics instructors, educators, lay health advisors, health educators, nurses, physicians, and peer volunteers. Further, the methods of delivery varied from individualized and group instruction, individual and group counseling, individual and group interactive activities (e.g., contests), classes and seminars, interviews, hands-on training/information, and the provision of FOBT kits. Finally, the spaces where interventions were conducted included exercise facilities, participants' homes, mammography vans, hospice care settings, worksites, screening facilities, and physician offices. The environment where an intervention takes place can dictate the intervention outcome. For example, Gritz suggested in Chapter 4 that most cancer-treatment centers maintain a frantic pace of diagnosis, treatment, and rapid discharge. Thus, teaching moments—that is, times when healthcare providers could intervene regarding patients' already compromised smoking habits and discuss cessation approaches— are lost.

Adjusting intervention delivery modes and locations is complex and should include not only the mode through which the intervention is delivered (e.g., telephone, in-person, or multimedia), but also the setting in which it takes place and the preparation and expertise of the professional who delivers the intervention. Additional complexities include considerations such as whether or not who delivers the intervention should be the same gender or ethnicity as the patients involved in a study. For example, whether or not it is more effective for a woman to intervene regarding prostate cancer screening for men is an issue likely to affect intervention enrollment, duration, and perhaps the adjustment of other intervention variables.

Literacy levels and skills are also a crucial variable. For example, although an interactive CD-ROM might be effective in one population, another study population might not have the skills necessary to use a computer or even have access to a computer with which to use the CD-ROM. Further, the mode of learning is a factor in how patients adopt an intervention technique. If an individual learns better through textual material, a print letter may work well. However, if an individual learns best through pictures and/or listening, a method of delivery other than a print letter may be necessary.

Although the studies summarized in the chapters here present a multiplicity of approaches related to the adjustment of intervention intensity, duration, and delivery, most of the research reported is still preliminary. Future research will have to address these complicated and often intertwined variables. Future work must pose questions related to how the length and duration of intervention intensity will influence the results among patients with different psychological or personal dispositions as well as the disease or treatment modalities either alone or together. Further, this same question of length and duration must be applied to how intervention intensity affects the desired results and how long those results are sustained.

Currently, some interventions are being targeted, tailored, and individualized based on the characteristics of patients. However, these developments have been confined almost exclusively to prevention trials. Further research needs to explore how the results of interventions vary according to their modes of delivery, the characteristics of the target audience, and the professionals who deliver the intervention. Rationales should be developed for how and why intervention delivery systems are combined. Employing an understanding of patients' literacy skills, family and community dynamics, and other variables into the intervention adjustment is a path for future research. None of the studies summarized here report on variations in intervention intensity or duration adjustment, if adjustment had an effect on outcomes, or if differences were achieved for different subgroups. Researchers may want to adjust the dosage so that patients with certain risk factors receive a more intense dosage of the intervention and analyze whether or not these patients do better than patients with similar factors but who receive a less intense dose.

The content of the intervention needs to be clarified in many descriptions of RCTs. Many interventions are only briefly described and the real matter remains in a "black box." This makes interventions difficult to understand and compare, and it is difficult to know what component(s) of the intervention might be most effective. Also, few studies have included attention controls, so it is difficult to know how attention control alone— rather than the substantive content of an intervention—might produce the outcome of interest.

Interventions, as do all treatment-related activities, have specific stop and start points. The length of the intervention has implications regarding outcomes. The summaries of studies here suggest that longer interventions and/or the inclusion of adequate follow-up periods are necessary to future research. Longer studies and extended follow-up periods will allow us to assess the long-term consequences of an intervention and assess related intervention-use variables, such as effectiveness and cost-effectiveness.

## THEORETICAL FRAMEWORKS AND OUTCOME ASSESSMENTS

As is obvious, the way intervention effects are anticipated and then measured influences the results. Although not all the studies summarized include a theoretical or conceptual framework, the theory that was reported in the studies included Cognitive Behavior Therapy, Self-control Therapy, self-care, Community Organization concepts, Diffusion of Innovation, stages of change, stress and coping, exercise training, and others.

The most commonly relied upon and reported theoretical constructs in the studies have been summarized in the book as well. The first is the Health Belief Model (HBM), which is applied primarily to prevention and screening interventions and not at all to treatment-related interventions. The HBM is used to explain and predict preventive health behaviors through a recognition of beliefs held by individuals, such as their understanding of a disease, their recognition of symptoms, the likelihood they will modify their behavior, and their readiness to act. The HBM helps researchers to understand which populations are at risk and to determine how those risks are perceived. This model then allows researchers to construct intervention approaches that may reduce the barriers to participation in health behaviors or to identify the actual and perceived levels of risk.

A second theoretical model relied upon—again primarily in prevention and screening interventions—was the Transtheoretical Model (TTM), which recognizes that change is a complicated process best understood as progress through a series of stages. Using the TTM as a framework to construct and deploy an intervention helps researchers to identify how, when, and under what conditions individuals will decide to engage in a behavior change.

Researchers also reported using Social Learning Theory (SLT), which recognizes and highlights the often complicated interplay among intrapersonal, social, and physical factors. Further, SLT helps to explore and explain how behaviors may or may not be learned through observation and modeling. SLT helps researchers design interventions that will appeal to their target patient audience and to create approaches that study participants will respond to, learn, and ideally undertake on their own.

A fourth theoretical approach included in some of the studies described in this book consists of the biobehavioral and cognitive-behavioral models. Andersen described, in Chapter 6, the biobehavioral model as including psychological (stress and quality of life), behavioral (health behaviors and compliance), and biologic (neuroendocrine and immune) factors. The model aids healthcare practitioners in identifying the pathways by which health outcomes (e.g., disease endpoints like recurrence or a disease-free interval) might be affected. This model recognizes the complex experience of cancer-related effects, including those that affect patients' cognition and behavior. The cognitive-behavioral model complements the biobehavioral model and allows for the identification of particularly stressful cancer-related effects. It also helps researchers and interventionists provide decision-making support, depression intervention, compliance with treatment encouragement, coping-skills development, and emotional expression activities.

Finally, theories of self-care are relied upon primarily in Chapter 7, "The PRO-SELF© Program: A Self-Care Intervention Program," although patient ability to perform care tasks is addressed across chapters. Self-care is essentially the activities individuals undertake to maintain life-quality variables and healthy functioning; these activities range from feeding oneself to maintaining a healthy balance between solitude and social interaction. Participating in self-care activities requires the agency or ability to do so; an individual must be able to both initiate and perform these tasks. Interventions that rely upon self-care models aid patients in learning and undertaking self-care tasks through information delivery, skill development, and provision of support. Much self-care theory is based upon Orem's theory of self-care, which suggests that all adults have basic self-care behaviors, but that certain diseases and disease factors can interrupt self-care or introduce new self-care requirements.

Although these five theoretical perspectives provided the framework for interventions, the outcome measurement approaches reported in the studies summarized here were quite diverse. Rarely was the sensitivity and specificity of measures addressed, and few studies addressed sensitivity to change or attempted to identify how clinically important changes might correspond with statistically significant changes. The end points and decay periods for outcome measurements varied significantly across interventions. Future research should analyze postintervention effects, which patients retained the changes that were achieved, how long an intervention effect continues, and when the greatest losses are likely to occur. Following these questions, research should determine whether or not patients with more severe disease or treatment-related risks revert to their status prior to the intervention more rapidly than those persons or patients who do not appear to be at risk. Second, research must explore whether intensity, duration, and/or modes of delivering the intervention have an effect on which patients experience greater decay of the psychological or behavioral changes resulting from the intervention. These issues have not been addressed in any systematic manner in the research described.

Three aspects of outcomes need to be clarified through future research: the type of outcome, when it will occur following implementation of the intervention, and how long the predetermined outcome can be sustained. Depending upon where the behavioral intervention is targeted along the cancer trajectory, widely varying expectations will be anticipated with respect to outcomes. Preventive and screening interventions have very precise types of outcomes that relate to whether or not the procedure or test has been obtained. However, in many circumstances along the cancer trajectory, if the intervention does not have a precise outcome goal or deadline, if the intervention has multiple outcome points, or if the intervention is expected to change behaviors over the coming years or even decades, then the issue of sustainability is quite different and more complex. Further, patient conditions may change over interventions; they may get better or worse during the study.

The consequences of outcome measurement are crucial to behavioral interventions; measurement marks important levels of change and allows researchers to discern how much of a dose or a certain intervention—delivered in a certain manner to patients at certain risks—produces enough change to achieve some level of outcome. Related questions to be addressed include whether or not behavioral interventions allow (for physical or psychological reasons) patients to continue treatment, or whether or not behavioral interventions reduce hospitalizations. Such outcomes have been largely ignored in trials of behavioral interventions, but deserve careful consideration. For example, does an intervention that addresses behavioral management of one or more symptoms enable patients to continue treatment with fewer dose reductions or eliminations? Do these interventions reduce the need for psychotropic medications or other supportive-care drugs? Does the intervention affect length of care? Prevent hospitalizations? Decrease the costs of care? These and other questions that link the impact of behavioral interventions with clinical outcomes deserve careful evaluation and inclusion as secondary outcomes in future trials.

Theoretical support for interventions varied across studies and across the cancer trajectory. Future work should be attentive to the development and refinement of which aspects of a theory are most effective in guiding specific intervention strategies and how these approaches can inform additional theoretical development.

Finally, future work needs to improve the precision with which interventions are implemented. Research must better address whether or not interventions specify effect sizes and when sample sizes are large enough to detect a significant difference. Although not widely described in the literature reviewed here, it seems reasonable to assume that many of the studies reviewed were inadequately powered to detect the desired effects; many studies had small and homogeneous samples. Whether or not the measures used were sensitive to the results of the intervention is a crucial query. A related concern is whether or not the timing of the measures was appropriate to both the intervention and to other aspects of treatment or care that patients might have received.

## CONCLUDING REMARKS

A carefully developed body of science that specifies which patients can benefit from behavioral interventions, the conditions under which the intervention will be effective, and the duration and magnitude of those effects is absolutely necessary for payers, practitioners, and the public at large to accept behavioral models of change. Beyond this, lobbying and other efforts will be necessary to move behavioral science into the realm of practice.

The discussions of recruitment issues, adjustment variables, and outcome assessments are obviously tightly interconnected with the research designs and the criteria introduced in the opening chapter: theory, research questions, bias, and precision. Each of these components contributes to the quality and robustness of a research framework upon which future studies can be built; these components help standardize the conduct of inquiry, sharpen comparisons, and increase confidence in conclusions.

The preceding chapters provide an impressive body of evidence indicating that behavioral interventions can affect important dimensions of patients' outcomes. Despite the strength of this evidence, behavioral interventions lie outside standard clinical practice. The reasons for this no doubt are complex. Central among the barriers to behavioral interventions is that insurers do not reimburse practitioners for the time they devote to implementing behavioral interventions. Perhaps third-party reimbursement is not available because little effort has been made to provide evidence that behavioral interventions save costs when used to augment conventional treatments, reduce hospitalizations, include the use of other services, or to reduce work lost for employers who purchase health care.

Behavioral research has not done an adequate job of translating and interpreting findings to gain credibility among practitioners or to stimulate a rise in consumer demand for these interventions. It is simply not enough to demonstrate improvements in quality of life. Third-party payers must be convinced that, in the course of improving their lives, patients require fewer other treatments, experience less morbidity, report fewer days lost from work, and experience lower levels of mortality related to the disease. At this time, only screening programs have shown that cancers diagnosed at earlier stages require less costly treatments and reduce subsequent mortality.

The studies summarized here and the careful analyses of the chapter authors help orient behavioral intervention research in directions that will bring it more toward the mainstream of cancer care, whether that be preventive, treatment-related, or end-of-life care. The ultimate goal is to develop evidence strong enough to convince payers, clinicians, and the public of the value added by behavioral interventions beyond traditional care alone.

Our goals in this book have been to synthesize state-of-the-science behavioral interventions for cancer care, to summarize interventions across the cancer trajectory, and to identify concerns and goals for future research. With this book, we hope to have contributed significantly to the relatively new but rapidly growing body of behavioral intervention science, which offers great promise as a viable complement to traditional therapy. Behavioral interventions can influence the manner in which patients seek care, select among treatment alternatives, and become better informed and involved in their own care during treatment and preparation for death. Future work needs to explore how these interventions can directly affect screening and treatment. In doing so, future efforts must also demonstrate the value-added effects of behaviorally centered care for personal as well as clinical and system-related outcomes for addressing care across the cancer trajectory.

# Index

abdominal cancer, acupuncture and, 324
acupuncture, 293, 322, **323,** 324
Adaptation for Aging Changes, colorectal
cancer screening and, 95
adjustment variables, behavioral oncology
research and, 410–415
aerobic exercise vs. fatigue, 261
African-Americans (*See also* minorities), 408
diet and, 26, 41
exercise and physical activity and, 47
screening and early detection of breast
cancer and, 79–80, 84–85, 94–96
age, end-of-life care and, 378
Agency for Healthcare Research and
Quality (AHRQ), smoking cessation
guidelines, 124–125
alcohol consumption, 21
alternative medical systems (Ayurveda,
homeopathic) in, 294, 322–324, 325
American Cancer Society (ACS), 3, 64
analgesics, 112
*Andersen, Barbara L.,* 179
anxiety (*See* stress management)
aroma therapy, 391
art therapy, 384, 391
Ask, Advise, Assess, Assist, Arrange (5 As),
smoking cessation, 125, **126**
attitude, in pain management, 274, 284
autogenic training, in end-of-life care, 384

barriers to implementation of behavioral
oncology, 418–419
Beck Depression Inventory (BDI), 185
behavioral oncology research, 1–13, 407–419
adjustment variables in, 410–415
barriers to implementation of, 418–419
bias and, in evaluation of, 10–12
cognitive-behavioral models and, 9, 416
content of interventions and, variations
in, 414–415
defining, 1

duration of interventions and, 411–415
end-of-life care and, 411–412
evidence supporting, 6–8
future research issues in, 6–10, 407–419
goals of, 1, 2
Health Belief Model (HBM) in, 415
history and development of, 3–13
interventions across cancer trajectory, 3–6
literacy and educational levels of
participants in, 413–415
measurements in, 417–418
mode of intervention delivery and, 412–413
outcome assessment in, 417–418
precision and, in evaluation of, 12–13
quality interventions and, four defining
features of, 8–13
recruitment issues in, 408–410
research questions in, 9–10
self-care and PRO-SELF programs, 416
social learning theory (SLT) in, 415–416
sociodemographic factors and, 408–410
targeted and tailored interventions in, 414
theoretical frameworks and outcome
assessments in, 8–9, 415–418
transtheoretical model (TTM) in, 415
behavior-based pain management, 274–275,
279–285, **280–283**
behavior-change interventions vs. decision
aids, 143–145, **143**
benefit-risk analysis in treatment, 144–145,
153–154
for hormone replacement therapy (HRT),
162–168, **163–166**
in prostate cancer, 148–149
benzodiazepines, 112
beta carotene (carotenoids), 20, 21
bias, in clinical trials, 10–12
biobehavioral model of cancer stress and
disease course, 179, **180**
biobehavioral model of nicotine addiction and
smoking, 124–125, **124**

421

CPSIA information can be obtained at www.ICGtesting.com
Printed in the USA
BVOW011151290412

288926BV00005B/24/A